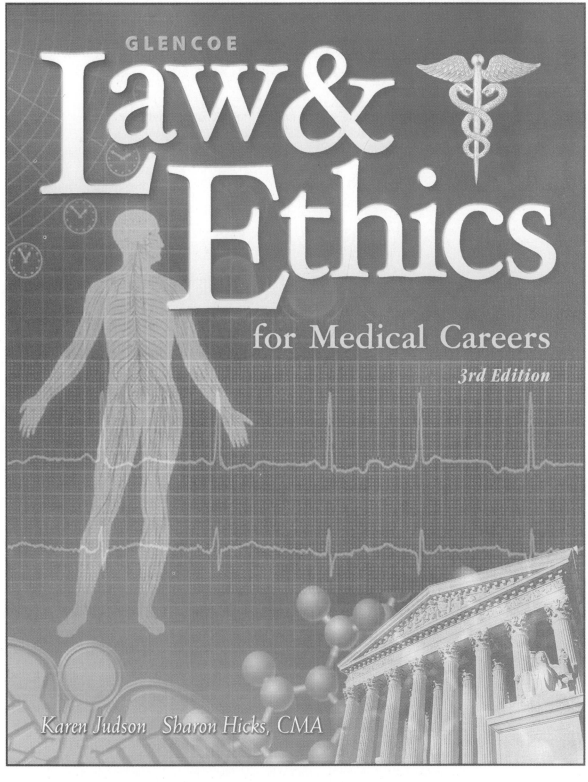

GLENCOE

Law & Ethics

for Medical Careers

3rd Edition

Karen Judson   Sharon Hicks, CMA

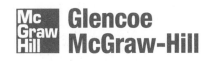

Glencoe
McGraw-Hill

New York, New York   Columbus, Ohio   Chicago, Illinois   Peoria, Illinois   Woodland Hills, California

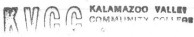

Library of Congress Cataloging-in-Publication Data

Judson, Karen, 1941-
  Law & ethics for medical careers / Karen Judson, Sharon Hicks.–3rd ed.
    p. cm.
  Includes index.
  ISBN 0-07-828940-8
  1. Medical ethics. 2. Medical jurisprudence. 3. Medical assistants–Professional ethics.
  4. Medical assistants–Legal status, laws, etc. I. Title: Law and ethics for medical
careers. II. Hicks, Sharon, 1953- III. Title.

  R725.5.J83 2002
  174'.2–dc21

                                                                    2002032673

Cover: (background)Bill Frymire/Masterfile; (t)Gary S. and Vivian Chapman/Getty Images; (b)file photo;

Interior Photos: **2** Pete Saloutos /CORBIS; **19** Ariel Skelley/Corbis Stock Market; **52** PhotoDisc; **114** Siede Preis/PhotoDisc; **84** PhotoDisc; **130** Digital Stock/CORBIS; **154** Digital Stock/CORBIS; **178** Nick Rowe/PhotoDisc; **200** Digital Stock/CORBIS; **222** Digital Stock/CORBIS; **252** Spike Mafford/PhotoDisc; **277** Digital Stock/CORBIS.

Glencoe/McGraw-Hill

A Division of The McGraw-Hill Companies

Law and Ethics for Medical Careers, Third Edition

ISBN 0-07-828940-8

1 2 3 4 5 6 7 8 9 **071** 07 06 05 04 03 02

Glencoe Law and Ethics for Medical Careers, Third Edition, is an educational tool, not a law practice book. Since the law is in constant change, no rule or statement of law in this text should be relied upon for any service to any client. The reader should always consult standard legal sources for the current rule or law. If legal counseling or other expert advice is needed, the services of appropriate professionals should be sought. Between the time that Web site information is gathered and published, it is not unusual for some sites to have closed. Also, the transcription of the URLs can result in typographical errors. Text changes will be made in reprints when possible.

TABLE OF CONTENTS

TABLE OF CONTENTS

CHAPTER 12

Death and Dying 277

TO THE STUDENT

As you study to become a health care practitioner, you have undoubtedly realized that patients are more than the sum of their medical problems. In fact, they are people with loved ones, professions, worries, and daily routines that are probably much like your own. Because patients' lives and well-being are at stake as they seek and receive health care, complex legal, moral, and ethical issues will arise that must be resolved.

Law and Ethics for Medical Careers, Third Edition, provides an overview of the laws and ethics you should know to help you give competent, compassionate care to patients that is within acceptable legal and ethical boundaries. The text can also serve as a guide to help you resolve the many legal and ethical questions you may reasonably expect to face as a student and, later, as a health care practitioner.

To derive maximum benefit from *Law and Ethics for Medical Careers, Third Edition:*

- Review the Objectives and Key Terms at the beginning of each chapter for an overview of the material included in the chapter.
- Complete all Check Your Progress questions as they appear in the chapter, and correct any incorrect answers.
- Review the legal cases to see how they apply to topics in the text, and try to determine why the court made its particular ruling.
- Complete the review questions at the end of the chapter, correct incorrect answers, and review the material again.
- Review case studies and use your critical-thinking skills to answer the questions.
- Complete the Internet Activities at the end of the chapter to become familiar with online resources and to see what additional information you can find about selected topics.
- Study each chapter until you can correctly answer questions posed by the Objectives, Check Your Progress, and Chapter Review.

Chapter Structure

Each chapter begins with a page that previews what you will be studying:

OBJECTIVES   The objectives describe the basic knowledge that can be acquired by studying the chapter.

KEY TERMS   This alphabetic list is of important vocabulary terms found in the chapter. The terms are printed in bold-faced type when they first appear in the chapter text and are defined in the margin of the page on which the term is introduced.

Several pages of exercises are found at the end of each chapter that will help you review, apply, and build the knowledge related to the chapter material:

CHAPTER REVIEW   Each review includes questions that review facts given and points made in the text. Use these questions to test your comprehension of the material, then review appropriate sections of the text as necessary to reinforce your learning.

CASE STUDIES   Each case study is followed by exercises that allow you to practice your critical-thinking skills and use knowledge gained from reading the text in order to decide how to resolve the real-life situations or theoretical scenarios presented.

INTERNET ACTIVITIES   Each activity includes exercises that are designed to increase your knowledge of topics related to chapter material and to gain expertise in using the Internet as a research tool. Keep a resource notebook to record useful Web sites as they are found. To locate new Web sites, conduct a subject search as needed to help you answer the questions that follow each activity.

Text Features

The following special features are found in the student text/workbook for *Law and Ethics for Medical Careers, Third Edition.* These features are designed to stimulate classroom discussion, provide supplementary facts and examples to the text material, introduce you to Internet research, and provide review of the text material covered.

CHECK YOUR PROGRESS   This feature is a short quiz that allows you to test your comprehension of the material just read. Answer the questions, correct incorrect answers, and then review appropriate sections to be sure you understand the material.

VOICE OF EXPERIENCE   This feature illustrates real-life experiences that are related to the text material. Each quotes health care practitioners in various locations throughout the United States as they encounter problems or situations relevant to the material discussed in the text.

YOU BE THE JUDGE   This feature presents real-life scenarios for your consideration. Study each situation, and then answer the questions, based on material presented in the text and your opinions.

FYI (FOR YOUR INFORMATION)   Each short feature contains information supplementary to the text material. It provides varied perspectives on issues discussed within the text.

COURT CASE   Each case summarizes a lawsuit that illustrates points made in the text. In each case, consider the relevance of the case to your health care specialty area and note the outcome. Determine why the court made its particular ruling. The legal citations at the end of each court case indicate where to find the complete text of a case. "Landmark" cases are those that established ongoing precedent.

How to Interpret Court Case Citations

The following steps describe how to interpret a court citation as published in legal case books (called reporters), using the example *Koher v. Dial,* 653 N.E.2d 524 (Ind. Ct. of App., July 26, 1995):

1. The italicized case name gives the names of the litigants, in this case, *Koher v. Dial.*

2. After the case name, the reporter in which the case report may be found is listed. Each reporter covers a specific geographic area of the country and is named for that area. Within the citation, the name of the reporter is usually abbreviated as indicated by the following examples of reporters and corresponding abbreviations: Northeast (N.E.) Reporter, New York Supplement (N.Y.S.), Northwest (N.W.) Reporter, Southern (So.) Reporter, Southwestern (S.W.) Reporter, Atlantic (A.) Reporter, Pacific (P.) Reporter. (Sometimes in case citations the periods are omitted; for example, NE, NYS, NW, and so on.) Since each reporter consists of many volumes, the case citation specifies the volume number of the reporter, a series number (when applicable), and the page number on which the case report begins. The book for the example case is 653 of the Northeast Reporter 2d series, beginning on page 524.

3. The state indicates where the case was tried; sometimes the name of the court is also included in the citation. The example case was tried in an Indiana Court of Appeals.

4. At the end of the citation, the year (sometimes the complete date) that the decision was made is provided. The decision in *Kohr v. Dial* was reached on July 26, 1995.

Citations for cases available on the Internet from a subscription service called Lexis-Nexis will contain the Lexis file number instead of a reporter reference; for example, *Samuel v. Baton Rouge General Medical Center,* 2000 La.App. Lexis 321 (Court of Appeal of Louisiana, First Circuit, February 18, 2000).

AAMA Role Delineation Study Areas of Competence (1997) Correlation Chart

Areas of Competence	Student Edition Chapters
CLINICAL *Patient Care*	
• Maintain medication and immunizition records.	6
GENERAL (TRANSDISCIPLINARY) *Professionalism*	
• Project a professional manner and image.	1
• Adhere to ethical principles.	1, 10, 11
• Work as a team member.	2
• Adapt to change.	1
Communication Skills	
• Treat all patients with compassion and empathy.	1, 10, 11, 12
• Use professional telephone technique.	4
• Use effective and correct verbal and written communication.	4
• Serve as a liaison.	3, 4, 6
Legal Concepts	
• Maintain confidentiality.	1, 2, 4, 5, 6, 11
• Practice within the scope of education, training, and personal capabilities.	1, 2, 4
• Prepare and maintain medical records.	5, 6, 11
• Document accurately.	4, 5, 6, 11
• Use appropriate guidelines when releasing information.	6
• Follow employer's established policies dealing with the health care contract.	3
• Maintain and dispose of regulated substances in compliance with government guidelines.	8
• Comply with established risk management and safety procedures.	2, 8
• Recognize professional credentialing criteria.	2
• Participate in the development and maintenance of personnel, policy, and procedure manuals.	4, 9
Instruction	
• Locate community resources and disseminate information.	8
Operational Functions	
• Apply computer techniques to support office operations.	6

ACKNOWLEDGMENTS

We are grateful to the following individuals for their input into the third edition of *Law & Ethics for Medical Careers.* We appreciate their reviews, ideas, and suggestions.

Clyde L. Brumfield
Medical Careers Institute
Newport News, Virginia

Carol Demagall, RN, MSN
Central Carolina Community College
Sanford, North Carolina

Michael Dorich, CST-CAHI
Western School of Health and Business
Monroeville, Pennsylvania

Beth K. Elder, CMA
South Piedmont Community College
Polkton, North Carolina

Sharon Gibson, RN, BSN, C, CHES
Hawaii Business College
Honolulu, HI

Carlene Harrison, BS, MPA, CMA
International College
Naples, Florida

Dorothy Kiel, CMA-C
Lima Technical College
Lima, Ohio

Alice Oyakawa, RN, CMA
National College of Business & Technology
Danville, Virginia

Kathy Trawick, EdD, MAEd, RHIA
University of Arkansas for Medical Sciences
Little Rock, Arkansas

THE FOUNDATIONS OF LAW AND ETHICS

CHAPTER

1
Introduction to Law and Ethics

2
Working in Health Care

3
Law, the Courts, and Contracts

INTRODUCTION TO LAW AND ETHICS

Objectives

After studying this chapter, you should be able to:

1. Explain why knowledge of law and ethics is important to health care practitioners.
2. Recognize the importance of professional codes of ethics.
3. Trace the history of medical ethics from the earliest written code to the current medical guidelines.
4. Distinguish among law, ethics, bioethics, etiquette, and protocol.
5. Define *moral values* and explain how they relate to law, ethics, and etiquette.
6. In a generalized sense, state the consequences of illegal and unethical behavior.
7. List and discuss at least five bioethical issues of concern to medical practitioners.

Key Terms

- *American Medical Association Principles*
- bioethics
- code of ethics
- ethics
- ethics committees
- etiquette
- fraud

- health care practitioners
- Hippocratic oath
- law
- litigious
- moral values
- protocol
- summary judgment

Why Study Law and Ethics?

health care practitioners
Those who are trained to administer medical or health care to patients.

litigious *Prone to engage in lawsuits.*

There are two important reasons for you to study law and ethics. The first is to help you function at the highest possible professional level, providing competent, compassionate health care to patients. The second reason is to help you avoid legal entanglements that can threaten your ability to earn a living as a successful **health care practitioner**—one who is trained to administer medical or health care to patients.

We live in a **litigious** society, where patients, relatives, and others are inclined to sue health care practitioners, health care facilities, manufacturers of medical equipment and products, and others when medical outcomes are not acceptable. This means that every person responsible for health care delivery is at risk of being involved in a health care–related lawsuit. It is important, therefore, for you to know the basics of law and ethics as they apply to health care, so you can recognize and avoid those situations that might not serve your patients well, or might put you at risk of legal liability.

In addition to keeping you at your professional best and helping you avoid litigation, a knowledge of law and ethics can also help you gain perspective in the following three areas:

1. *The rights, responsibilities, and concerns of health care consumers.* Health care practitioners not only need to be concerned about how law and ethics impact their respective professions; they must also understand how legal and ethical issues affect the patients they treat. With the increased complexity of medicine has come the desire of consumers to know more about their options and rights and more about the responsibilities of health care providers. Today's health care consumers are likely to consider themselves partners with health care practitioners in the healing process and to question fees and treatment modes. They may ask such questions as, Do I need to see a specialist? If so, which specialist can best treat my condition? Will I be given complete information about my condition? How much will medical treatment cost? Will a physician treat me if I have no health insurance?

   In addition, as medical technology has advanced, patients have come to expect favorable outcomes from medical treatment, and when expectations are not met, lawsuits may result.

2. *The legal and ethical issues facing society, patients, and health care practitioners as the world changes.* Nearly every day the media report news events concerning individuals who face legal and ethical dilemmas over biological/medical issues. For example, a grief-stricken husband must give consent for an abortion in order to save the life of his critically ill and unconscious wife. Parents must argue in court their decision to terminate life-support measures for a daughter whose injured brain no longer functions. Patients with HIV/AIDS fight to retain their right to confidentiality.

   Whereas the situations that make news headlines often deal with larger social issues, legal and ethical questions are resolved daily, on a smaller scale, each time a patient visits his or her physician, dentist, physical therapist, or other health care practitioner. Questions that must often be resolved include these: Who can legally give consent if the patient cannot? Can patients be assured of confidentiality, especially since telecommunication has become a way of life? Can a physician or other health care practitioner refuse to treat a patient? Who may legally examine a patient's medical records?

Rapid advances in medical technology have also influenced laws and ethics for health care practitioners. For example, recent court cases have debated these issues: Does the husband or the wife have ownership rights to a divorced couple's frozen embryos? Will a surrogate mother have legal visitation rights to the child she carried to term? Should modern technology be used to keep those patients alive who are diagnosed as brain-dead and have no hope of recovery? How should parenthood disputes be resolved for children resulting from reproductive technology?

3. *The impact of rising costs on the laws and ethics of health care delivery.* Rising costs, both of health care insurance and of medical treatment in general, lead to questions concerning access to health care services and allocation of medical treatment. For instance, should the uninsured or underinsured receive government help to pay for health insurance? And should everyone, regardless of age or lifestyle, have the same access to scarce medical commodities, such as organs for transplantation or highly expensive drugs?

◆ ◆ ◆ ◆ ## Court Cases Illustrate Risk of Litigation

As illustrated in the following three court cases, a wide variety of legal questions can arise for those engaged directly in providing health care services, whether in a hospital or medical office setting, or in an emergency situation. As the heart valve case indicates, health care equipment and product dealers and manufacturers can be held indirectly responsible for defective medical devices and products through charges of:

- Breach of warranty.

- Statements made by the manufacturer about the device or product that are found to be untrue.

- Strict liability, for cases in which defective products threaten the personal safety of consumers.

fraud *Dishonest or deceitful practices in depriving, or attempting to deprive, another of his or her rights.*

- **Fraud** or intentional deceit. (Fraud is discussed in further detail in Chapter 3.)

summary judgment *A decsion made by a court in a lawsuit in response to a motion that pleads there is no basis for a trial.*

Court cases appear throughout each chapter of the text, to illustrate how the legal system has decided complaints brought by or against health care service providers and product manufacturers. Some of these cases, such as those found on pages 5 and 6 in this chapter, involve **summary judgment.** Summary judgment is the legal term for a decision made by a court in a lawsuit in response to a motion that pleads there is no basis for a trial because there is no genuine issue of material fact. In other words, a motion for summary judgment states that one party is entitled to win as a matter of law. Summary judgment is available only in a civil action. (Chapter 3 distinguishes between criminal and civil actions.)

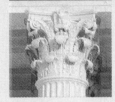

Patient Sues Hospital

In August 1997 a patient admitted to a Louisiana medical center for the treatment of bronchitis and back pain called the nurses' station to ask for someone to fix the television set and the window blinds. In response, two maintenance workers came to the patient's room and removed the television set. The workers examined the blinds but informed the patient they could not fix them. The workers then left, promising to replace the television set but not commenting on the window blinds.

The patient continued to ask for someone to adjust the window blinds to keep out the sun. She said that when she was in pain, light was unpleasant to her. No one came to fix the blinds.

The patient eventually tried to close the blinds herself. Dressed in street clothes and sandals, she climbed on a recliner chair with lockable wheels located in her room and reached high above her head in an attempt to turn the slats of the blinds. The patient fell off the chair and sustained an injury to her left shoulder, upper back, and cervical spine.

The patient then sued the medical center for the injuries she suffered. An appeals court overturned a circuit court's decision to dismiss and sent the case back for further proceedings. The appeals court determined: "It is not unforeseeable that a patient experiencing discomfort due to bright light entering the room, and who has obtained no relief through repeated requests for aid, might decide to take matters into her own hands and attempt to close the broken blinds. Furthermore, because the top of the blinds is located above the easy reach of the average person, it is not unforeseeable that the patient would attempt to use a chair to reach the top of the blinds."

Lichti v. Schumpert Medical Center, 2000 La.App. Lexis 61 (La. Ct. of App., 2d Cir., January 26, 2000).

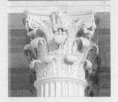

County Liable in Ambulance Delay

In 1991 an Indiana man suffered a heart attack while mowing the lawn. He took two nitroglycerin tablets while his wife called an ambulance. The emergency operator took the wife's call at 2:10 P.M. and said an ambulance would be dispatched. Seven minutes later the ambulance had not arrived, so the wife called a nearby fire station where the local branch of the emergency medical squad was holding a meeting. An ambulance was sent immediately when this call was received, and it arrived at the patient's house in one minute.

The patient later learned that the emergency operator who was first called had never dispatched an ambulance to his home. The chief deputy sheriff of the county explained that the officer taking emergency calls was inexperienced as a dispatcher. The officer had been the only one assigned to monitor the emergency line that day because the sheriff's department was having its annual picnic.

The patient sued the county for negligence in operating the 911 emergency service. He claimed he had suffered permanent heart damage because of the operator's failure to dispatch an ambulance promptly.

The county moved for summary judgment based on the fact that it had no relationship with the man that created a duty of care to him. The trial court granted the motion, but an appellate court reversed the judgment. It held that the call to the emergency operator, in which the man's wife spoke of her husband's heart attack and the immediate need for an ambulance, was sufficient to establish knowledge that inaction could be harmful.

When the operator said an ambulance would be dispatched, he established that the county explicitly agreed to assist the patient. Accordingly, the court held, the county had assumed a private duty to the man and could be held liable for failure to dispatch an ambulance.

Koher v. Dial, 653 N.E.2d 524 (Ind. Ct. of App., July 26, 1995).

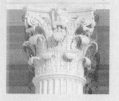

Landmark Case: Heart Valve Defect Creates Cause of Action

A federal appellate court for Pennsylvania held that a patient who was implanted with a heart valve could recover damages for fraud and breach of express warranty from the manufacturer of the defective valve.

In 1982 the patient had surgery to replace a defective mitral valve in her heart with an artificial Shiley valve. The surgery was successful, and the valve functioned properly.

In the late 1980s the patient learned that strut fractures had occurred in about 1 percent of all implanted Shiley valves. In almost every case in which fractures occurred, the patient died. The patient sued the manufacturer of Shiley valves for negligent manufacture and design, strict product liability, breach of implied warranty, breach of express warranty, and fraud.

At trial, summary judgment was granted to the manufacturer based on the 1976 Medical Devices Amendments of the Food, Drug, and Cosmetics Act of 1938 that extended to the federal government control of "therapeutic devices." The amendments required manufacturers of medical devices to register with the Food and Drug Administration (FDA) and follow quality control procedures.

On appeal, the court denied the patient's claims for negligent manufacture and design, strict product liability, and breach of implied warranty. However, the appeals court reversed the grant of summary judgment on the breach of express warranty and fraud claims. It found that genuine issues of material fact existed as to whether:

1. the manufacturer was liable under the terms of its warranty for physical and emotional trauma occasioned by the need to take the valve from the patient, and
2. the manufacturer engaged in fraud when it misrepresented the performance level of the Shiley valve in its advertisements and letters to physicians.

Michael v. Shiley, Inc., 46 F.3d 1316 (C.A.3., Pa., Feb. 7, 1995).

Comparing Aspects of Law and Ethics

In order to understand the complexities of law and ethics better, it is helpful to define and compare a few basic related terms. Table 1-1 summarizes the terms described in the following sections.

◆ ◆ ◆ ◆ **Law**

law *Rule of conduct or action prescribed or formally recognized as binding or enforced by a controlling authority.*

A **law** is defined as a rule of conduct or action prescribed or formally recognized as binding or enforced by a controlling authority. Governments enact laws to keep society running smoothly and to control behavior that could threaten public safety. Laws are considered the minimum standard necessary to keep society functioning.

Enforcement of laws is made possible by penalties for disobedience, which are decided by a court of law or are mandatory as written into the law. Penalties vary with the severity of the crime. Lawbreakers may be fined, imprisoned, or both. Sometimes lawbreakers are sentenced to probation. Other penalties, appropriate to the crime, may be handed down by the sentencing authority, as when offenders must perform a specified

Table 1-1   **COMPARING ASPECTS OF LAW AND ETHICS**

	Law	Ethics	Moral Values
Definition	Set of governing rules.	Principles, standards, guide to conduct.	Beliefs formed through the influence of family, culture, and society.
Main Purpose	To protect the public.	To elevate standard of competence.	To serve as a guide for personal ethical conduct.
Standards	Minimal—promotes smooth functioning of society.	Builds values and ideals.	Serves as a basis for forming a personal code of ethics.
Penalties for Violation	Civil or criminal liability. Upon conviction: fine, imprisonment, revocation of license, or other penalty as determined by courts.	Suspension or eviction from medical society membership, as decided by peers.	Difficulty in getting along with others.
	Bioethics	**Etiquette**	**Protocol**
Definition	Discipline relating to ethics concerning biological research, especially as applied to medicine.	Courtesy and manners.	Rules of etiquette applicable to one's place of employment.
Main Purpose	To allow scientific progress in a manner that benefits society in all possible ways.	To get along with others.	To get along with others engaged in the same profession.
Standards	Leads to highest standards possible in applying research to medical care.	Leads to pleasant interaction.	Promotes smooth functioning of workplace routines.
Penalties for Violation	Penalties can include all those listed under "Law," "Ethics," and "Etiquette." As current standards are applied and as new laws and ethical standards evolve to govern medical research and development, penalties may change.	Ostracism from chosen groups.	Disapproval of one's professional colleagues; possible loss of business.

number of hours of volunteer community service or are ordered to repair public facilities they have damaged.

Many laws affect health care practitioners, including criminal and civil statutes as well as state medical practice acts. Medical practice acts apply specifically to the practice of medicine in a certain state. Licensed health care professionals convicted of violating criminal, civil, or medical practice laws may lose their license to practice. (Medical practice acts are discussed further in Chapter 2. Laws and the court system are discussed in more detail in Chapter 3.)

Ethics

An illegal act by a health care practitioner is always unethical, but an unethical act is not necessarily illegal. **Ethics** are concerned with standards of behavior and the concept of right and wrong, over and above that which is legal in a given situation. **Moral values**—formed through the influence of the family, culture, and society—serve as the basis for ethical conduct. In our culture, acting morally toward others usually requires that you put yourself in their place. When you are a patient in a physician's office, how do you like to be treated? As a health care provider, can you give care to a person whose conduct or professed beliefs differ radically from your own? In an emergency, can you provide for the patient's welfare without reservation?

Check Your Progress

1. Name two important reasons for studying law and ethics.

   _____

   _____

2. Which state laws apply specifically to the practice of medicine?

   _____

3. What purpose do laws serve?

   _____

   _____

4. How is the enforcement of laws made possible?

   _____

   _____

Codes of Ethics

While most individuals can rely on a well-developed personal value system, organizations for the health occupations also have formalized **codes of ethics** to govern behavior of members and to increase the level of competence and standards of care within the group. Included among these are the American Nurses' Association Code for Nurses, American Medical Association's *Code of Medical Ethics: Current Opinions with Annotations*, American Society of Radiologic Technologists Code of Ethics, and the Code of Ethics of the American Association of Medical Assistants. Many additional professional organizations for health care practitioners publish a code of ethics for members.

One of the earliest medical codes of ethics, the code of Hammurabi, was written by the Babylonians around 2250 B.C. This document discussed the conduct expected of physicians at that time, including fees that could be charged.

I swear by Apollo, the physician, and Aesculapius, and Health, and Allheal, and all the gods and goddesses, that, according to my ability and judgment, I will keep this oath and stipulation, to reckon him who taught me this art equally dear to me as my parents, to share my substance with him and relieve his necessities if required; to regard his offspring as on the same footing with my own brothers, and to teach them this art if they should wish to learn it, without fee or stipulation, and that by precept, lecture, and every other mode of instruction, I will impart a knowledge of the art to my own sons and to those of my teachers, and to disciples bound by a stipulation and oath, according to the law of medicine, but to none other.

I will follow that method of treatment which, according to my ability and judgment, I consider for the benefit of my patients, and abstain from whatever is deleterious and mischievous. I will give no deadly medicine to anyone if asked, nor suggest any such counsel; furthermore, I will not give to a woman an instrument to produce abortion.

With purity and holiness I will pass my life and practice my art. I will not cut a person who is suffering with a stone, but will leave this to be done by practitioners of the work. Into whatever houses I enter I will go into them for the benefit of the sick and will abstain from every voluntary act of mischief and corruption; and further from the seduction of females or males, bond or free.

Whatever, in connection with my professional practice, or not in connection with it, I may see or hear in the lives of men which ought not to be spoken abroad, I will not divulge, as reckoning that all such should be kept secret.

While I continue to keep this oath unviolated, may it be granted to me to enjoy life and the practice of the art, respected by all men at all times, but should I trespass and violate this oath, may the reverse be my lot.

Figure 1-1
Hippocratic Oath

Hippocratic oath A pledge for physicians, developed by the Greek physician Hippocrates circa 400 B.C.

Sometime around 400 B.C., Hippocrates, the Greek physician known as the Father of Medicine, created the **Hippocratic oath,** a pledge for physicians that remains influential today (see Figure 1-1).

Percival's Medical Ethics, written by the English physician and philosopher Thomas Percival in 1803, superseded earlier codes to become the definitive guide for a physician's professional conduct.

When the American Medical Association met for the first time in Philadelphia in 1847, the group devised a code of ethics for members based on Percival's code. The resulting *American Medical Association Principles,* currently called the *American Medical Association Principles of Medical Ethics,* have been revised and updated periodically to keep pace with changing times (see Figure 1-2 on p. 10). The *American Medical Association Principles of Medical Ethics* briefly summarizes the AMA's position on ethical treatment of patients, while the more extensive *Code of Medical Ethics: Current Opinions with Annotations* provides more detailed coverage.

American Medical Association Principles A code of ethics for members of the American Medical Association, written in 1847.

Adopted in 1980, the Code of Ethics of the American Association of Medical Assistants lists ethical standards for medical assistants (see Figure 1-3 on p. 11).

When members of professional associations such as the AMA and the AAMA are accused of unethical conduct, they are subject to peer council

Preamble. The medical profession has long subscribed to a body of ethical statements developed primarily for the benefit of the patient. As a member of this profession, a physician must recognize responsibility not only to patients but also to society, to other health professionals, and to self. The following Principles adopted by the American Medical Association are not laws but standards of conduct that define the essentials of honorable behavior for the physician.

I. A physician shall be dedicated to providing competent medical service with compassion and respect for human dignity.

II. A physician shall deal honestly with patients and colleagues and strive to expose those physicians deficient in character or competence, or who engage in fraud or deception.

III. A physician shall respect the law and also recognize a responsibility to seek changes in those requirements which are contrary to the best interests of the patient.

IV. A physician shall respect the rights of patients, of colleagues, and of other health professionals and shall safeguard patient confidences within the constraints of the law.

V. A physician shall continue to study, apply, and advance scientific knowledge; make relevant information available to patients, colleagues, and the public; obtain consultation; and use the talents of other health professionals when indicated.

VI. A physician shall, in the provision of appropriate patient care, except in emergencies, be free to choose whom to serve, with whom to associate, and the environment in which to provide medical services.

VII. A physician shall recognize a responsibility to participate in activities contributing to an improved community.

Figure 1-2
American Medical Association Principles of Medical Ethics

review and may be censured by the organization. Although a professional group cannot revoke a member's license to practice, unethical members may be expelled from the group, suspended for a period of time, or ostracized by other members. Unethical behavior by a medical practitioner can result in loss of income and eventually the loss of a practice if, as a result of that behavior, patients choose another practitioner.

◆ ◆ ◆ ◆ **Bioethics**

bioethics *A discipline dealing with the ethical implications of biological research methods and results, especially in medicine.*

Bioethics is a discipline dealing with the ethical implications of biological research methods and results, especially in medicine. As biological research has led to unprecedented progress in medicine, medical practitioners have had to grapple with issues such as:

• What ethics should guide biomedical research? Do individuals own all rights to their body cells, or should scientists own cells they have altered? Is human experimentation essential, or even permissible, to advance biomedical research?

The Code of Ethics of AAMA shall set forth principles of ethical and moral conduct as they relate to the medical profession and the particular practice of medical assisting.

Members of AAMA dedicated to the conscientious pursuit of their profession and thus desiring to merit the high regard of the entire medical profession and the respect of the general public which they serve, do pledge themselves to strive always to:

A. render service with full respect for the dignity of humanity;

B. respect confidential information obtained through employment unless legally authorized or required by responsible performance of duty to divulge such information;

C. uphold the honor and high principles of the profession and accept its disciplines;

D. seek to continually improve the knowledge and skills of medical assistants for the benefit of patients and professional colleagues;

E. participate in additional service activities aimed toward improving the health and well-being of the community.

CREED

• I believe in the principles and purposes of the profession of medical assisting.

• I endeavor to be more effective.

• I aspire to render greater service.

• I protect the confidence entrusted to me.

• I am dedicated to the care and well-being of all people.

• I am loyal to my employer.

• I am true to the ethics of my profession.

• I am strengthened by compassion, courage, and faith.

Figure 1-3
Code of Ethics of the American Association of Medical Assistants

• What ethics should guide organ transplants? Although organs suitable for transplant are in short supply, is the search for organs dehumanizing? Should certain categories of people have lower priority than others for organ transplants?

• What ethics should guide fetal tissue research? Some say such research, especially stem cell research, offers hope to disease victims, while others argue that it is immoral.

• Do reproductive technologies offer hope to the childless, or are they unethical? Are the multiple births that sometimes result from taking fertility drugs an acceptable aspect of reproductive technology, or are those multiple births too risky for women and their fetuses and even immoral in an allegedly overpopulated world?

• Should animals ever be used in research?

• How ethical is genetic research? Should genetic research be restricted to medical therapy? Should the government regulate it? Will genetic testing benefit those at risk for genetic disease, or will it lead to discrimination?

You Be the Judge

A physician admitted an elderly patient to the hospital, where she was treated for an irregular heartbeat and chest pain. The patient was competent to make her own decisions about a course of treatment, but her opinionated and outspoken daughter repeatedly second-guessed the physician's recommendations with medical information she had obtained from the Internet.

In your opinion, what responsibilities, if any, does a physician or other health care practitioner have toward difficult family members or other third parties who interfere with a patient's medical care?

_____

_____

_____

_____

What might the physician in the above situation have said to her patient's daughter to help resolve the situation?

_____

_____

_____

_____

Should the cloning of human organs for transplantation be permitted? Should cloning of human beings ever be permitted?

Society is attempting to address these questions, but because the issues are complicated, many questions may never be completely resolved. (Bioethical issues as they relate to medical professions are discussed in further detail in Chapter 10.)

The Role of Ethics Committees ◆ ◆ ◆ ◆

Health care practitioners may be able to resolve the majority of the ethical issues they face in the workplace from their own intuitive sense of moral values and ethics. However, some ethical dilemmas are not so much a question of right or wrong, but more "which of these alternatives will do the most good and the least harm?" In these more ambiguous situations, health care practitioners may want to ask the advice of a medical ethicist or members of an institutional ethics committee.

—continued

Etiquette

Whereas professional codes of ethics focus on the protection of the patient and his or her right to appropriate, competent, and humane treatment, **etiquette** refers to standards of behavior considered good manners within a profession. Every culture has its own ideas of common courtesy. Behavior considered good manners in one culture may be bad manners in another. For example, in some Middle Eastern countries it is extremely discourteous for one male acquaintance to ask another, "How is your wife?" In Western culture, such a question is well received. Similarly, within nearly every profession, there are recognized practices considered good manners for members.

Most health care facilities have their own policies concerning professional etiquette that staff members are expected to follow. Policy manuals written especially for the facility can serve as permanent records and as guidelines for employees in these matters.

Medical ethicists or bioethicists are specialists who consult with physicians, researchers, and others to help them make difficult decisions, such as whether to resuscitate brain-damaged premature infants, or what ethics should govern privacy in genetic testing. Hospital or medical center **ethics committees** usually consist of physicians, nurses, social workers, clergy, a patient's family, members of the community, and other individuals involved with the patient's medical care. A medical ethicist may also sit on the ethics committee if such a specialist is available. When difficult decisions need to be made, any one of the individuals involved in a patient's medical care can ask for a consultation with the ethics committee.

When a difficult case is referred to the ethics committee, the members meet and review the case. The committee does not make binding decisions, but helps the physician, nurse, patient, patient's family, or others clarify the issue and understand the medical facts of the case and the alternatives available to resolve the situation. Ethics committees may also help with conflict resolution among parties involved with a case, but they do not function as institutional review boards or morals police looking for health care workers who have committed unethical acts.

By the same token, health care practitioners are expected to know **protocol,** standard rules of etiquette applicable specifically to their place of employment. For example, when another physician telephones, does the receptionist put the call through without delay? Is a physician who is also a patient billed at the same rate as other patients who are not physicians?

Within the health care environment, all health care practitioners are, of course, expected to treat patients with the same respect and courtesy afforded others in the course of day-to-day living. Politeness and appropriate dress are mandatory.

Qualities of Successful Health Care Practitioners

Successful health care practitioners have a knowledge of techniques and principles that includes an understanding of legal and ethical issues. They must also acquire a working knowledge of and tolerance for human nature and individual characteristics, since daily contact with a wide variety of individuals with a host of problems and concerns is a significant part of the work. Courtesy, compassion, and common sense are often cited as the "three C's" most vital to the professional success of health care practitioners.

Additional capabilities that are helpful to those who choose to work in the health care field include:

- A relaxed attitude when meeting new people.

- A willingness to learn new skills and techniques.

- An aptitude for working with the hands.

- An understanding of and empathy for others.

- Computer literacy.

- Good communication skills, including writing, speaking, and listening.

- Patience in dealing with others and the ability to work as a member of a health care team.

- Proficiency in English, science, and mathematics.

- Tact.

- The ability to impart information clearly and accurately.

- The ability to keep information confidential.

- The ability to leave private concerns at home.

- Trustworthiness and a sense of responsibility.

The health care practitioner who demonstrates the above qualities, coupled with a working knowledge of law and ethics, is most likely to find success and job satisfaction in his or her chosen profession.

5. Tell how each of the following characteristics relates to law and ethics in the health care professions:

The ability to be a good communicator and listener.

_____
_____
_____

The ability to keep information confidential.

_____
_____
_____
_____

The ability to impart information clearly and accurately.

_____
_____
_____
_____

VOICE OF EXPERIENCE
A "Big Mouth" an Ethical Concern

Loretta, a certified medical assistant (CMA) in a clinic, often advises new employees to "keep your mouth shut and your ears open," because remarks overheard can be taken out of context.

For instance, a medical assistant noticed that a patient had forgotten to pick up his prescription after his visit, so she called to him across a busy waiting room, "Mr. Smith, you forgot your prescription for Dilantin." (Dilantin is commonly used to control seizures.) The patient, a local banker, had kept his epilepsy a secret. Others in the waiting room overheard the medical assistant's remark, and soon the word about Mr. Smith's condition was out. He sued his physician for breach of confidentiality and won.

Applying Knowledge

Answer the following questions in the spaces provided.

1. List three areas where health care practitioners can gain insight through studying law and ethics.

   _____

   _____

   _____

2. Define *summary judgment*.

   _____

   _____

3. Define *bioethics*.

   _____

   _____

4. Define *law*.

   _____

   _____

5. Define *ethics*.

   _____

   _____

6. How is unethical behabior punished?

   _____

   _____

7. Define *etiquette*.

   _____

   _____

8. How are violations of etiquette handled?

   _____

   _____

   _____

9. What is the purpose of a professional code of ethics?

   _____

   _____

   _____

Review and Case Studies

10. Name five biothical issues of concern in today's society.

_____

_____

_____

_____

_____

Write "T" or "F" in the blank to indicate whether you think the statement is true or false.

_____**11.** Written codes of ethics for health care practitioners evolved primarily to serve as moral guide-lines for those who provided care to the sick.

_____**12.** Percival was a Greek physician who is known as the Father of Medicine.

_____**13.** The Hippocratic oath is a pledge for physicians that remains influential today.

_____**14.** *Percival's Medical Ethics* superseded earlier codes to become the definitive guide for a physi-cian's professional conduct.

_____**15.** Unethical behavior is always illegal.

_____**16.** Unlawful acts are always unethical.

_____**17.** Violation of a professional organization's formalized code of ethics leads automatically to expul-sion from the organization.

_____**18.** Law is the minimum standard necessary to keep society functioning smoothly.

_____**19.** Conviction of a crime cannot result in loss of license unless ethical violations also exist.

_____**20.** One's morals serve as the basis for ethical conduct.

_____**21.** Sellers and manufacturers cannot be held legally responsible for defective medical devices and products through charges of fraud.

_____**22.** Hospitals are immune from lawsuits brought by patients.

_____**23.** Formalized codes of ethics are as enforceable as laws in governing the behavior of an organiza-tion's members.

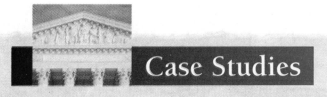

Case Studies

Use your critical-thinking skills to answer the questions that follow each of the case studies. Indicate whether each situation is a question of law, ethics, protocol, or etiquette.

You are employed as a dental assistant in a dentist's office. Your neighbor asks you to find out for him how much another patient was charged for a procedure performed by the dentist who employs you.

24. What should you say?

_____

_____

_____

_____

A physician employs you as a medical assistant. Another physician comes into the medical office where you work and asks to speak with your physician/employer.

25. Should you seat the physician in the waiting room, or show her to your employer's private office? Why?

_____

_____

_____

You are employed as a licensed practical/vocational nurse. A woman visits the clinic where you work, complaining of "sore" eyes that are obviously red and matted. She says she recently came in contact with a child who had the same symptoms, and she asks, "What did this child see the doctor for, and what was his diagnosis?" You explain that you cannot give out this information, but another LPN (licensed practical nurse) overhears, pulls the boy's chart, and gives the woman the information she requested.

26. Did both LPNs in this scenario act ethically and responsibly? Explain your answer.

_____

_____

_____

_____

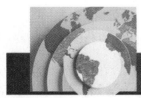

Internet Activities

Complete the activities and answer the questions that follow.

27. Use a search engine to conduct a search for Web sites on the Internet concerned with bioethics. Name two of those sites you think are reliable sources of information. Explain your choices. How does each site define the term *bioethics?*

_____

_____

_____

_____

28. Locate the Web site for the organization that represents the health care profession you intend to practice. Does the site provide guidance on ethics? If so, how? Does the site link to other sites concerning ethics? If so, list, then explore, three ethics links.

_____

_____

_____

_____

29. Visit the Web site for the American Medical Association. Find the ethics column and briefly summarize below one recent ethical issue discussed at the site. Do you agree or disagree with the conclusions reached about the issue? Explain your answer.

_____

_____

_____

_____

2

WORKING IN HEALTH CARE

Objectives

After studying this chapter, you should be able to:

1. Define *licensure, certification, registration,* and *accreditation.*
2. Explain the purpose of the medical practice acts.
3. Explain the purpose of medical boards.
4. Identify licensing requirements for physicians.
5. Cite reasons for which a physician may lose his or her license.
6. Discuss the doctrine of *respondeat superior.*
7. Define four types of medical practice management systems.
8. Discuss three important provisions for health care found in HIPAA.
9. Discuss two federal acts that prohibit fraud and abuse in health care billing.
10. Explain the purpose of a quality improvement and risk manager within a health care facility.
11. Define three types of managed care health plans.
12. Define *telemedicine, cybermedicine,* and *e-health,* and discuss their role in today's health care environment.

Key Terms

- accreditation
- ambulatory-care setting
- associate practice
- certification
- corporation
- cybermedicine
- e-health
- endorsement
- Federal False Claims Act
- gatekeeper physician
- group practice

- Health Care Quality Improvement Act of 1986 (HCQIA)
- Health Insurance Portability and Accountability Act of 1996 (HIPAA)
- Healthcare Integrity and Protection Data Bank (HIPDB)
- health maintenance organization (HMO)
- indemnity
- individual (or independent) practice association (IPA)
- licensure
- managed care
- medical boards

- medical practice acts

- National Practitioner Data Bank (NPDB)

- partnership

- physician-hospital organization (PHO)

- point-of-service (POS) plan

- preferred provider organization (PPO), or preferred provider association (PPA)

- primary care physician (PCP)

- quality improvement (QI) (or quality assurance)

- reciprocity

- registration

- *respondeat superior*

- risk management

- sole proprietorship

- telemedicine

Licensure, Certification, and Registration

With increased medical specialization have come more exacting professional requirements for health care practitioners. Members of the health care team today are usually licensed, registered, or certified to perform specific duties, depending on job classification and state requirements. Furthermore, programs for educating health care practitioners are often accredited, a process that implies that certain standards have been met. Managed care plans may also earn accreditation or certification for excellence.

licensure *A mandatory credentialing process established by law, usually at the state level, that grants the right to practice certain skills and endeavors.*

Licensure is a mandatory credentialing process established by law, usually at the state level. Licenses to practice are required in every state for all physicians and nurses and for many other health care practitioners as well. Individuals who do not have the required license are prohibited by law from practicing certain health care professions.

certification *A voluntary credentialing process whereby applicants who meet specific requirements may receive a certificate.*

Certification is a voluntary credentialing process, usually national in scope, and is most often sponsored by a nongovernmental, private sector group. Certification by a professional organization, usually through an examination, signifies that an applicant has attained a certain level of knowledge and skill. Since the process is voluntary, lack of certification does not prevent an employee from practicing the profession for which he or she is otherwise qualified.

registration *An entry in an official registry or record, listing the names of persons in a certain occupation who have satisfied specific requirements.*

Registration is an entry in an official registry or record, listing the names of persons in a certain occupation who have satisfied specific requirements. The list is usually made available to health care providers. One way to become registered is simply to add one's name to the list in the registry. Under this method of registration, unregistered persons are not prevented from working in a field for which they are otherwise qualified.

A second way to become registered in a health occupation is to attain a certain level of education and/or pay a registration fee. Under this second method, when there are specific requirements for registration, unregistered individuals may be prevented from working in a field for which they are otherwise qualified.

Under no circumstances can persons claim to be licensed, certified, or registered if they are not.

Accreditation is the process by which health care practitioner education programs, health care facilities, and managed care plans are officially authorized. Two examples of accrediting agencies for health care practitioner education programs are the Commission on Accreditation of Allied Health Education Programs (CAAHEP), discussed in more detail on page 26, and the Accrediting Bureau of Health Education Schools (ABHES). Accreditation is usually voluntary, but accredited programs for various disciplines must maintain certain standards to earn and keep accreditation. Most accredited programs for health care education also include an internship or externship (practical work experience) that lasts for a specified period of time.

The Joint Commission on Accreditation of Healthcare Organizations (JCAHO) accredits health care organizations that meet certain standards. As of 2001, the Joint Commission evaluated and accredited nearly 18,000 health care organizations and programs in the United States, including:

- General, psychiatric, children's, and rehabilitation hospitals
- Health care networks, including health maintenance organizations (HMOs)
- Home care organizations
- Long-term care facilities
- Assisted living facilities
- Behavioral health care organizations
- Ambulatory care providers
- Clinical laboratories

To earn and maintain JCAHO accreditation, an organization must undergo an on-site survey by a JCAHO survey team at least every three years. Laboratories must be surveyed every two years.

A recognized accrediting agency for managed care plans is the National Commission for Quality Assurance (NCQA), an independent, nonprofit organization that evaluates and reports on the quality of the nation's managed care organizations. NCQA evaluates managed care programs in three ways:

1. Through on-site review of key clinical and administrative processes.
2. Through the Health Plan Employer Data and Information Set (HEDIS)— data used to measure performance in areas such as immunization and mammography screening rates.
3. Through use of member satisfaction surveys.

Participation in NCQA accreditation and certification programs is voluntary, but the organization reported in 2001 that more than half of the nation's HMOs were participating.

Reciprocity

For those professions that require a state license, such as physician, registered nurse, or licensed practical/vocational nurse, **reciprocity** may be granted. This means that a state licensing authority will accept a person's valid license from another state as proof of competency without requiring reexamination.

1. Define *registration.*

_____

_____

_____

2. Define *licensure.*

_____

_____

_____

3. Define *certification.*

_____

_____

_____

4. Define *accreditation.*

_____

_____

_____

5. Define *reciprocity.*

_____

_____

_____

If a state license is required and reciprocity is not granted when moving to another state, the health care practitioner must apply to the state licensing authority to take the required examinations in order to obtain a valid license to practice in the new state.

Medical Practice Acts and Medical Boards

medical practice acts *State laws written for the express purpose of governing the practice of medicine.*

In all 50 states **medical practice acts** have been established by statute to govern the practice of medicine. They define what is meant by "practice of medicine" in each state, explain requirements and methods for licensure, provide for the establishment of medical licensing boards, establish grounds for suspension or revocation of license, and give conditions for license renewal.

Medical practice acts were first passed in colonial times but were repealed in the 1800s when citizens decided that the United States Constitution gave anyone the right to practice medicine. Quackery became rampant, and for the protection of the public, medical practice acts were reenacted.

You Be the Judge

Physician's assistants (PAs) are employed in physicians' offices throughout the United States. Although the PA provides direct patient care, he or she is always under the supervision of a licensed physician. Duties include taking patients' medical histories, performing physical examinations, ordering diagnostic and therapeutic procedures, providing follow-up care, and teaching and counseling patients. In some states PAs may write prescriptions. The PA may be the only health care practitioner a patient sees during his or her visit to the physician's office. Therefore, patients sometimes refer to a PA as "the doctor." Ned, a physician's assistant for five years, says he is often addressed as "doctor" by the patients he sees.

Similarly, Marie, a long-time employee of a physician in private practice in a rural area, is often referred to as "the doctor's nurse." Although Marie has never had the training necessary to become a certified medical assistant or a registered nurse, she sometimes refers to herself as the "office nurse."

What legal and ethical considerations are evident in these situations?

_____

_____

_____

Should Ned allow his patients to call him "doctor"? Explain your answer.

_____

_____

_____

Should Marie use the title "nurse" or allow others to call her that? Explain.

_____

_____

_____

What would you do in either Ned's or Marie's situation?

_____

_____

_____

Note: A health care practitioner is held to the standard of care practiced by a reasonably competent person of the same profession. A physician's assistant using the title "doctor" and a medical assistant using the title "nurse" may be held to the standard of care of a physician and a nurse, respectively, and may be accused of practicing without the appropriate license.

Although laws are in place to protect consumers against medical quackery, even today unscrupulous people attempt to circumvent the law by hawking devices, potions, and treatments they say are "guaranteed" to cure any ailment or infirmity. Each state periodically revises its medical practice acts to keep them current with the times. Medical practice acts can be found in each state's state code, which consists of laws for that state. A copy of the state code is available in most public libraries, in some university libraries, and in some cases on the Internet.

Each state's medical practice acts also mandate the establishment of **medical boards,** whose purpose is to protect the health, safety, and welfare of health care consumers through proper licensing and regulation of physicians and, in some jurisdictions, other health care practitioners. Board membership is composed of physicians and others who are, in most cases, appointed by the state's governor. Some boards act independently, exercising all licensing and disciplinary powers, whereas others are part of larger agencies, such as the department of health. Funding for state medical boards comes from licensing and registration fees. Most boards include an executive officer, attorneys, and investigators. Some legal services may be provided by the state's office of the attorney general.

Through licensing, each state medical board ensures that all health care practitioners who work in areas for which licensing is required have adequate and appropriate education and training and that they follow high standards of professional conduct while caring for patients. Applicants for license must generally:

- Provide proof of education and training.

- Provide details about work history.

- Pass an examination designed to assess their knowledge and ability to apply that knowledge and other concepts and principles important to ensure safe and effective patient care.

- Reveal information about past medical history (including alcohol and drug abuse), arrests, and convictions.

Each state's medical practice acts also define unprofessional conduct for medical professionals. Laws vary from state to state, but examples of unprofessional conduct include:

- Physical abuse of a patient.

- Inadequate record keeping.

- Failure to recognize or act on common symptoms.

- The prescribing of drugs in excessive amounts or without legitimate reason.

- Impaired ability to practice due to addiction or physical or mental illness.

- Failure to meet continuing education requirements.

- The performance of duties beyond the scope of a license.

- Dishonesty.

- Conviction of a felony.

- The delegation of the practice of medicine to an unlicensed individual.

Minor disagreements and poor customer service do not fall under the heading of misconduct.

See Appendix 1 for a list of medical board addresses and telephone numbers in all 50 states. Facsimile (fax) numbers and Web site or e-mail addresses are included where available.

Check Your Progress

6. Define *medical practice acts.*

_____

_____

_____

7. Where can you find the medical practice acts for your state?

_____

_____

_____

8. What is the primary responsibility of state medical boards?

_____

_____

_____

Court Case

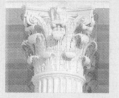

Physician Disciplined by Board of Medical Examiners

A state's Board of Medical Examiners disciplined a physician under its jurisdiction for excessively prescribing controlled drugs. The physician sought judicial review of the disciplinary act. The case reached the state Supreme Court, which held:

1. Disciplinary provisions in state medical practice acts were not unconstitutionally vague.

2. The Medical Board's executive director did not impermissibly combine prosecutorial and adjudicatory functions.

3. The preponderance of the evidence standard was sufficient to satisfy due process and did not violate equal protection guarantees.

4. Evidence was sufficient to support the finding that the physician had excessively prescribed controlled drugs.

Eaves v. Board of Medical Examiners, 467 N.W.2d 234 (Iowa 1991).

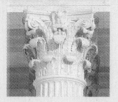
Health Care Professions

Today a growing number of specialized medical practitioners work with physicians as part of the health care team. Nonphysician members of the health care team, sometimes called allied health care practitioners:

- Share responsibility for delivery of health services.

- Have generally received a certificate, associate's degree, bachelor's degree, master's degree, doctoral degree, or postbaccalaureate training in a science related to health care and have met all state requirements concerning licensure, certification, and registration.

Listed below are a few of the licensed, certified, and registered health care practitioners who work with physicians, dentists, and other professionals in providing services to patients in medical offices, dental offices, hospitals, clinics, hospices, extended-care facilities, community programs, schools, and other health care settings. A brief description of each profession is given. When both technicians and technologists are included in the description of a profession, technologists perform duties at a higher level of expertise than technicians. They have either taken a more extensive course of study than technicians or have acquired qualifying experience. Since educational and credentialing requirements are subject to change, this information should be obtained from national organizations representing the profession or from state credentialing authorities.

The Commission on Accreditation of Allied Health Education Programs (CAAHEP) was established in 1994. CAAHEP currently accredits programs in 18 allied health professions and provides information concerning duties, education requirements, and sources for further information about the profession and the location of schools offering the accredited programs. Professions marked with an asterisk are currently included in the list of CAAHEP accredited programs.

*ANESTHESIOLOGIST ASSISTANT   The anesthesiologist assistant assists the anesthesiologist in developing and implementing an anesthesia care plan. Duties can include preoperative and postoperative tasks, as well as operating room assistance.

*ATHLETIC TRAINER   The athletic trainer works with attending or consulting physicians as an integral part of the health care team associated with physical training and sports.

AUDIOLOGIST   Audiologists are educated in the science of hearing and are qualified to test patients' hearing and to prescribe some types of therapy for hearing problems.

*CARDIOVASCULAR TECHNOLOGIST   The cardiovascular technologist works under the supervision of physicians to perform diagnostic and therapeutic examinations in the cardiology (heart) and vascular (circulation) areas.

*CYTOTECHNOLOGIST   Cytology is the study of the structure and function of cells. Cytotechnologists work with pathologists to microscopically examine body cells in order to detect changes that may help diagnose cancer and other diseases.

DENTAL HYGIENIST   Dental hygienists perform clinical and educational duties related to hygiene of the mouth and teeth, usually for dentist/employers within a dental office. They may work for one dentist or dental clinic or for several dentists at varying locations.

*DIAGNOSTIC MEDICAL SONOGRAPHER   The diagnostic medical sonographer administers ultrasound examinations under the supervision of a physician responsible for the use and interpretation of ultrasound procedures.

DIETICIAN AND NUTRITIONIST   Dieticians and nutritionists work closely with physicians and other medical practitioners to educate and assist patients with special dietary and nutritional needs.

ECG TECHNICIAN   Electrical activity of the heart is measured and recorded by electrocardiographic equipment operated by ECG (electrocardiogram) technicians under the supervision of physicians.

EEG TECHNICIAN AND TECHNOLOGIST   Electroencephalography is the recording and study of the electrical activity of the brain. EEG (electroencephalogram) technicians and technologists work under the supervision of physicians to operate EEG equipment used to perform patient diagnostic tests.

*ELECTRONEURODIAGNOSTIC TECHNOLOGIST   Electroneurodiagnostic technology involves the study and recording of the electrical activity of the brain and nervous system. Electroneurodiagnostic technologists work in collaboration with EEG technicians and technologists.

*EMERGENCY MEDICAL TECHNICIAN/PARAMEDIC   Emergency medical technicians (EMTs), or paramedics, most often work from an ambulance or in a hospital emergency room, providing life-support care to critically ill and injured patients.

*HEALTH INFORMATION ADMINISTRATOR/HEALTH INFORMATION TECHNICIAN AND TECHNOLOGIST   Health information specialists may have full responsibility for managing health information of medical offices, clinics, hospitals, or other health care institutions. Duties include organizing, analyzing, and preparing health information about patients, usually for use by patients, patients' physicians, and the health care facility, as well as handling the coding and billing for reimbursement for the health care facility.

*KINESIOTHERAPIST   Kinesiology is the study of muscles and muscle movement. Kinesiotherapists work under a physician's supervision, using therapeutic exercise and education to treat the effects of disease, injury, and congenital disorders on body movement.

LPN/LVN   Licensed practical nurses (LPNs) or licensed vocational nurses (LVNs) perform many of the same duties as registered nurses, with some exceptions, depending on state law. LPNs and LVNs work under the supervision of physicians and registered nurses.

ambulatory-care setting
Medical care provided in a facility such as a medical office, clinic, or out-patient surgical center for patients who can walk and are not bedridden.

*MEDICAL ASSISTANT   Medical assistants perform administrative and clinical duties for physicians/employers, usually within an **ambulatory-care setting,** such as a medical office, clinic, or outpatient surgical center. The certified medical assistant (CMA) credential is earned through the certifying board of the American Association of Medical Assistants. The registered medical assistant (RMA) credential is obtained through the American Medical Technologists (AMT) organization. Both credentials involve specific educational requirements and require applicants to pass an examination assessing knowledge and skills.

*MEDICAL ILLUSTRATOR   Medical illustrators must be knowledgeable in the biological sciences, anatomy, physiology, pathology, general medical knowledge, and the visual arts. They create illustrations for science and medical texts and other publications, and they also function in administrative, consultative, and advisory capacities.

MEDICAL LABORATORY TECHNICIAN AND MEDICAL TECHNOLOGIST
Duties of medical technicians include performing simple tests in hematology, serology, blood banking, urinalysis, microbiology, and clinical chemistry. Medical technologists have completed a longer training course than laboratory technicians. They supervise technicians and assistants and perform more complicated analytical laboratory tests.

MEDICAL TRANSCRIPTIONIST   Medical transcriptionists key material dictated by physicians, to be placed with patients' medical records. They must have preparation in English grammar, anatomy and physiology, and pharmacology. Many work out of their homes, but they may also work in medical records departments in hospitals, managed care plan facilities, nursing homes, and ambulatory-care facilities such as clinics, medical offices, and outpatient surgical centers.

NURSE PRACTITIONER   Those individuals who have earned a registered nurse (RN) license may be admitted to university programs to become nurse practitioners. Nurse practitioners are skilled in physical diagnosis, psychosocial assessment, and primary health care management. They may work independently, in collaboration with a physician, or under the supervision of a physician.

NURSING ASSISTANT   Nursing assistants provide basic patient care under the supervision of registered nurses. Routine duties include changing bed linens; taking temperature, respiratory, and blood pressure readings for patients; bathing patients and helping with personal care; helping patients with eating, walking, and exercise programs; and supporting patients when they are allowed to get out of bed. Employment opportunities exist in hospitals, long-term care facilities, and other health care institutions.

OCCUPATIONAL THERAPIST   A baccalaureate degree is required to enter the course of study for occupational therapy. Occupational therapists (OTs) work with clients who are mentally, physically, developmentally, or emotionally disabled to help these individuals become more independent and productive.

*OPHTHALMIC MEDICAL TECHNICIAN/TECHNOLOGIST   Ophthalmic medical technicians and technologists assist ophthalmologists (medical doctors who specialize in diseases and conditions of the eye) by performing such tasks as collecting data, administering diagnostic tests, and administering some treatments ordered by the supervising ophthalmologist. They may also maintain surgical instruments and office equipment.

OPTICIAN   Opticians are licensed specifically to sell or construct optical materials.

OPTOMETRIST   Optometrists are trained and licensed to examine the eyes in order to determine the presence of vision problems and to prescribe and adapt lenses to preserve or restore maximum efficiency of vision.

*ORTHOTIST AND PROSTHETIST   Orthotists and prosthetists work directly with physicians and others to rehabilitate people with disabilities. The orthotist designs and fits devices (orthoses) for patients with disabling conditions of the limbs and spine. The prosthetist designs and fits devices (prostheses) for patients who have partial or total absence of a limb.

*PERFUSIONIST   A perfusionist operates transfusion equipment when necessary and consults with physicians in selecting the appropriate equipment, techniques, and transfusion media to be used, depending on the patient's condition.

PHLEBOTOMIST   Phlebotomists are trained to draw blood from patients or donors for diagnostic testing or other medical purposes. They may also perform related tasks, such as preparing stains and reagents and cleaning and sterilizing equipment; taking patients' blood pressure, pulse, and respiration rates; performing ECGs; and billing, entering data, and answering telephones.

PHYSICAL THERAPIST   Physical therapists (PTs) must complete a baccalaureate degree program in physical therapy. They help patients restore function to muscles, nerves, joints, and bones after impairment due to illness or injury.

*PHYSICIAN'S ASSISTANT   Physicians employ physician's assistants (PAs) to perform many of the routine diagnostic and treatment procedures related to patient care. They can legally perform more procedures than registered nurses and can prescribe some medications, but they are not licensed to perform all the duties of a physician.

RADIOLOGIC OR MEDICAL IMAGING TECHNOLOGIST   Radiologic technologists are qualified to position patients for X rays, operate the X-ray equipment, prepare X-ray films for viewing, and maintain records and images for each patient. In addition to X-ray imaging, these technologists may be trained in other types of imaging, such as ultrasound and magnetic resonance scans. They cannot interpret images, nor can they inject or otherwise administer drugs necessary for some diagnostic imaging procedures.

REGISTERED NURSE   Registered nurses perform a variety of patient-care duties, such as administering drugs prescribed by the supervising physician, monitoring the cardiovascular and pulmonary status of the critically ill, caring for newborns and their mothers, and assisting surgeons in the operating room. They also supervise LPNs, LVNs, nursing assistants, and other medical office, clinic, or hospital personnel. In addition, they document patient care for physicians and other heath care team members.

*RESPIRATORY THERAPIST AND RESPIRATORY THERAPY TECHNICIAN   Respiratory therapists assume primary responsibility for all respiratory patient-care procedures to help patients with breathing disorders. They also supervise respiratory therapy technicians.

*SPECIALIST IN BLOOD BANK TECHNOLOGY   These specialists must have a bachelor's degree and certification in medical technology and must have completed the required course of study in blood bank technology. They perform both routine and specialized tests in blood bank immunohematology and perform transfusion services.

*SURGICAL TECHNOLOGIST   Surgical technologists work closely with surgeons, anesthesiologists, nurses, and other surgical personnel before, during, and after surgery. They may function as scrub, circulating, or first or second assisting surgical technologist. Duties vary according to assignment.

Although a variety of health care practitioners often work together as a team to provide medical care to patients, each individual is legally able to perform only those duties mandated by professional and statutory guidelines. Each health care practitioner is responsible for understanding the laws and rules pertaining to his or her job and for knowing requirements concerning renewal of licenses, recertification, and payment of fees for licensure, certification, and registration.

The Physician's License and Responsibilities

Each state's medical board has the authority to grant or to revoke a physician's license. The federal government has no medical licensing authority except for the permit issued by the Drug Enforcement Administration (DEA) for any physician who dispenses, prescribes, or administers narcotics (see Chapter 7).

The following criteria must be met before a physician can be granted a state license to practice medicine. He or she must:

- Have reached the age of majority, generally 21.

- Be of good moral character.

- Have completed required preliminary education, including graduation from an approved medical school.

- Have completed an approved residency program.

- Be a U.S. citizen or have filed a declaration of intent to become a citizen. (Some states have dropped this requirement.)

- Be a state resident.

- Have passed all examinations administered by the state board of medical examiners or the board of registration.

When these conditions are satisfied and a license is granted, the physician who moves out of the licensing state may obtain a license in his or her new state of residence by:

- Reciprocity—The process by which a valid license from out of state is accepted as the basis for issuing a license in a second state if prior agreement to grant reciprocity has been reached between those states.

- **Endorsement**—The process by which a license may be awarded based on individual credentials judged to meet licensing requirements in the new state of residence.

In some situations, physicians do not need a valid license to practice medicine in a specific state. These situations include:

- When responding to emergencies.

- While establishing state residency requirements in order to obtain a license.

- When employed by the U.S. Armed Forces, Public Health Service, Veterans Administration, or other federal facility.

- When engaged solely in research and not treating patients.

Physicians may be licensed in more than one state. Periodic license renewal is necessary, which usually requires simply paying a fee. However, many states require proof of continuing education units for license renewal.

endorsement *The process by which a license may be awarded based on individual credentials judged to meet licensing requirements in a new state.*

A Physician's Education

Before he or she can become licensed to practice medicine, a physician must complete a course of education that consists of:

- Graduation with a bachelor's degree from a four-year, premedicine course—usually with a concentration in the sciences.
- Graduation from a four-year medical school—in the United States a school accredited by the Liaison Committee on Medical Education. Upon graduation from medical school, students are awarded the MD degree (doctor of medicine).
- Passing the U.S. Medical Licensing Examination (USMLE), commonly called medical boards. After the first year of medical school, student physicians take Part 1 of the exam. Students take Part 2 of the exam during the fourth year of medical school, and Part 3 during the first or second year of postgraduate medical training.
- Completion of a residency—a period of practical postgraduate training in a hospital. The first year of residency is called an internship.
- Certification by the National Board of Medical Examiners (NBME), after completion of the internship and passing the medical boards. The physician is now certified as an NBME Diplomate.

—continued

License Revocation or Suspension

To specialize, physicians must complete an additional two to six years of residency in the chosen specialty. When the residency is completed, specialists can then apply to the American Board of Medical Specialties (ABMS) to take an exam in their specialty. After passing the exam, physicians are board-certified in their area of specialization; for example, a specialist in oncology becomes a board-certified oncologist, and so on.

A person educated in a foreign medical school who wishes to practice in the United States must serve a residency and must take the Clinical Skills Assessment Exam (CSAE) before being licensed. The CSAE evaluates a candidate's ability to take medical histories, interact with patients and treat a case, and use the English language.

A physician's license can be revoked (canceled) or suspended (temporarily recalled) for conviction of a felony, unprofessional conduct, or personal or professional incapacity.

A felony is a crime that is punishable by death or a year or more in prison. Conviction of a felony is grounds for revocation or suspension of the license to practice medicine. Felonies include such crimes as murder, rape, larceny, manslaughter, robbery, arson, burglary, violations of narcotic laws, and tax evasion.

Unprofessional conduct is also cause for revoking or suspending a physician's license. Some states substitute the term *gross immorality* for *unprofessional conduct,* but offenses in either category are considered serious breaches of ethics and may also be illegal. Conduct deemed unprofessional includes falsifying records, using unprofessional methods to treat a disease, betrayal of patient confidentiality, fee splitting, coding and billing fraud, and sexual misconduct.

Personal or professional incapacity may be due to senility, injury, illness, chronic alcoholism, drug abuse, or other conditions that impair a physician's ability to practice.

Court Case

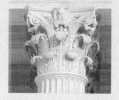

Nurse's License Revoked

A nurse's license to practice was properly revoked for drug use and other violations of professional responsibility, the Iowa Supreme Court ruled.

The Iowa Board of Nursing found that the nurse misappropriated a narcotic from the hospital where she worked, failed to report her use of prescription medications to the board, showed behavior indicative of a substance abuse problem, and had applied for employment as a registered nurse under a suspended license.

Hartwig v. Board of Nursing of the State of Iowa, 448 N.W.2d 321 (Iowa Sup. Ct., Nov. 22, 1989).

Fraud may, in some states, be considered unprofessional conduct, or it may be separately specified as grounds for revoking a physician's license. A physician is considered guilty of fraud if "intent to deceive" can be shown. Acts generally classified as fraud include:

- Falsifying medical diplomas, applications for licenses, licenses, or other credentials.

- Billing a governmental agency for services not rendered.

- Falsifying medical reports.

- Falsely advertising or misrepresenting to a patient "secret cures" or special powers to cure an ailment.

Revocations and suspensions of license are never automatic. A physician is always entitled to a written description of charges against him or her and a hearing before the appropriate state agency. Decisions are usually subject to appeal through the state's court system.

An honest mistake or a single incident of alleged incompetence or negligence is not usually sufficient grounds for license revocation.

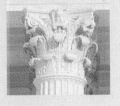
Check Your Progress

9. Name three types of unprofessional conduct for which a physician may lose his or her license.

_____

_____

_____

Fill in the blanks to accurately complete the following statements:

10. A physician is licensed by the _____ in which he or she wishes to practice.

11. The federal government's authority regarding medical licensing extends only to _____

_____

12. Revocations and suspensions of medical licenses are never _____ .

13. Name four situations in which physicians do not need a valid license to practice in a specific state:

_____

_____

_____

_____

◆ ◆ ◆ ◆ Respondeat Superior

respondeat superior *Literally, "Let the master answer." A doctrine under which an employer is legally liable for the acts of his or her employees, if such acts were performed within the scope of the employees' duties.*

Under the doctrine of ***respondeat superior,*** which is Latin for "Let the master answer," physicians are legally responsible (liable) for their own acts of negligence and for negligent acts of employees working within the scope of their employment.

The test used to determine whether an employee was or was not acting within the scope of employment when a negligent act was committed is whether or not the employee's behavior serves the interest of the employer or in some way furthers the employer's business.

For example, after a patient's initial visit for treatment of a hand injury, a physician allows the medical assistant to change the dressings and check the wound over a period of several weeks. The medical assistant fails to recognize early signs of infection, and complications develop that eventually cost the patient the full use of his hand. The patient sues the physician and wins, since the physician/employer is legally responsible for the negligence of the employee while the employee is acting within the interest of the employer's business.

The physician is vicariously responsible for negligence in the above example, but the medical assistant remains responsible for negligent actions as well. Even though licensed physicians employ medical assistants, dental assistants, nurses, and other health care practitioners, these individuals are liable for their own acts of negligence and can be sued for malpractice as well.

The concept of *respondeat superior* is based on the law of agency, which is discussed in further detail in Chapter 3.

Medical Practice Management Systems

There are four basic types of medical practice:

- Sole proprietorship
- Partnership
- Professional corporation
- Group practice

Laws governing the various types of practices vary, but medical office personnel should be aware of those laws that apply to their employer's practice management system.

◆ ◆ ◆ ◆ Sole Proprietorship

sole proprietorship *A form of medical practice management in which a physician practices alone, assuming all benefits and liabilities for the business.*

In medicine's bygone days, physicians most often practiced alone, providing all patient services from receptionist, to medical treatment, to billing, to house calls. They were engaged in a "solo practice," and they took all the profits and bore all the risks associated with the **sole proprietorship.** Today, some physicians still practice alone (with the help of employees to perform receptionist, billing, and some patient care tasks), but they are in the minority.

associate practice *A medical management system in which two or more physicians share office space and employees but practice individually.*

Two or more physicians may decide to practice individually but agree to share office space and employees. This arrangement is called an **associate practice** and allows a sharing of expenses, not a sharing of profits and liability.

◆ ◆ ◆ ◆ Partnership

When two or more physicians decide to practice together, they may form a **partnership,** based on a legal written agreement specifying the rights, obligations, and responsibilities of each partner.

partnership *A form of medical practice management system whereby two or more parties practice together under a written agreement specifying the rights, obligations, and responsibilities of each partner.*

Advantages of partnerships include sharing the workload and expenses, and pooling profits and assets. A major disadvantage is that each partner has equal liability for the acts, conduct, losses, and deficits of the partnership, unless specific provisions are made for these contingencies in the initial agreement.

◆ ◆ ◆ ◆ Professional Corporation

corporation *A body formed and authorized by law to act as a single person.*

A **corporation** is a body formed and authorized by law to act as a single person, although constituted by one or more persons and legally endowed with various rights and duties. State law governs corporations, so requirements for incorporation may vary. The corporation may own, mortgage, or sell property; manage its own business affairs; and sue or be sued.

Physicians who form corporations are shareholders and employees of the organization. There are income and tax advantages to forming a corporation, and fringe benefits to employees may be more generous than with a sole proprietorship or partnership.

◆ ◆ ◆ ◆ Group Practice

group practice *A medical management system in which three or more licensed physicians share the collective income, expenses, facilities, equipment, records, and personnel for the business.*

The **group practice** may function as a corporation or as a partnership. A medical group practice is the provision of health care services by a group of three or more licensed physicians, engaged full time in a formally organized and legally recognized entity. They share the group's income and expenses in a systematic manner and also share facilities, equipment, records, and personnel involved in both patient care and business management.

Physicians in group practice may be engaged in the same specialty, calling themselves, for example, Urology Associates. They may provide care in two or three related specialties, for example, obstetrics-gynecology and pediatrics. Alternatively, they may offer a variety of services, for example, obstetrics-gynecology, pediatrics, family practice, and internal medicine.

For physicians in group practice, advantages are much the same as they are for those in a corporation, with the added benefit that the legal implications are not as far-reaching or complicated.

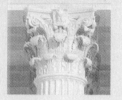
Types of Managed Care

managed care *A system in which financing, administration, and delivery of health care are combined to provide medical services to subscribers for a prepaid fee.*

Managed care health plans are corporations that pay for and deliver health care to subscribers for a set fee using a network of physicians and other health care providers. The network coordinates and refers patients to its health care providers and hospitals and monitors the amount and patterns of care delivered. The plans usually limit the services subscribers may receive under the plan. Managed care plans make agreed-upon payments to providers (hospitals or physicians) for providing health care services to subscribers to the health plan. The payment from a managed care plan to providers may be one of several types, including contracted fee schedules, percentages of billed charges, capitation, and others. (Capitation is a set advance payment made to providers, based on the calculated cost of medical care of a specific population of subscribers.)

Before managed care plans, private health insurance policies were traditionally written as third-party indemnity health insurance. *Third party* means that the insurance company reimburses health care practitioners for medical care provided to policy holders. **Indemnity** means the insured person is covered against a potential loss of money from medical expenses for an illness or accident. Indemnity insurance benefits are paid in a predetermined amount of money rather than in specific services.

indemnity *A traditional form of health insurance that covers the insured against a potential loss of money from medical expenses for an illness or accident.*

In an attempt to confront increasing health care costs, traditional fee-for-service health insurance companies now incorporate elements of managed care into their plans. Consequently, virtually all insured Americans have become familiar with such cost containment/managed care measures as coinsurance, co-payment fees, deductibles, formularies, gatekeeper or primary care physicians, and utilization review.

- *Coinsurance* refers to the amount of money that insurance plan members must pay out of pocket, after the insurance plan pays its share. For example, a plan may agree to pay 80% of the cost for a surgical procedure, and the subscriber must pay the remaining 20%.

- *Co-payment fees* are flat fees paid by insurance plan subscribers for certain medical services. For example, a subscriber might be required to pay $20 for each visit to a physician's office.

- *Deductible* amounts are specified by the insurance plan for each subscriber. For instance, the deductible for a single subscriber might be $250 a calendar year. In other words, the plan does not begin to pay benefits until the $250 deductible has been satisfied.

- *Formularies* are a plan's list of approved prescription medications for which it will reimburse subscribers.

- *Utilization review* is the method used by a health plan to measure the amount and appropriateness of health services used by its members.

◆ ◆ ◆ ◆   Health Maintenance Organizations

health maintenance organization (HMO) *A health plan that combines coverage of health care costs and delivery of health care for a prepaid premium.*

Health maintenance organizations (HMOs) are one of several types of managed care organizations providing health care services to subscribers within the United States. HMOs and preferred provider organizations (see below) are the most common types of managed care plans. Under HMO plans all health services are delivered and paid for through one organization. The three general types of HMOs are group model HMOs, staff model HMOs, and individual (or independent) practice associations (IPAs).

Group model HMOs contract with independent groups of physicians to provide coordinated care for large numbers of HMO patients for a fixed, per-member fee. They often provide medical care for members of several HMOs. Group model HMOs include prepaid group practices (PGPs). Physicians in PGPs are salaried employees of the HMO, usually practice in facilities provided by the HMO, and share in profits at the end of the year.

Staff model HMOs employ salaried physicians and other allied health professionals who provide care solely for members of one HMO. Subscribers to staff model HMOs can often see their doctors, get laboratory tests and X rays, have prescriptions filled, and even order glasses or contact lenses all in one location. Staff model HMOs also employ specialists or contract with outside specialists in some cases.

individual (or independent) practice association (IPA) *A type of HMO that contracts with groups of physicians who practice in their own offices and receive a per-member payment from participating HMOs to provide a full range of health services for members.*

An **individual (or independent) practice association (IPA)** is an association of physicians, hospitals, and other health care providers that contracts with an HMO to provide medical services to subscribers. Health care practitioners who are members of an IPA may usually still see patients outside of the contracting HMO. The providers who contract with an IPA practice in their own offices and receive a per-member payment, or capitation, from participating HMOs to provide a full range of health services for HMO members. These providers often care for members of several HMOs, which gives them a larger patient and income base than staff model HMOs.

Preferred Provider Organizations or Preferred Provider Associations

preferred provider organization (PPO), or preferred provider association (PPA) *A network of independent physicians, hospitals, and other health care providers who contract with an insurance carrier to provide medical care at a discount rate to patients who are part of the insurer's plan.*

Preferred provider organizations (PPOs), also called **preferred provider associations (PPAs),** are managed care plans that contract with a network of doctors, hospitals, and other health care providers who provide services for set fees. Subscribers may choose their primary health provider from an approved list and must pay higher out-of-pocket costs for care provided by health care practitioners outside the PPO group.

Physician-Hospital Organizations

physician-hospital organization (PHO) *A health care plan in which physicians join with hospitals to provide a medical care delivery system and then contract for insurance with a commercial carrier or an HMO.*

Physician-hospital organizations (PHOs) are another type of managed care plan. PHOs are organizations that include physicians, hospitals, surgery centers, nursing homes, laboratories, and other medical service providers that contract with one or more HMOs, insurance plans, or directly with employers to provide health care services.

Other Variations in Managed Care Plans

Managed care plans may also include the following identifying features:

gatekeeper physician *The primary care physician who directs the medical care of managed care health plan members.*

primary care physician (PCP) *The physician responsible for directing all of a patient's medical care and determining whether the patient should be referred for specialty care.*

- **Gatekeeper or primary care plan.** The insured must designate a **primary care physician (PCP).** The **gatekeeper physician** or primary care physician directs all of a patient's medical care and generates any referrals to specialists or other health care practitioners.

- **Point-of-Service (POS). Point-of-service plans** allow plan members to seek health care from nonnetwork physicians, but the plan pays the highest benefits for care when it is given by the PCP or via a referral from the PCP. When care is provided without a referral, but still within the network, the plan pays benefits at a reduced level. Members also have out-of-network benefits, but at greatly reduced payment levels.

point-of-service (POS) plan *A health care plan that allows members to seek health care from nonnetwork physicians but pays the highest benefits for care when it is given by the PCP or via a referral from the PCP.*

- **Open Access.** Subscribers may see any in-network health care provider without a referral.

Managed care plans differ from each other in some respects, but all are designed to cut the cost of health care delivery. The impact of cost-cutting measures on the quality of health care remains a major point of contention. Advocates claim that managed care plans can deliver medical services more efficiently and at much less expense than traditional fee-for-service plans. Critics argue that necessary, quality medical services are often sacrificed for profit margins and attention to the bottom line.

Of special concern to patients enrolled in managed care plans are such questions as:

- Will the most knowledgeable and experienced physician treat my medical conditions and those of my family?

- Is my physician too concerned with saving money?

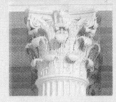

Court Rules HMO Must Cover High-Dose Chemotherapy Treatment

A Georgia HMO refused to authorize recommended high-dose chemotherapy and a bone marrow transplantation procedure called peripheral stem cell rescue for a 51-year-old patient with metastatic breast cancer. The patient sued in state court, and the case was transferred to federal court, which decided in her favor.

The HMO denied coverage on the grounds that the treatment was "experimental," and bone marrow transplant was excluded under the HMO contract. The patient could not afford the recommended care without coverage. She sought to force coverage by requesting a preliminary injunction against the HMO.

An urgency was imposed on the proceeding, due to the woman's condition. The plaintiff was able to show that the proposed treatment was not experimental and was not excluded by language of the coverage contract. The temporary injunction was granted and the woman began high-dose chemotherapy.

Mattive v. Health Source of Savannah Inc., 893 F.Sudd. 1559 (D.C., Ga., July 11, 1995).

- Must I fight to get routine procedures from my HMO?
- What if my HMO refuses to pay for a procedure I need?

In addition, physicians and other medical professionals, administrators of managed care plans, government officials, and HMO members are concerned with such issues as:

- Do managed health care and competition actually drive costs down?
- Do regulations exist regarding patient rights in managed care plans?
- Do quality ratings for HMOs help consumers?
- Does managed health care provide higher quality care than fee-for-service medicine?

Managed care is a fixture of modern medicine, but health care consumers and practitioners continue to debate its advantages and disadvantages and may do so for many years to come.

Check Your Progress

14. Define *managed care*.

_____

_____

15. Name and distinguish among three types of managed care plans.

_____

_____

_____

Legislation Affecting Health Care Plans

Congress has passed legislation intended to improve the quality of health care in the United States, to reduce fraud, and to help assure managed care and other types of health insurance subscribers that they will not be summarily dropped or otherwise be unfairly or unlawfully discriminated against by insurance providers. Two of the most significant health care laws passed in recent years are the Health Care Quality Improvement Act of 1986 and the Health Insurance Portability and Accountability Act of 1996.

◆ ◆ ◆ ◆ Health Care Quality Improvement Act of 1986

Health Care Quality Improvement Act of 1986 (HCQIA) *A federal statute passed to improve the quality of medical care nationwide. One provision established the National Practitioner Data Bank.*

In creating the **Health Care Quality Improvement Act of 1986 (HCQIA),** Congress found that "The increasing occurrence of medical malpractice and the need to improve the quality of medical care have become nationwide problems that warrant greater efforts than those that can be undertaken by any individual state." Accordingly, the act requires that professional peer review action be taken in some cases, limits the damages for professional review, and protects from liability those who provide information to professional review bodies.

National Practitioner Data Bank (NPDB) *A repository of information about health care practitioners, established by the Health Care Quality Improvement Act of 1986.*

One of the most important provisions of the HCQIA was the establishment of the **National Practitioner Data Bank (NPDB).** Use of the NPDB was intended to improve the quality of medical care nationwide by encouraging effective professional peer review of physicians and dentists. Information that must be reported to the NPDB includes medical malpractice payments, adverse licensure actions, adverse clinical privilege actions, and adverse professional society membership actions. The NPDB is a resource to assist state licensing boards, hospitals, and other health care entities in investigating qualifications of physicians, dentists, and other health care practitioners.

NPDB queries are mandatory for hospitals when a physician applies for privileges and every two years for physicians already on the medical staff who wish to maintain their privileges. They are voluntary for hospitals conducting professional review, other health care entities with formal peer review programs, state licensing boards at any time, those who wish to self-query, and plaintiffs' attorneys under certain circumstances. The NPDB may not disclose information to a medical malpractice insurer, defense attorney, or member of the general public.

◆ ◆ ◆ ◆ Health Insurance Portability and Accountability Act of 1996

Health Insurance Portability and Accountability Act of 1996 (HIPAA) *Helps workers keep continuous health insurance coverage for themselves and their dependents when they change jobs, protects confidential medical information from unauthorized disclosure or use, and helps curb the rising cost of fraud and abuse.*

The **Health Insurance Portability and Accountability Act of 1996 (HIPAA)** was an ambitious attempt by Congress to reform the American health care system. The HIPAA helps workers keep continuous health insurance coverage for themselves and their dependents when they change jobs, but its many provisions go far beyond this mandate. In addition to protecting insurance coverage for some working Americans and their families, the act was designed to:

- Improve the efficiency and effectiveness of the health care industry.

- Protect confidential medical information that identifies patients from unauthorized disclosure or use.

- Curb the rising cost of fraud and abuse.

Most important for the health care industry, the HIPAA provides for standardizing the interchange of electronic data for certain administrative and financial transactions, in order to protect the security and confidentiality of electronically stored and transmitted health information that identifies patients. Before passage of the act, there was no common standard for the transfer of information between health care providers and payers. For providers who submit claims to hundreds of payers, this made programming computer systems a difficult and expensive process. When all providers have met standardizing requirements, the act's provisions will:

- Accelerate billing processes and reduce paperwork.

- Reduce health care billing fraud.

- Reduce the risk of privacy violations.

- Facilitate tracking of health information.

- Improve accuracy and reliability of shared data.

- Increase access to computer networks within health care facilities.

The HIPAA also provides for significant criminal and civil penalties for noncompliance and serious liability risks for unauthorized disclosure of confidential medical information.

Healthcare Integrity and Protection Data Bank (HIPDB)
Established by HIPAA. A national health care fraud and abuse data collection program for the reporting and disclosure of certain adverse actions taken against health care providers, suppliers, or practitioners.

The HIPAA also provided for the creation of the **Healthcare Integrity and Protection Data Bank (HIPDB).** The HIPDB is a national health care fraud and abuse data collection program for the reporting and disclosure of certain adverse actions taken against health care providers, suppliers, or practitioners. Data from the HIPDB is available to federal and state government agencies and to health plans, but is not available to the general public.

◆ ◆ ◆ ◆ **Controlling Health Care Fraud and Abuse**

Partly because of the rising costs of health care, fraud and abuse within the industry have become major issues in recent years. As a result, legislation has been passed to control three types of illegal conduct:

1. False claims in billing
2. Kickbacks
3. Self-referrals

Federal False Claims Act *A law that allows for individuals to bring civil actions on behalf of the United States government for false claims made to the federal government, under a provision of the law called qui tam (from Latin meaning "to bring an action for the king and for one's self").*

Several federal and state statutes prohibit false claims. The HIPAA, discussed above, and the federal False Claims Act are two examples of laws that prohibit false claims and detail the penalties that can be levied against violators.

The **Federal False Claims Act** allows for individuals to bring civil actions on behalf of the United States government for false claims made to the federal government, under a provision of the law called *qui tam* (from Latin meaning "to bring an action for the king and for one's self"). These individuals, commonly known as whistleblowers, are referred to as *qui tam relators* and can share in any court-awarded damages.

Suits brought under the False Claims Act are most often related to the health care and defense industries. The act prohibits:

- Making a false record or statement to get a false or fraudulent claim paid by the government.

- Conspiring to have a false or fraudulent claim paid by the government.

- Withholding property of the government with the intent to defraud the government or to willfully conceal it from the government.

- Making or delivering a receipt for government property that is false or fraudulent.

- Buying government property from someone who is not authorized to sell the property.

- Making a false statement to avoid or deceive an obligation to pay money or property to the government.

- Causing someone else to submit a false claim by submitting false information.

Kickbacks, or giving financial incentives to a health care provider for referring patients or for recommending services or products, are prohibited under the federal Anti-Kickback Law, and by state laws.

Self-referrals, or referring patients to any service or facility where the health provider has a financial interest, are prohibited by the federal Ethics in Patient Referral Act, as well as other federal and state laws.

Violations of laws against health care fraud and abuse can result in imprisonment and fines, loss of license, loss of health care facility staff privileges, and exclusion from participation in federal health care programs.

The Patients' Bill of Rights Act of 1999

Concerns about the quality of medical care patients receive under managed care plans prompted Congress to first consider a Patients' Bill of Rights Act in 1999. The act contained provisions applicable to managed care plans for

Court Case

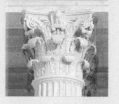

Physician's Records Called

A Maryland appellate court ruled that a physician's professional corporation could be compelled to produce records of all purchases of medical equipment and supplies.

The Medicaid Fraud Control Unit subpoenaed the records for a criminal investigation based on the allegation that the physician did not purchase enough medical supplies to justify the number of laboratory tests he billed to Medicaid. The physician asserted his Fifth Amendment privilege against self-incrimination and refused to produce the records.

A trial court compelled him to produce the records, and the appellate court affirmed. The court held that the records in question were corporate records, not the physician's individual records, and he could not assert a Fifth Amendment privilege on behalf of the corporation.

In re Criminal Investigation No. 465, 563 A.2d 1117 (Md. Ct. of Special App., Sept. 27, 1989).

access to care, quality assurance, patient information and securing privacy, grievances and appeals procedures, protecting the doctor-patient relationship, and promoting good medical practice. In late 2001 the act had stalled in Congress as members debated the rights of patients to file lawsuits against managed care plans in federal or state courts, and whether or not awards in such lawsuits should be limited by law to certain amounts.

Risk Management

risk management *Steps taken to minimize danger, hazard, and liability.*

Since liability is a major factor in health care delivery, and since health care delivery systems and practitioners seek to minimize liability whenever possible, **risk management** has become a necessary practice component. Risk management is one approach to reducing the likelihood of a malpractice lawsuit. Risk management involves identifying problem practices or behaviors, then eliminating or controlling them. Risk management activities that may help avoid litigation include providing written job descriptions for health care practice employees and providing office procedures manuals and employee handbooks that can help avoid misunderstandings and mistakes that lead to liability risks. Other common health care facility activities that may affect the likelihood or course of litigation include medical record charting, patient scheduling, writing prescriptions, and communicating with patients.

quality improvement (QI) (or quality assurance) *Measures taken by health care providers and practitioners to uphold the quality of patient care.*

Measures used to manage risk are part of **quality improvement (QI), or quality assurance,** practices performed by health care providers and practitioners to uphold the quality of patient care and to reduce liability risk.

Most health care facilities and plans employ quality improvement and risk managers to oversee risk and quality issues relating to physicians and support staff. Quality improvement and risk managers may also assume responsibility for compliance with federal, state, and other health care regulatory agencies. A compliance plan is developed to help assure that all governmental regulations are followed. Such a plan is especially beneficial for seeing that coding and billing regulations for Medicare, Medicaid, and other government plans are followed.

Health care institutions and organizations employ individuals who are responsible for credentialing. Credentialing may be done by risk management staff or by other departments within a health care organization. Credentialing is the process of verifying a health care provider's credentials. The process may be performed by an insurance company before a provider is admitted to the network, by medical offices prior to granting hospital privileges, or by other groups who routinely employ or contract with health care providers. Credentialing usually consists of these steps:

1. A provider fills out an application and attaches copies of his or her medical license, proof of malpractice insurance coverage, and other requested credentials.
2. The listed sources are asked to verify the information.
3. Medicare and Medicaid sanctions and malpractice history are checked via the National Practitioner Data Bank.
4. The findings are presented to a credentialing committee.
5. A peer review process completes the credentialing procedure.

Terri, a registered nurse, is the quality improvement and risk manager for 85 physicians at 35 different Midwestern locations. She supervises compliance with federal and state regulations and credentialing for physicians and their support staff. She also investigates complaints against staff members. She looks for troubling patterns and trends concerning staff conduct via adverse reports from hospitals, managed care organizations, patients, and lawsuits filed. In addition, she uses the National Practitioner Data Bank to verify licensure and credentialing information.

Terri's responsibilities also include identifying and preventing Medicare and Medicaid fraud and abuse. Staff members are cautioned to watch for billing for more expensive procedures than those that were performed or for tests or procedures that were not performed, codes without adequate documentation, and laboratory tests performed without substantiating diagnoses. She tells staff members, "If you know fraud is going on and you do nothing, you are as guilty as the physician or office manager."

Telemedicine

telemedicine *Remote consultation by patients with physicians or other health professionals via telephone, closed-circuit television, or the Internet.*

Telemedicine refers to remote consultation with physicians or other health care professionals via telephone, closed-circuit television, fax machine, or the Internet. When telemedicine was first used, it generally involved transmission of X rays, sonograms, or other medical data between two distant points. In some cases, usually through closed-circuit television, a physician could exam a patient at a distant location, thus allowing patients in rural areas more complete access to medical care. Today, transmitted medical data includes video, audio, and written or computerized patient data. In fact, increasing use of the Internet has made telemedicine an important component of the health care system.

Two additional aspects of telemedicine are cybermedicine and e-health. **Cybermedicine** involves direct contact between physician and patient. There are many Web sites on the Internet that allow patients to consult directly with a physician, usually for a fee. The physician may offer medical advice and even prescribe medication.

cybermedicine *A form of telemedicine that involves direct contact between patients and physicians over the Internet, usually for a fee.*

E-health is the term used for the increasing use of the Internet as a source of consumer information about health and medicine. E-health has become a popular aspect of telemedicine, as increasing numbers of patients query their doctors and other health care providers about where to find health information on the Internet and how to evaluate such information.

e-health *The term for the use of the Internet as a source of consumer information about health and medicine.*

Health-related Internet sites included under the category "e-health" most often provide:

- Consumer information services.

- Support groups.

- Prescription drug sales.

- Medical advice and diagnosis (cybermedicine).

- Contract health services as part of insurance plans for covered subscribers.

- Health business support services for health professionals and health care organizations.

Telemedicine fits the cost-cutting goals for managed care and offers possibilities for improving health care delivery, but there is currently no case law governing the role of telephysicians and their potential liability, since the few telemedicine suits brought have been settled out of court. Use of telemedicine in the United States has been steadily expanding, but legal questions currently unresolved include the following:

- Since physicians must be licensed in the state where they practice, do they need a license in every state where a patient resides? States have begun reviewing their medical practice acts, and since 1997 some have amended legislation or added provider licensing requirements for telemedicine. Most state laws and regulations, however, are vague on the issue, especially for situations in which a physician assumes a limited consulting role with an out-of-state patient. A national telemedicine license has been suggested that would be accepted in any state.

- How will providers be reimbursed for telemedical services? Medicare had begun to reimburse some types of telemedicine in 2001, under provisions for telehomecare, but for the most part, patients must have direct personal contact with a physician for services to be reimbursed by the government. An increasing number of private insurers now cover telehomecare and remote patient monitoring services.

- Can patient confidentiality be maintained? Physicians practicing telemedicine must comply with confidentiality laws in the state where the patient resides. The HIPAA will impact this issue as telecommunication standards mandated by the act are implemented.

- Does teleconsultation constitute a traditional physician-patient relationship under duty-of-care standards?

- How is informed consent affected? According to the Physician Insurers Association of America, the physician may be held to a higher standard in teleconsultation situations, since the courts may view telemedicine as experimental.

◆ ◆ ◆ ◆ Consumer Precautions Regarding Telemedicine

Individuals using the Internet for health care and medical information should evaluate Web sites for reliability, since there is currently no regulating body responsible for overseeing online health and medical information or services. Users should ask questions such as:

- Who is sponsoring the site? Sites linked with major medical centers and groups, government agencies, and medical professionals or major medical publications are most likely to present reliable information.

- Are several reliable Web sites offering similar information? If so, the information is most likely to be reliable.

- Does the site tout miracle cures or peculiar therapies? Users should discuss any claims made with a trusted health care practitioner before sending for materials or following such advice.

Clearly, technology has improved our ability to record, store, transfer, and share medical data electronically. It has also magnified privacy, security, and confidentiality concerns that normally pertain to patient medical records. Although the HIPAA has addressed the issue by mandating the development of far-reaching national standards for electronic health transactions, HIPAA rules do not necessarily cover all consumer-oriented Web sites that collect, store, and maintain personally identifiable consumer information. To address telemedicine privacy concerns, the industry has promoted self-regulation by developing standards for health-related Web sites. For example, some of the principles recommended by the Internet Healthcare Coalition are candor, honesty, quality, and informed consent. Principles adopted by the Health Internet Ethics Coalition include a commitment to adopt a privacy policy, enhanced privacy protection for health-related personal information, safeguarding consumer privacy in relationships with third parties, and disclosing ownership and sponsorship information.

Federal and state governments have introduced many bills addressing consumer privacy, but uniform legislation is needed that will sufficiently regulate telemedicine.

Court Case

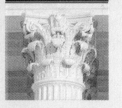

Electronic Prescription Program Raises Telemedicine Issues

Walgreen Company, the owner and operator of pharmacies in many states, created and tested a new computer system for the electronic transmission of prescriptions by ten physicians in Wisconsin. Walgreen provided the necessary software to the participating physicians and also supplied six of them with used computers and modems at no cost. Each electronically transmitted prescription contained the same information as a written or faxed prescription but did not include the physician's signature.

The Wisconsin Pharmacy Examining Board determined that Walgreen's system violated Wisconsin law requiring written prescriptions to be signed by physicians. Since Walgreen Company also supplied equipment to some physicians free of charge, the board also determined that the company had violated a state law prohibiting pharmacies from participating in "rebate or fee-splitting arrangements" with physicians.

Walgreen Company appealed the decision of the Wisconsin Pharmacy Examining Board. The trial court that heard the case reversed the board's ruling. A court of appeals affirmed, holding that electronic transmissions were more like oral or telephone transmissions and that no signature was required. The court also held that a more "reasonable interpretation" of the Wisconsin law against rebate or fee-splitting arrangements was that Walgreen Company's electronic prescription program had not violated the law.

Walgreen Co. v. Wisconsin Pharmacy Examining Board, 217 Wis.2d 290, 577 (unpublished opinion).

Applying Knowledge

Write "L" for licensure, "C" for certification, "R" for registration, or "A" for accreditation in the space provided to indicate which are applicable in the following descriptions (more than one may apply).

_____ **1.** Involves a mandatory credentialing process established by law, usually at the state level.

_____ **2.** Involves simply paying a fee.

_____ **3.** Involves a voluntary credentialing process, usually national in scope, most often sponsored by a private-sector group.

_____ **4.** Required of all physicians, dentists, and nurses in every state.

_____ **5.** Consists simply of an entry in an official record.

_____ **6.** A process that implies that health care facilities or HMOs have met certain standards.

Match each of the following managed care or insurance terms with the correct description by writing the appropriate letter in the space provided.

a. physician-hospital organization (PHO)

b. point-of-service

c. gatekeeper or primary care physician

d. gatekeeper or primary care plan

e. preferred provider organization (PPO)

_____ **7.** Under this plan insured patients must designate a primary care physician (PCP).

_____ **8.** This plan allows members to seek health care from non-HMO physicians, but the plan pays the highest benefits when care is provided by the PCP or via a referral from the PCP.

_____ **9.** Under this plan insurer payments are higher if health providers are not chosen from a list provided to patients.

_____ **10.** This individual determines whether patients enrolled in a designated managed care plan should be referred to medical specialists.

_____ **11.** Physicians, hospitals, surgery centers, nursing homes, laboratories, and other medical service providers contract with one or more HMOs, insurance plans, or directly with employers to provide health care services.

Review and Case Studies

Match each term below with its correct definition by writing the appropriate letter in the space provided.

_____12. Doctrine that is Latin for "Let the master answer."

_____13. The concept in question 11 is based on this law.

_____14. An insurance term indicating the fee paid by patients over and above that paid by the insurance company.

_____15. A mandatory process, established by law and required of certain health care practitioners.

_____16. The term for the process by which a health care provider's license and other credentials are checked before he or she is employed by a managed care plan.

a. licensure

b. *respondeat superior*

c. credentialing

d. co-payment

e. law of agency

Answer the following questions in the spaces provided.

17. What is the purpose of medical practice acts?

_____

_____

18. List four requirements that must be met before a physician can be granted a license to practice medicine.

_____

_____

_____

_____

19. List four instances in which a physician might not need a license.

_____

_____

_____

_____

20. Name three circumstances under which a physician's license may be revoked.

_____

_____

_____

21. Who has the authority to revoke a physician's license?

_____

_____

_____

22. Give one advantage and one disadvantage for each of the following practice management systems:

    Sole proprietorship

    Advantage: _____

    Disadvantage: _____

    Partnership

    Advantage: _____

    Disadvantage: _____

    Corporation

    Advantage: _____

    Disadvantage: _____

23. List three types of managed care health care plans.

    _____

    _____

    _____

24. Name three major types of provisions provided under the Health Insurance Portability and Accountability Act of 1996 (HIPAA).

    _____

    _____

    _____

25. Name the "whistleblower" statute that deals with fraud and abuse in health care.

    _____

26. Define *risk management.*

    _____

    _____

27. Distinguish among the terms *telemedicine, cybermedicine,* and *e-health.*

    _____

    _____

    _____

28. What problems of legality must currently be resolved for telemedicine to be used more extensively in medical practice?

    _____

    _____

    _____

    _____

    _____

29. What is the sole authority granted the federal government concerning the licensing of physicians?

    _____

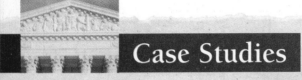

Case Studies

Use your critical-thinking skills to answer the questions that follow the case study.

A patient complained to the state medical board that her health care plan physician turned her away from a scheduled office visit because she did not have her checkbook with her and thus could not make the required $20 advance co-payment. She complained that, because she was ill, it was unfeeling and unrealistic of the physician to expect her to go home and get her checkbook. She pointed out that the physician's office had a record of her insurance coverage and her payment record was good. When she asked her physician to make an exception to his rule requiring co-payments in advance, he replied, "You would bring your checkbook with you if you went to the supermarket, wouldn't you?"

30. **In your opinion, should the physician have made an exception to his payment rule? Why or why not?**

     _____

     _____

     _____

     _____

31. **Is the comparison of a medical office to a supermarket appropriate? Explain your answer.**

     _____

     _____

     _____

     _____

32. **If you believe the physician was at fault, should he be reprimanded or sanctioned in some way? If so, what would you recommend?**

     _____

     _____

     _____

     _____

33. **How could the physician's payment policy be adjusted to avoid future difficulty?**

     _____

     _____

     _____

     _____

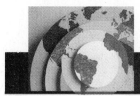

Complete the activities and answer the questions that follow.

34. Conduct a Web search for the Clinical Skills Assessment Exam. Who must take the exam, and when is it administered?

_____

_____

_____

_____

35. Find the Web site for the Federation of State Medical Boards of the United States (FSMB). What purpose does the federation serve? Have recent FSMB actions affected medical practice in your state? If so, how?

_____

_____

_____

_____

_____

_____

36. Locate the Web sites on the Internet for the Internet Healthcare Coalition and the Health Internet Ethics Coalition. Summarize their respective positions on the issue of electronic privacy.

_____

_____

_____

_____

_____

LAW, THE COURTS, AND CONTRACTS

3

Objectives

After studying this chapter, you should be able to:

1. Discuss the three primary sources of law.
2. Differentiate between criminal law and civil law.
3. Define intentional and unintentional torts.
4. Explain the unintentional tort of negligence.
5. List and discuss the four essential elements of a contract.
6. Differentiate between expressed contracts and implied contracts.
7. Discuss the contractual rights and responsibilities of both physicians and patients.
8. Relate how the law of agency and the doctrine of *respondeat superior* apply to health care contracts.

Key Terms

- administrative law
- agent
- breach of contract
- case law
- common law
- contract
- criminal law
- defendant
- expressed contract
- Fair Debt Collection Practices Act
- felony
- jurisdiction
- implied contract
- law of agency

- legal precedents
- minor
- misdemeanor
- negligence
- plaintiff
- prosecution
- Statute of Frauds
- statutory law
- substantive law
- third party payor contract
- tort
- tortfeasor
- void
- voidable

The Basis for Laws

Federal laws governing the administration of health care and all other national matters derive from powers and responsibilities delegated to the three branches of government by the United States Constitution. As you probably recall from basic government classes, the three branches of government are legislative, executive, and judicial. Here is a quick review of the three branches' composition and responsibilities:

- The *legislative branch* consists of the two houses of Congress—the Senate and the House of Representatives. Congress originates legislation that becomes federal law.

- The *executive branch* includes the President of the United States as chief executive and his or her various appointed assistants and hired employees. The executive branch of government is responsible for administering the law.

    Through his or her ability to issue executive orders, the President has limited legislative powers. Executive orders become law without the prior approval of Congress. They are usually issued for one of three purposes: to create administrative agencies or change the practices of an existing agency, to enforce laws passed by Congress, or to make treaties with foreign powers.

- The United States Supreme Court heads the *judicial branch* of government, which also includes federal judges and courts in every state. The judicial branch interprets the law and oversees the enforcement of laws.

The division of powers and responsibilities among three branches of government ensures that a system of checks and balances will keep any one branch from assuming too much power (see Figure 3-1).

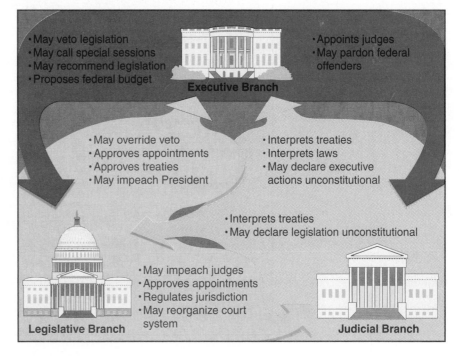

Figure 3-1
System of Checks and Balances

Sources of Law

case law *Law established through common law and legal precedent.*

common law *The body of unwritten law developed in England, primarily from judicial decisions based on custom and tradition.*

legal precedents *Decisions made by judges in various courts that become rule of law and apply to future cases, even though they were not enacted by legislation.*

statutory law *Law passed by the U.S. Congress or state legislatures.*

Laws are classified into three types—case law, statutory law, and administrative law—based on source.

Case law is law set by legal precedent. Case law began with **common law.** In the early days in America, laws derived from those originating in England, and they were not often written down. Matters of law were decided based on the customs and traditions of the people. Judges shared their decisions with other judges, and these decisions became common law.

Later court decisions were written down, and judges could now refer to past cases to help them make current decisions. These written cases were then used as **legal precedents.** When deciding cases with similar circumstances, judges were required to follow these earlier cases or legal precedents. Today legal precedents are the rule of law, applying to future cases, even though they were not enacted by legislation. Precedents can be changed only by the court that originally decided a case or by a higher court.

Statutory law refers to laws enacted by state or federal legislatures. Individual laws in this body of law are called statutes. (Laws passed by city governments are called municipal ordinances.) Statutes begin as bills at the federal or state levels. The bills may become laws, or presidents or governors may veto them. Once passed, the laws may be amended, repealed, revised, or superseded by legislatures. The courts can review statutes for constitutionality, application, interpretation, and other legal questions. (See Figure 3-2.)

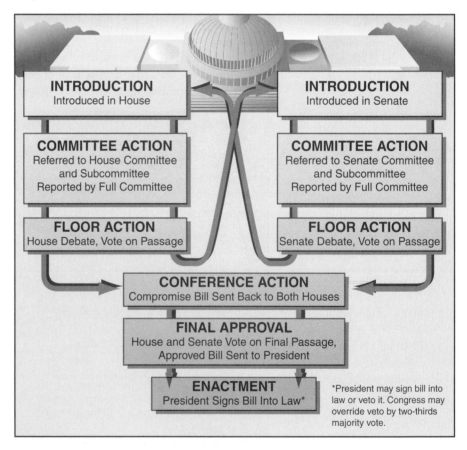

Figure 3-2
How a Federal Bill Becomes a Law

administrative law *Enabling statutes enacted to define powers and procedures when an agency is created.*

substantive law *Regulations passed by an agency that pertain specifically to the functions of that agency.*

Administrative law includes statutes enacted to define specific powers and procedures when agencies are created. Administrative agencies are created by Congress, the President, or state legislatures. Regulations may be passed that pertain specifically to the functions of one agency, such as the Internal Revenue Service (IRS), Social Security Administration (SSA), or Occupational Safety and Health Administration (OSHA). These regulations are called **substantive law.**

Check Your Progress

1. What are the three types of law, based on source?

_____

_____

_____

2. Which of the three types of law began with common law?

_____

3. Briefly define *substantive law.*

_____

Classifications of Law

After laws are created through case, statutory, or administrative law, they are classified as to type, such as criminal, civil, military, or international. Since criminal and civil laws are most likely to pertain to health care practitioners, they are discussed in more detail below.

◆ ◆ ◆ ◆ Criminal Law

criminal law *Law that involves crimes against the state.*

A crime is an offense against the state or sovereignty, committed or omitted, in violation of a public law forbidding or commanding it. Thus the body of **criminal law** involves crimes against the state. When a state or federal criminal law is violated, the government brings criminal charges against the alleged offender (for example, *New York v. John Doe*).

State criminal laws prohibit such crimes as murder, burglary, robbery, arson, rape, sodomy, larceny, mayhem (needless or willful damage or violence), and practicing medicine without a license. Federal criminal offenses include matters affecting national security (treason), crimes involving the country's borders, and illegal activities that cross state lines, such as kidnapping or hijacking.

felony *An offense punishable by death or by imprisonment in a state or federal prison for more than one year.*

A criminal act may be classified as a felony or a misdemeanor. A **felony** is a crime punishable by death or by imprisonment in a state or

Can Knowledge Make You Guilty?

Persons who commit crimes are, of course, the principals in criminal proceedings. However, those individuals who have knowledge of a crime may, in certain circumstances, also be subject to prosecution. An *accessory* is one who contributes to or aids in the commission of a crime, either by a direct act, by an indirect act (such as encouragement), by watching and not giving aid, or by concealing the criminal's crime.

misdemeanor *A crime punishable by fine or by imprisonment in a facility other than a prison for less than one year.*

plaintiff *The complaining party in a lawsuit.*

prosecution *The government as plaintiff in a criminal case.*

defendant *The person or party against whom charges are brought in a criminal or civil lawsuit.*

federal prison for more than one year. Felonies include abuse (child, elder, or domestic violence), arson, burglary, conspiracy, embezzlement, fraud, illegal drug dealing, grand larceny, manslaughter, mayhem, murder or attempted murder, rape, robbery, sodomy, tax evasion, and practicing medicine without a license.

Misdemeanors are less serious crimes than felonies. They are punishable by fines or by imprisonment in a facility other than a prison for one year or less. Examples of misdemeanors include some traffic violations, thefts under a certain dollar amount, attempted burglary, and disturbing the peace.

Figure 3-3 identifies the different participants in court and the roles they play.

Civil Law ◆ ◆ ◆ ◆

Whereas criminal law involves crimes against the state, civil law involves crimes against persons. Under civil law, a person can sue another person, a business, or the government. Civil disputes often arise over issues of contract violation, slander, libel, trespassing, product liability, or automobile accidents. Many civil suits involve family matters such as divorce, child support, and child custody. Court judgments in civil cases often require the payment of a sum of money to the injured party.

When criminal and civil cases go to court, a complaining party—the **plaintiff**—must show that he or she was wronged or injured. The government—the **prosecution**—is the plaintiff in criminal cases. A private individual is the plaintiff in civil cases. The **defendant,** who is charged with an offense, must dispute the complaint.

Officers of the court are responsible for carrying out courtroom duties:

- Judges are elected or appointed to preside over the court and in most states must be licensed attorneys. They rule on points of law about trial procedure, presentation of evidence, and all laws that apply to the case. If there is no jury, the judge determines the facts in the case. Judges hand down sentences after a verdict is rendered.

- Attorneys represent plaintiffs and defendants, presenting evidence so that the jury or the judge can reach a verdict.

- Court clerks keep court records and seals, enter court orders and judgments into the record, and keep the papers of the court.

- Bailiffs keep order in the courtroom and may remove disruptive persons from the court upon the judge's request.

- Court reporters make a running account of all court proceedings, using a stenotype machine that types shorthand symbols onto a tape.

- Juries are most often selected from lists of registered voters. Six or twelve jurors are chosen to hear the evidence presented in court and render a verdict.

Figure 3-3
Players in the Court Scene

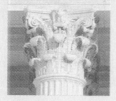

Group Guilty of Practicing Medicine Without a License

A California trial court found a religious association guilty of engaging in the illegal practice of medicine. The group made diagnoses, gave physical examinations, gave advice on physical conditions, and claimed that a water-only fast could cure illness. At least three persons were harmed as a result of undertaking the water-only fasts supervised by the religious group.

The court said the fasting constituted the practice of medicine without a license and was not faith healing as the group maintained. The trial court granted an injunction against the group's activities, and the appellate court affirmed.

Board of Medical Quality Assurance v. Andrews, 260 Cal. Rptr. 113 (Cal. Ct. of App., June 29, 1989).

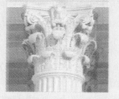

Disorderly Conduct in Emergency Room Leads to Criminal Trial

A security guard on duty in the emergency room of a large city hospital heard a woman having an "extremely loud" conversation with a group of people later identified as the woman's family members. The guard asked the woman to "hold it down," since there were approximately 60 people in the emergency room at the time. The woman confronted the security guard, shouting, "You can't tell me what to do, I'll do what I want."

As the situation escalated, the security guard attempted to escort the woman from the emergency room. The woman dropped to the floor, kicked chairs, and yelled and screamed. The security guard requested assistance, and it took four officers to physically carry the screaming woman from the emergency room. City police were called, and the officer who responded tried to calm the woman in order to remove her from the hospital. The woman refused to calm down, refused to sign a citation issued by the police officer, and insisted on going to jail. She was then arrested and taken to jail.

At trial the woman said she spoke loudly in the emergency room because her mother is hard of hearing. She said she was attempting to calm her agitated mother when the hospital security officer approached her. The woman said she began to cry and scream when the security officer took her arm and tried to remove her from the hospital emergency room. She charged that while she was in the security office a rag was stuffed in her mouth.

The trial court found the woman guilty of disorderly conduct. She appealed to the state Court of Criminal Appeals. The appeals court upheld the trial court decision, stating in part: "[The defendant's] behavior was so disruptive that it was necessary for emergency room nurses to call security for assistance. . . . Emergency room business was disrupted. We believe there was sufficient evidence for the trial court to reasonably conclude that [defendant] created unreasonable noise that prevented others from carrying on lawful activities."

State of Tennessee v. Alice Cook, 2000 Tenn. Crim. App. Lexis 135 (Ct. of Criminal App. of Tennessee, Middle Section, at Nashville, Feb. 4, 2000).

Tort Liability

Civil law includes a general category of law known as torts. A **tort** is broadly defined as a civil wrong committed against a person or property, excluding breach of contract. The act, committed without just cause, may have caused physical injury, resulted in damage to someone's property, or deprived someone of his or her personal liberty and freedom. Torts may be intentional (willful) or unintentional (accidental).

◆ ◆ ◆ ◆ Intentional Torts

Some torts involve intentional misconduct. When one person intentionally harms another, the law allows the injured party to seek a remedy in a civil suit. The injured party can be financially compensated for any harm done by the **tortfeasor** (person guilty of committing a tort.) If the conduct is judged to be malicious, punitive damages may also be awarded. Examples of intentional torts include the following:

ASSAULT   Assault is the open threat of bodily harm to another, or acting in such a way as to put another in the "reasonable apprehension of bodily harm."

BATTERY   Battery is an action that causes bodily harm to another. It is broadly defined as any bodily contact made without permission. Battery may or may not result from the threat of assault. In health care delivery, battery may be charged for any unauthorized touching of a patient, including such actions as suturing a wound, administering an injection, or performing a physical examination.

DEFAMATION OF CHARACTER   Damaging a person's reputation by making public statements that are both false and malicious is considered defamation of character. Defamation can take the form of libel or slander. Libel is expressing in published print, writing, pictures, or signed statements that injure the reputation of another. Libel also includes reading statements aloud or broadcasting for the public to hear. Slander is speaking defamatory or damaging words intended to prejudice others against an individual in a manner that jeopardizes his or her reputation or means of livelihood.

FALSE IMPRISONMENT   False imprisonment is the intentional, unlawful restraint or confinement of one person by another. The offense is treated as a crime in some states. Refusing to dismiss a patient from a health care facility upon his or her request or preventing an employee or patient from leaving the facility might be seen as false imprisonment.

FRAUD   Fraud consists of deceitful practices in depriving or attempting to deprive another of his or her rights. Health care practitioners might be accused of fraud for promising patients "miracle cures" or for accepting fees from patients for using mystical or spiritual powers to heal.

INVASION OF PRIVACY   Invasion of privacy is an intrusion into a person's seclusion or private affairs, public disclosure of private facts about a person, false publicity about a person, or use of a person's name or likeness without permission. Improper use of or breaching the confidentiality of medical records may be seen as invasion of privacy.

Intentional torts may also be crimes. Therefore, some civil actions may also be prosecuted as criminal acts in separate court actions. See Table 3-1 for a summary of intentional torts.

Table 3-1

INTENTIONAL TORTS

Tort	Description
Assault	Threatening to strike or harm with a weapon or physical movement, resulting in fear.
Battery	Unlawful, unprivileged touching of another person.
Trespass	Wrongful injury or interference with the property of another.
Nuisance	Anything that interferes with the enjoyment of life or property.
Interference with contractual relations	Intentionally causing one person not to enter into or to break a contract with another.
Deceit	False statement or deceptive practice done with intent to injure another.
Conversion	Unauthorized taking or borrowing of personal property of another for the use of the taker.
False imprisonment (false arrest)	Unlawful restraint of a person, whether in prison or otherwise.
Defamation	Wrongful act of injuring another's reputation by making false statements.
Invasion of privacy	Interference with a person's right to be left alone.
Misuse of legal procedure	Bringing legal action with malice and without probable cause.
Infliction of emotional distress	Intentionally or recklessly causing emotional or mental suffering to others.
Fraud	Dishonest or deceitful practices in depriving, or attempting to deprive, another of his or her rights.

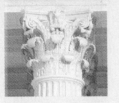

Court Case

Patient Sues for Invasion of Privacy

A patient was undergoing a medical examination as part of a workers' compensation claim. During the course of the exam, the patient told the nurse he was HIV positive, so that she could be especially careful in handling samples and contaminated medical instruments. His admission was not related to his claim. The examining physician reported the information to the patient's employer, and the patient sued. The court found against the defendant and upheld the patient's "reasonable expectation of privacy."

Estate of Ubaniak v. Newton, No. A.D. 45593 (Cal. Ct. of App. 1st Dist., Jan. 14, 1991).

The more common torts within the health care delivery system are those committed unintentionally. Unintentional torts are acts that are not intended to cause harm but are committed unreasonably or with a disregard for the consequences. In legal terms, this constitutes **negligence.**

negligence *An unintentional tort alleged when one may have performed or failed to perform an act that a reasonable person would or would not have done in similar circumstances.*

Negligence is charged when a health care practitioner fails to exercise ordinary care and a patient is injured. The accused may have performed an act or failed to perform an act that a reasonable person, in similar circumstances, would or would not have performed. "Didn't intend to do it" or "should have known better" best describe a negligent act. Under principles of negligence, civil liability exists only in cases in which the act is judicially determined to be wrongful. A health care practitioner, for example, is not necessarily liable for a poor-quality outcome in delivering health care. He or she becomes liable only when his or her conduct is determined to be malpractice, the negligent delivery of professional services.

Negligence and defenses to liability suits are discussed in detail in Chapters 4 and 5, respectively.

Court Case

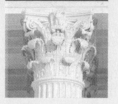

Bad Outcome Alone Not Sufficient to Prove Negligence

A patient was to have mucous membranes from his sinuses removed. An otolaryngologist performed the surgery, after reassuring the patient that he had performed the surgery several times. The next day, physicians saw that the patient was not recovering properly. A consulting neurosurgeon determined that the patient had suffered brain damage due to surgical penetration into the cranial cavity during surgery. The patient ultimately died, and his estate sued the otolaryngologist for negligence. The claim was brought before the Health Claims Arbitration Panel, whose members decided for the physician. The estate filed a motion to nullify the ruling, and the case proceeded to trial. After expert testimony on both sides, the court concluded that negligence cannot automatically be deduced from an unsuccessful medical treatment and ruled for the otolaryngologist. An appellate court affirmed.

Kennelly v. Burgess, 636 A. 2d 32 (Md. Ct. of App., Jan. 27, 1994).

Court Case

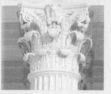

No Injury, No Award

While performing a procedure to treat esophageal cancer, a Colorado surgeon penetrated a patient's heart wall with a central venous catheter. The patient sued the physician for negligence, and after a jury trial a judgment was entered in favor of the surgeon, who was awarded costs.

On appeal, the court agreed that there was no evidence the patient suffered an injury as a result of the surgeon's alleged negligence. Without evidence of such injury, the patient could not recover damages but was entitled to a hearing on the award of costs to the surgeon.

Dunlap v. Long, 902 P.2d 446 (Colo. Ct. of App., Jan. 19, 1995; rehearing denied March 2, 1995; *certiorari* denied Sept. 5, 1995).

[A *certiorari* is a writ (written order) issued by a superior court to call up the records of a lower court or of a body acting in a quasi-judicial capacity.]

4. Which type of law involves crimes against the state? _____

5. Which type of law involves crimes against persons? _____

6. Torts are wrongs committed against _____ .

7. The two broad types of torts are _____ and _____ .

8. The type of torts most likely to concern health care practitioners is _____ .

Court Case

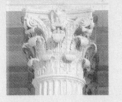

Patient Fails to Prove Physician Negligence

A patient was diagnosed with scabies, a skin condition. Her physician subsequently prescribed lindane for topical treatment of the condition. The patient applied the lindane for three days and her scabies was cured.

On the day following the last application of lindane, the patient sought treatment for tingling and numbness in her face. Several physicians failed to determine the cause of the symptoms and diagnosed atypical facial pain.

The patient brought an action for malpractice against the physician who prescribed lindane. No testimony was entered listing lindane as the cause of the patient's symptoms.

The trial court determined that there was insufficient evidence to submit the case to the jury for verdict and granted a directed verdict for the physician.

The patient appealed, but the fact remained that the patient failed to introduce expert testimony as to how the physician's alleged negligence had caused her injuries. The trial court's judgment was allowed to stand.

Reynolds v. Warthan, 896 S.W.2d 813 (Texas Ct. of App., March 17, 1995).

The Court System

The type of court that tries a case depends on the state law or federal law that was allegedly violated. The federal court system, with some exceptions, hears cases involving federal matters. State court systems are independent of one another, and each system has its own rules and regulations. Generally, state courts decide cases involving matters occurring within their own state borders.

◆ ◆ ◆ ◆ **Federal Courts**

jurisdiction *The power and authority given to a court to hear a case and to make a judgment.*

Jurisdiction is the power and authority given to a court to hear a case and to make a judgment. Examples of cases over which federal courts have jurisdiction include federal crimes, federal antitrust law, bankruptcy, patents, copyrights, trademarks, suits against the United States, and areas of admiralty law (pertaining to the sea).

State Courts

Each state has its own court system, but the general structure is the same in all states. The bottom tier consists of local courts. The next highest tier includes trial courts, followed by appellate courts, and then the state supreme court, which is the highest state court. As with the federal court system, there are also special state courts with jurisdiction in certain kinds of cases.

Figure 3-4 shows the various federal and state court systems in the United States.

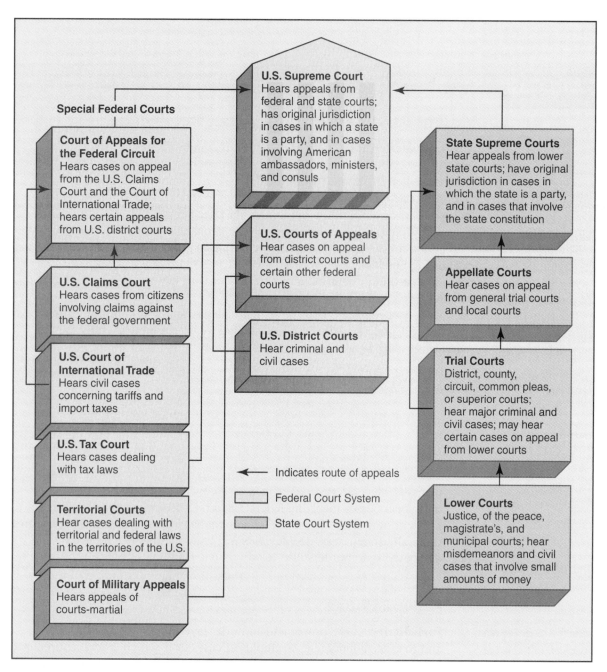

Figure 3-4
Court Systems in the United States

A physician was notified that the extension he had built on his house to serve as his office violated the town's zoning law. Has he committed a crime? If so, what kind?

_____

Does a patient have the legal right to leave the hospital, even though his or her physician believes treatment is incomplete?

_____

Does a patient have the right to ask a physician whether he or she has ever been charged with negligence?

_____

Contracts

contract _A voluntary agreement between two parties in which specific promises are made for a consideration._

A **contract** is a voluntary agreement between two parties in which specific promises are made for a consideration. The elements of a contract are important to health care practitioners because health care delivery takes place under various types of contracts. To be legally binding, four elements must be present in a contract:

1. _Agreement_—One party makes an offer and another party accepts it. Certain conditions pertain to the offer:
   - It can relate to the present or the future.
   - It must be communicated.
   - It must be made in good faith and not under duress or as a joke.
   - It must be clear enough to be understood by both parties.
   - It must define what both parties will do if the offer is accepted.

   For example, a physician offers his or her services to the public by obtaining a license to practice medicine and opening for business. Patients accept the physician's offer by scheduling appointments, submitting to physical examinations, and allowing the physician to prescribe or perform medical treatment. The contract is complete when the physician's fee is paid.

2. _Consideration_—Something of value is bargained for as part of the agreement. In the above example, the physician's consideration is providing his or her services; the patient's consideration is payment of the physician's fee.

3. _Legal subject matter_—Contracts are not valid and enforceable in court unless they are for legal services or purposes. For example, a contract entered into by a patient to pay for services of a physician in private practice would be **void** (not legally enforceable) if the physician was

void _Without legal force or effect._

Law, the Courts, and Contracts **63**

breach of contract *May be charged if either party fails to comply with the terms of a legally valid contract.*

not duly licensed to practice medicine. **Breach of contract** may be charged if either party fails to comply with the terms of a legally valid contract.

4. *Contractual capacity*—Parties who enter into the agreement must be capable of fully understanding all of its terms and conditions. A mentally incompetent person cannot enter into a legal contract. For example, persons declared legally insane, persons in a drug altered mental state, and in some cases, persons under extreme duress are considered incapable of entering into a contract. Exceptions may be made for situations in which a contract is necessary to sustain life.

voidable *Able to be set aside or to be revalidated at a later date.*

If either of the concerned parties is incompetent at the time a contract is made, the agreement may be **voidable,** that is, able to be set aside or to be validated at a later date. Say, for example, a patient enters into a contract while under the effects of a medication that can interfere with judgment. After the effects of the medication have worn off, the patient may say, "No, I don't want the contract enforced," or "Yes, I want the contract enforced."

minor *Anyone under the age of majority—18 in most states, 21 in some jurisdictions.*

Of special concern to health care providers is the physician-patient contract as applied to minors. Because of the risk of being accused of battery or assault, health care practitioners cannot treat a minor without the consent of a responsible parent or legal guardian. A **minor** is defined as anyone under the age of majority, which is 18 in most states, 21 in some jurisdictions. See Chapter 9 for a more extensive discussion of minors and the administration of medical services.

Court Case

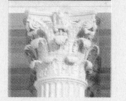

Surgeon Must Face Suit Over Contract

A Virginia cosmetic surgeon asked a federal trial court in Massachusetts to dismiss a breach-of-contract claim filed against him.

The patient bringing suit saw the cosmetic surgeon's advertisement in a Washington, D.C., newspaper while she was living in Massachusetts. She later moved to Maryland.

The patient consulted with the cosmetic surgeon and decided to have surgery. Presurgery tests were done at a Massachusetts hospital. The surgeon operated on the patient in his Virginia office. The operation was not successful. Another operation was performed, which also was unsuccessful.

The patient then moved back to Massachusetts. Several months later, the cosmetic surgeon wrote to her, offering to pay for a different surgeon to perform a third operation, if the patient would release him from any potential claims. She agreed, in writing, and the third operation was performed.

Afterward, the patient tried to recover the cost of the third operation from the surgeon who had agreed to pay for the procedure, but he refused. She sued him for breach of contract.

The physician moved to have the case dismissed, based on lack of personal jurisdiction and improper venue, but his petition was denied. The court held that although the surgeon practiced medicine in another state, his contractual dealings with the patient and his advertising activities made him subject to the jurisdiction of Massachusetts courts, where the breach-of-contract suit would be decided.

Salpoglou v. Widder, MD, PA, 899 F.Supp. 835 (D.C. Mass., Sept. 26, 1995).

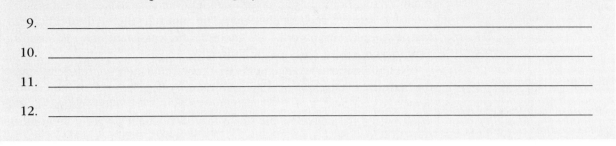
List the four elements present in a legally valid contract.

9. _____

10. _____

11. _____

12. _____

Types of Contracts

expressed contract *Explicitly stated in written or spoken words.*

implied contract *Unspoken or unwritten agreements whose terms result from actions of the involved parties.*

The two main types of contracts are expressed contracts and implied contracts. **Expressed contracts** are explicitly stated in written or spoken words. **Implied contracts** are unspoken. Their terms result from actions of the involved parties.

◆ ◆ ◆ ◆

Expressed Contracts

An expressed contract may be written or oral, but all terms of the contract are explicitly stated. In the medical office some contracts, in order to be legally valid, must be in writing. In each state the **Statute of Frauds,** derived from the Statute for the Prevention of Frauds and Perjuries formulated in England in 1677, states which contracts must be in writing to be enforced.

Statute of Frauds *State legislation governing written contracts.*

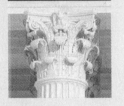

Court Case

Upset or Incompetent?

Emotional upsets do not necessarily make a patient incompetent to consent to medical treatment. During a fight with his son, a Seattle man felt chest discomfort and thought he was having a heart attack. At the hospital he was given four drugs, including a narcotic pain medication. The suspected heart attack was diagnosed as a muscle strain, but while he was hospitalized the man agreed to surgery on his nose. The nose surgery turned out badly, and the man sued, claiming that he had been in a drug-induced state and could not make an intelligent decision about having the nose surgery. If he had not been competent, then the man had not actually consented to the surgery, and the surgeon committed assault.

A judge dismissed the case. The law presumed that the patient in this case had been competent, because a legally competent person is one who can understand his or her illness, the proposed treatment, and the risks in either accepting or refusing it. The patient met these criteria.

Grannum v. Berard, 70 Wash.2d 304; 422 P.2d 812 (1967), annot. 25 A.L.R.3d 1434.

A type of contract often used in the medical office that falls under the Statute of Frauds is the **third party payor contract.** These contracts are agreements by a third party to pay for services rendered to another. Such contracts must be in writing to be enforced and should be signed before health care services are rendered. For example, suppose Susan becomes ill while visiting her aunt in a distant city, and the aunt makes an appointment for Susan to see her physician. The aunt tells the medical office assistant, "I will pay Susan's bill." The medical office assistant may ask Susan's aunt to sign a third party payor contract.

Not all financial arrangements that require written contracts fall under the Statute of Frauds. Others are governed by Regulation Z of the Consumer Protection Act of 1968, also known as the Truth-in-Lending Act. For example, if a patient and a physician make a bilateral payment agreement (one in which both parties are mutually affected) that fees will be paid in four or more installments or will include finance charges, the agreement must be in writing and must contain the following information:

- Fees for services

- Amount of any down payment

- The date each payment is due

- The date of the final payment

- The amount of each payment

- Any interest charges to be made

The patient signs the agreement and is given a copy. A second copy is filed with the patient's records. Most physicians' offices do not levy finance charges, but it is legal and considered ethical to do so.

For agreements falling under the Truth-in-Lending Act, the medical office must supply the patient with a written disclosure statement. The primary purpose of this legislation is to protect consumers from fraudulent, or deceptive, hidden finance charges levied by creditors, but creditors can also use it to collect outstanding debts.

Written payment agreements (see Figure 3-5) do not fall under the Truth-in-Lending Act. If the patient makes a unilateral decision to pay a small amount of a bill monthly, the medical office continues to bill for the full amount and no interest charges are applied.

The federal **Fair Debt Collection Practices Act** requires debt collectors and creditors to treat debtors fairly. It ensures fair treatment by prohibiting certain methods of debt collection. Debt collection practices prohibited by the act include harassment, misrepresentation, threats, disseminating false information about the debtor, and engaging in unfair or illegal practices in attempting to collect a debt. Personal, family, and household debts are covered under the act. This includes money owed for the purchase of an automobile, medical care, and charge accounts.

Bruce Whiting, MD
310 Madison Avenue
Anderson, Indiana 46027

I agree to pay $_____ per week/month on my account balance of $_____.

Payments are due by the_____ of each _____ and will begin _____.
$\qquad$ (week/month) $\qquad$ (date)

Interest will/will not be charged on the outstanding balance (see Truth-in-Lending form below for rate of interest).

I agree that if payments are not made in the full amount stated above or if payments are not received on time, the entire account balance will be considered delinquent and will be due and payable immediately.

I agree to be responsible for any reasonable collection costs or attorney fees incurred in collecting a delinquent account.

_____   _____
Date   Signature

<hr>

This disclosure is in compliance with the Truth-in-Lending Act.

_____   _____
Patient's Name   Address

_____   _____
Responsible Party (if other than patient) City, State, Zip Code

1. Cash Price (Medical and/or Surgical Fee)   _____
    Less Cash Down Payment (Advance)   _____
2. Unpaid Balance of Cash Price   _____
3. Amount Financed   _____
4. FINANCE CHARGE   _____
5. Total of Payments (3 + 4)   _____
6. Deferred Payment Price (1 + 4)   _____
7. ANNUAL PERCENTAGE RATE   _____

The "Total of Payments" shown above is payable to Bruce Whiting, MD, at the address shown above in _____ monthly installments of $_____, the first installment being payable _____ and all subsequent installments are due on the same day of
$\qquad$ (date)
each consecutive month until paid in full.

_____   _____
Date   Signature

Figure 3-5
Truth-in-Lending Payment Agreement

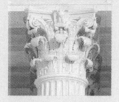
◆ ◆ ◆ ◆ Implied Contracts

Implied contracts are those in which the conduct of the parties, rather than expressed words, creates the contract. Most contracts in the medical office are implied. For example, suppose a patient comes to a clinic complaining of a sore throat and asks to see a physician. The physician does not literally say, "I offer to treat your condition," to the patient, but by making his or her services available, he or she has made an offer to treat. A patient does not state to the physician, "I accept your offer to provide medical care." Acceptance is implied by the patient's actions in allowing the physician to examine him or her and prescribe treatment. The physician's consideration is providing services. The patient's consideration is payment of the physician's fee. The contract is valid if both parties understand the offer, both are competent, and the services provided are legal.

A physician who provides emergency treatment to a patient in a situation not covered by a special arrangement, such as an emergency room, is limited to providing treatment at the site of the emergency. In such a situation, an implied limited contract between the physician and the patient is created, based on the patient's implied request for and consent to emergency treatment. The patient's promise to pay for the physician's services is also implied. In this case, the physician's obligation for care does not extend to treatment after the emergency situation has been resolved.

Check Your Progress

List three federal laws governing collections in the medical office.

13. _____

14. _____

15. _____

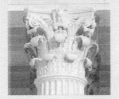
The Physician-Patient Contract and Managed Care

Managed care plans have added a third element to the physician-patient contract. Physicians still have contracts with their patients, but they may also have contracted with managed care programs to deliver medical services. This arrangement makes physicians employees of the managed care plan. Such contracts with managed care plans can interfere with patient care in some situations. For example, if physicians' contracts with the managed care plan can be terminated without due process, or if doctors' earnings are based on capitation (a uniform per capita payment or fee), this can cause a conflict between physicians' responsibilities to their patients and their economic motivation.

The physician's contract with an employing managed care organization also affects the release of patients' medical records. The member's enrollment form usually includes a statement allowing the managed care organization to access the member's medical records. The records are used for utilization review, quality management, inpatient stay review, and review by case managers. The records are also used routinely to check the care enrollees are receiving and to identify ways to prevent illness and disease. Managed care plans also exchange the information with firms hired to review treatment plans.

The Physician's Rights and Responsibilities

A physician has the right, after agreeing to accept an individual as his or her patient, to make reasonable limitations on the relationship. The physician is under no legal obligation to treat patients who may wish to exceed those limitations. Under the provisions of the physician-patient contract, both parties have certain rights and responsibilities. A physician has the right to:

- Set up practice within the boundaries of his or her license to practice

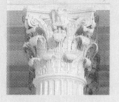

Court Affirms Vicarious Liability of HMO for Physician's Malpractice

After her husband died from testicular cancer, Mrs. D. filed a malpractice suit against two urologists and a primary care physician employed by her HMO. The suit alleged that the HMO was also liable, both for the negligence committed by the physicians and for a contractual breach. The deceased patient had first seen his primary care physician for a mass in his right testicle. He was treated with antibiotics for epididymitis. During subsequent visits, the patient did not receive tests to determine whether the persistent mass was cancerous. By the time cancer was finally diagnosed, it had spread to the liver. The cancer was so advanced that the patient's life could not be saved.

Since the physicians who treated Mrs. D.'s husband were paid by the HMO on a per capita basis, based on the number of subscribers to the HMO, they were not free to accept or reject a particular patient and thus were agents of the HMO. The court ruled that where the physician is a direct employee of the HMO, *respondeat superior* may be applied. The jury returned a verdict in favor of the plaintiff against the physicians and the employing HMO in the amount of $2,904,240.54.

Dunn v. Praiss, Marmar, South Jersey Urologic Associates, Brumbaugh, Health Care Plan of New Jersey, 256 N.J. Super. 180; 606 A.2d 862.

medicine. A specialist, for instance, does not have to practice outside the area of specialty and, in fact, would be severely criticized for doing so, except in an emergency in which no other physician is available.

- Set up an office wherever he or she chooses and to establish office hours.

- Specialize.

- Decide which services he or she will provide and how those services will be provided.

While practicing within the context of an implied contract with the patient, the physician is not bound to:

- Treat every patient who seeks medical care. The physician is free to use his or her own discretion, with one exception. If a physician is hired specifically to treat patients in one area or locale, such as a hospital emergency room, he or she must treat every patient who comes to the emergency room.

- Restore the patient to his or her original state of health. The fact that a patient grows progressively worse while under a physician's care and shows improvement when care is withdrawn does not necessarily constitute liability.

- Possess the highest skills possible within the profession or the maximum education attainable.

- Effect a recovery with every patient. The physician who fails to heal a patient cannot be condemned for lack of skill.

- Be familiar with the various reactions of patients to anesthetics or drugs of any kind. However, the physician is bound to note any allergic or adverse reactions to medications reported by the patient before treatment is administered.

- Be as skilled as a specialist if he or she is a general practitioner.

- Make a correct diagnosis in every case.

- Be free from mistakes of judgment in difficult cases.

- Display infallibility of judgment.

- Continue services after being discharged by the patient or by some responsible person, even if harm should come to the patient.

- Guarantee the successful result of any treatment or operation. In fact, guarantees of "cures" may constitute fraud on the part of the physician.

Under an implied contract with the patient, the physician has the obligation to:

- Use the same due care, skill, judgment, and diligence in treating patients that other physicians of the same practice usually exercise in similar locations and under similar circumstances.

- Stay informed about the best methods of diagnosis and treatment.

- Perform to the best of his or her ability, whether or not he or she is to receive a fee.

- Exercise his or her best professional judgment in all cases, particularly those in which considerable doubt is involved.

- Consider the established, customary treatment administered by members of the medical profession in similar cases.

- Abstain from performing experiments on a patient without first securing the patient's complete understanding and approval.

- Provide proper instructions for a patient's care to the person responsible for such care, so that proper treatment will be administered to the patient in the doctor's absence.

- Furnish complete information and instructions to the patient about diagnosis, options and methods of treatment, and fees for services.

- Take every precaution to prevent the spread of contagious disease.

- Advise patients against needless or unwise operations.

The Patient's Rights and Responsibilities

In the United States, patients generally have the right to choose the physician they will see, although some managed care plans may limit choices. They also have the right to terminate a physician's services if they wish. To help define patients' rights, most states have adopted a version of the American Hospital Association's Patients' Bill of Rights, created in 1973 and revised in 1992. In summary, the statement guarantees the patient's right to:

- Receive considerate and respectful care.
- Receive complete, current information concerning his or her diagnosis, treatment, and prognosis.
- Know the identity of physicians, nurses, and others involved with their care, as well as when those involved are students, residents, or trainees.
- Know the immediate and long-term costs of treatment choices.
- Have an advance directive concerning treatment or choice of a surrogate decision maker (as discussed in Chapter 12).
- Receive information necessary to give informed consent prior to the start of any procedure or treatment.
- Refuse treatment to the extent permitted by law.
- Receive every consideration of his or her privacy.
- Be assured of confidentiality.
- Obtain reasonable responses to requests for services.
- Obtain information about his or her health care and be allowed to review his or her medical record and to have any information explained or interpreted.
- Know whether treatment is experimental and be able to consent or decline to participate in proposed research studies or human experimentation.
- Expect reasonable continuity of care.
- Ask and be informed of the existence of business relationships among the hospital and others that may influence the client's treatment and care.
- Know which hospital policies and practices relate to client care, treatment, and responsibilities.
- Be informed of available resources for resolving disputes, grievances, and conflicts, such as ethics committees, patient representatives, or other mechanisms available in the facility.
- Examine his or her bill and have it explained, and be informed of available payment methods.

The patient also has certain implied duties to:

- Follow any instructions given by the physician and cooperate as much as possible.
- Give all relevant information to the physician in order to reach a correct diagnosis. If an incorrect diagnosis is made because the patient fails to give the physician the proper information, the physician is not liable.
- Follow the physician's orders for treatment, provided the treatment is similar to that administered by members of the system or school of medicine to which the physician belongs. If a patient willfully or negligently fails to follow the physician's instructions, that patient has little legal recourse.
- Pay the fees charged for services rendered.

This Patients' Bill of Rights was not legislated as law, but was intended simply to provide guidelines for patients receiving medical care. A legislated Patients' Bill of Rights Act was proposed in 1999 and is discussed in Chapter 2.

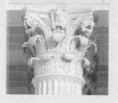

Incorrect Diagnosis Leads to Patient Award

A patient went to a hospital's emergency department complaining of foot pain. A physician diagnosed an ankle sprain. Two days later the patient returned to the emergency department and received the same diagnosis. One week later the patient returned, was diagnosed with ischemia, and was admitted to the hospital. A thrombectomy was performed on the patient's leg, but the procedure was unsuccessful. Three weeks later the leg was amputated below the knee.

A few months later the patient informed the hospital of his intent to sue, and that he had obtained a supporting affidavit from a general surgeon. The hospital denied liability and also supplied a general surgeon's affidavit. The case went to trial and the court granted summary judgment to the hospital.

On appeal the court reversed the trial court's decision and remanded the matter for further consideration. The appeals court held that the trial court had erred in granting summary judgment on the ground that the patient's expert had failed in his affidavit to set forth facts describing the hospital's alleged acts of negligence. It was sufficient, the court held, to notify the hospital, as the patient's expert had done, that the patient's medical records had been reviewed and that the expert believed that the hospital had been negligent in its treatment of the patient.

Maldonado v. EMSA Limited Partnership, 645 So.2d 86 (Fla. Dist. Ct. of App., Nov. 9, 1994).

Check Your Progress

Write "T" or "F" in the blank to indicate whether you think the statement is true or false.

Under terms of an implied contract:

_____**16.** A physician is *not* obligated to effect a recovery with every patient.

_____**17.** A physician is obligated to use due care, skill, and diligence in treating each patient.

_____**18.** A physician is obligated to note allergic or adverse reactions to medications reported by a specific patient.

_____**19.** A physician is *not* obligated to be as skilled as a specialist if he or she is a general practitioner.

_____**20.** A physician is *not* obligated to consider established, customary treatment (standard of care) when treating a patient.

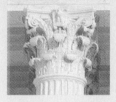
Termination of Contracts

The contract between a physician and a patient is usually terminated (ended) when all treatment has been completed and the bill has been paid. Situations may arise, however, in which premature termination of the contract takes place, such as in the following situations:

FAILURE TO PAY FOR SERVICES   A physician may stop treatment of a patient and end the physician-patient relationship if the patient habitually does not pay or fails to make satisfactory arrangements to pay for medical services, but only if adequate notice is given to the patient.

FAILURE TO KEEP SCHEDULED APPOINTMENTS   To protect the physician from charges of abandonment, all missed appointments should be noted on the patient's chart.

FAILURE TO FOLLOW THE PHYSICIAN'S INSTRUCTIONS   It makes no difference whether the failure is due to a patient's willfulness or negligence.

A PATIENT'S SEEKING THE SERVICES OF ANOTHER PHYSICIAN   Whenever a patient acknowledges, orally or in writing, that he or she will seek medical care from another physician, the medical office employee should document this on the patient's chart and then send a letter to the patient verifying the termination. A copy of the letter should be filed with the patient's records.

A patient may terminate a physician-patient relationship at any time. After a physician agrees to treat a patient, however, his or her responsibilities to the patient continue until the relationship is properly terminated. If a physician suddenly withdraws from treatment while the patient is still in need of medical care, fails to visit a hospitalized patient, or otherwise abandons the patient without arranging for substitute care, he or she may be charged with abandonment. Depending on the circumstances, the physician may also be charged with breach of contract or negligence.

Court Case

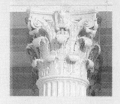

Physician Sued for Abandonment

A patient entered the emergency room of a hospital complaining of rectal bleeding and was admitted as a patient of her regular attending physician. Two diagnostic procedures were completed and three more were scheduled. The patient refused to sign consent forms for the three procedures, saying she didn't want to be anesthetized. Her physician discussed these concerns with the patient and told her to sign the consent forms or sign herself out of the hospital. The physician told the patient he would release her from his services. At that time, the patient was given a list of other physicians she could contact. The patient selected another physician and discharged herself from the hospital. She then charged the original physician with abandonment.

A superior court entered summary judgment for the physician. The plaintiff appealed, but the appeals court held the physician was not guilty of abandonment. Supplying the patient, who was not in need of immediate medical attention, with a list of substitute physicians to replace the attending physician was a reasonable means of severing the physician-patient relationship.

Miller v. Greater Southeast Community Hospital, 508 A.2d 927 (D.C. Ct. App. 1986).

To properly terminate the physician-patient relationship, the physician must give the patient formal written notice that he or she is withdrawing from the case. The physician should also note any need for the patient to receive continued medical care. In addition, the patient must be given time to find another physician. The notice of discharge of withdrawal should be sent by certified mail, return receipt requested, and a copy should be filed with the patient's records. Figure 3-6 illustrates a notice of termination.

Lane Medical Center
310 Lane Road
Bedford, Idaho 83210

October 10, 2005

Ted Rowe
Box 1041A
Bedford, Idaho 83210

Dear Mr. Rowe:

This is to inform you of our intent to discontinue medical care to you and the members of your family, due to habitual and continued nonpayment of medical bills. This will go into effect 30 days from the date of this letter, to allow you sufficient time to locate another physician. During this 30-day period, we will require you to pay cash for any care extended to your family. This includes our satellite offices.

We will be happy to forward your medical records to the physician of your choice. There is also 24-hour medical care available to you at the hospital.

If you need assistance in locating a new physician, please contact the Idaho Medical Society at 1-800-666-7777.

Sincerely,

P. White

Patricia White, M.D.

Figure 3-6
Physician's Letter of Dismissal for Nonpayment

Law of Agency

law of agency *The law that governs the relationship between a principal and his or her agent.*

agent *In performing workplace duties, the employee acts as the agent, or authorized representative, of the employer.*

By law, employers are liable for the actions of their employees when employees perform said actions as part of their work under the supervision of the employer. This is called the **law of agency.** In performing workplace duties, the employee acts as the **agent** of the employer.

Agency may be expressed or implied. In the medical office, it is most often implied. Medical office employees act as the physician's agent when they schedule appointments, speak with patients and other individuals, order supplies for the office, or otherwise perform duties ordered by and supervised by the employing physician in the conduct of his or her business.

Under the doctrine of *respondent superior,* or "Let the master answer," physicians are liable for the acts of their employees performed "within the course and scope" of employment. Therefore, heath care practitioners must avoid making promises their employer cannot keep.

Applying Knowledge

Answer the following questions in the spaces provided.

1. List and define three sources of law.

   _____

   _____

   _____

2. Define *common law.*

   _____

   _____

3. Define *substantive law.*

   _____

   _____

4. Decisions made by judges in the various courts and used as a guide for future decisions are called:

   _____.

5. Distinguish between criminal and civil law.

   _____

   _____

6. May a civil offense also be a crime? Explain your answer.

   _____

   _____

7. Define *jurisdiction.*

   _____

8. Define *tort.*

   _____

9. Define *tortfeasor.*

   _____

10. Distinguish between intentional and unintentional torts.

    _____

    _____

    _____

11. An unintentional tort charged when a health care practitioner fails to exercise ordinary care is called

    _____.

12. If a physician examines a patient without consent, can he or she be charged with an offense? Explain your answer.

_____

13. Are health care practitioners legally liable for all unsatisfactory medical outcomes? Explain your answer.

_____

_____

_____

14. Define *contract*.

_____

_____

15. List and briefly define the four essential elements of a contract.

_____

_____

_____

_____

16. List those situations in which a contract may be voidable.

_____

_____

17. Under what circumstances may breach of contract be charged?

_____

_____

18. Briefly explain the purpose of the Statute of Frauds.

_____

_____

19. Define *third party payor contract*.

_____

_____

20. Regulation Z of the Consumer Protection Act of 1968 requires that certain financial arrangements be in writing. These include:

_____

_____

_____

21. What is the Fair Debt Collection Practices Act?

_____

_____

_____

22. Give an example of an implied limited contract.

_____

_____

Review and Case Studies

23. List ten items to which a physician is *not* bound contractually in the context of an implied physician-patient contract.

_____   _____
_____   _____
_____   _____
_____   _____
_____   _____

24. List ten items to which a physician is obligated in an implied physician-patient contract.

_____   _____
_____   _____
_____   _____
_____   _____
_____   _____

25. List five responsibilities borne by the patient in an implied contract.

_____
_____
_____
_____
_____

26. Name four situations in which premature termination of the physician-patient contract may occur.

_____
_____
_____
_____

27. Why must a physician give the patient ample notice when withdrawing from a case?

_____
_____

28. Briefly explain how the law of agency applies to health care practitioners.

_____
_____

29. Name two ways in which managed care agreements have changed the physician-patient contract.

_____
_____

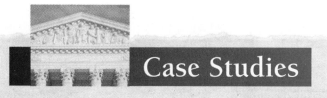

Case Studies

Use your critical-thinking skills to answer the questions that follow the case study.

Dan, a medical office assistant in a busy clinic, is a sympathetic and understanding employee. Therefore, when an elderly patient complanied to him that she "felt terrible most of the time," Dan consoled her. "Don't worry, Mrs. Smith," he told the woman. "Dr. Jones will make you feel better in no time."

30. **Has Dan, acting as Dr. Jones's agent, created an implied contract with Mrs. Smith? Explain your answer.**

_____

_____

_____

31. **If so, can Dr. Jones be sued by Mrs. Smith if he fails to fulfill the "terms" of the contract? Explain your answer.**

_____

_____

_____

32. **How might you respond to a patient under similar circumstances?**

_____

_____

_____

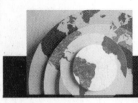

Internet Activities

Complete the activities and answer the questions that follow.

33. Find a Web site that defines the term "affidavit." Briefly explain the term and define a situation in which a health care professional may have to give an affidavit.

_____

_____

_____

_____

34. Visit the Web site for the U.S. House of Representatives. List any health care legislation currently pending before the House.

_____

_____

_____

_____

35. List two additional Web sites where information about health care legislation can be found.

_____

_____

_____

_____

PART

2

LEGAL ISSUES FOR WORKING HEALTH CARE PRACTITIONERS

CHAPTER

4
Professional Liability and Medical Malpractice

5
Defenses to Liability Suits

6
Medical Records and Informed Consent

4

PROFESSIONAL LIABILITY AND MEDICAL MALPRACTICE

Objectives

After studying this chapter, you should be able to:

1. Identify three areas of general liability for which a physician/employer is responsible.

2. Describe the reasonable-person standard.

3. Discuss the concept of standard of care.

4. Discuss the responsibilities of health care practitioners concerning privacy, confidentiality, and privileged communication.

5. Identify and explain the four elements necessary to prove negligence (the four Ds).

6. Name three advantages to alternative dispute resolution.

Key Terms

- alternative dispute resolution (ADR)

- confidentiality

- damages

- deposition

- interrogatory

- liable

- malfeasance

- misfeasance

- nonfeasance

- privileged communication

- *res ipsa loquitur*

- subpoena

- subpoena *duces tecum*

- summons

- testimony

- wrongful death statutes

Liability

All competent adults are **liable,** or legally responsible, for their own acts, both on the job and in their private lives. As homeowners and operators of automobiles, we carry liability insurance in case someone is injured in our homes or we are involved in a car accident. In the workplace, employers carry liability insurance to cover situations in which employees, or anyone else on the premises, may be injured or harmed.

As employers, physicians have general liability for the following areas:

THE PRACTICE'S BUILDING AND GROUNDS Adequate upkeep will help ensure that employees and patients are not injured on the premises. Employers must provide protection against theft, fire, and burglary in the building and must take all precautions to ensure that patients' records are protected. Theft, fire, and liability insurance to cover the workplace is a must for the physician/employer.

AUTOMOBILES If employees must use their own or the physician's automobile in the performance of their daily work (such as dropping off or picking up mail or supplies), the employer must be adequately insured for liability in the event of an accident.

EMPLOYEE SAFETY Employers must provide a reasonably comfortable and safe work environment for employees. State (and in some instances federal) regulations apply, but they vary from state to state. Employees should check with the state agency governing safety in the workplace, with workers' compensation laws, and with state medical societies to determine safety rules, rights, and responsibilities. A general safety procedure book for medical office workers should include guidelines for the handling of hazardous laboratory wastes and materials.

In addition to general liability, physicians and other health care providers also have certain professional liabilities.

Court Case

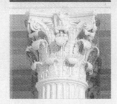

Patient Hurt in Parking Lot Sues

A patient stubbed her toe on something protruding from the ground in a hospital parking lot. She fell, breaking her foot, and subsequently sued the hospital. A jury returned a $70,000 verdict for the patient, and the Mississippi Supreme Court affirmed.

Biloxi Regional Medical Center v. David, 555 So.2d 53 (Miss. Sup. Ct., Dec. 13, 1989).

Standard of Care

As explained in Chapter 3, we are responsible for our actions (or our failure to act) under the reasonable-person standard. That is, we may be charged with negligence if someone is injured because we failed to perform an act that a reasonable person, in similar circumstances, would perform or if we commit an act that a reasonable person would not commit. Professionals—those individuals who are specially trained to perform specific tasks—are held to a higher standard of care than nonprofessionals (laypersons). If a patient is injured because a health care professional failed to exercise the care and expertise that under the circumstances could reasonably be expected of a professional with similar experience and training, then that person may be liable for negligence. (See the section below titled "Physicians" for the distinction between "standard of care" and "duty of care.")

Court Case

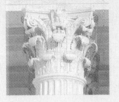

Medical Technologist Liable

A patient was admitted to a hospital in 1980 with the diagnosis of a possible pulmonary embolus. The patient's physician prescribed heparin, a clot-preventing drug. After a medical technologist drew blood from a vein in the patient's right arm, the arm began to swell and discolor. The patient later sued the hospital, claiming the negligent acts of hospital employees caused permanent disability in her arm and hand.

An appeals court held that failure of the medical technologist to take proper precautions in drawing blood had caused the patient's injury. The hospital's liability was vicarious, based on substandard conduct of a nurse and the medical technologist. The court said that nurses and medical technologists have their own duty of care and liability for their actions, as do physicians. The hospital has a standard-of-care duty that requires that patients be protected from dangers that may result from a particular medical condition or that a reasonable person under the circumstances would anticipate.

The court found for the plaintiff.

Belmon v. St. Frances Cabrini Hospital, 427 So.2d 541 (La. App. 3 Cir., 1983).

◆ ◆ ◆ ◆ Physicians

A physician in general practice is expected to conform to the standards of other general practitioners in his or her own or a comparable community. A specialist is held to a higher standard of care than is a general practitioner. The standard of care for a specialist is generally the same as for those of like specialists, wherever they practice.

Standard of care refers to the level of performance expected of a health care practitioner in carrying out his or her professional duties. *Duty of care* is the obligation of health care workers to patients and, in some cases, nonpatients. Physicians have a duty of care to patients with whom they have established a doctor/patient relationship, but they may also be held to a duty of care toward people who are not patients, such as the patient's family members, former patients, and even office personnel.

Generally, if actions or omissions within the scope of a health care practitioner's job could cause harm to someone, that person is owed a duty of care.

For example, medical facility custodians are nonpatients to whom a duty of care is owed. Various drugs, equipment, and supplies are used and discarded daily in a medical facility. Procedures for the proper disposal of drugs and potentially hazardous materials should be detailed in a facility's safety manual so that employees who handle these materials do not accidentally prick themselves with used needles or otherwise injure themselves. In some instances, depending on the situation and state law, physicians may have a duty under standard of care to warn nonpatients of danger, as in the case of a psychiatric patient who threatens harm to others or in the case of a patient with a communicable sexually transmitted disease.

Court Case

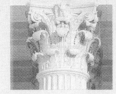

A Nonmedical Employee Sues

A hospital employee claimed he reinjured his back when a physician insisted that he move a piece of heavy equipment, even though the employee told the physician he had a bad back and showed him his surgery scar. The employee said he relied on the physician's knowledge of medical matters and he feared discipline by the hospital should he disobey the physician's order.

The employee filed suit against the physician. A Florida trial court dismissed the complaint, but a state appellate court reversed the decision. The court said the physician owed the employee a duty of care, and the employee had a cause of action.

Bengston v. Giroud, 559 So.2d 380 (Fla. Dist. Ct. of App., April 6, 1990).

Courts have generally held that informal consultations among physicians do not create a doctor-patient relationship and thus do not create a duty of care, as in the Grossman case discussed below.

Court Case

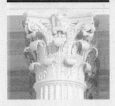

Landmark Case: Consultation Did Not Establish a Duty of Care

The doctrine that informal physician consultations do not create a doctor-patient relationship was established in 1973 in the California decision *Ranier vs. Grossman.* Morton Grossman was a professor of gastroenterology who often lectured physicians at their hospitals, then offered to review their cases with them. After one such lecture, a physician presented the X rays and medical history for a patient who suffered from ulcerative colitis. Grossman advised surgery without examining the patient. The surgery was subsequently performed and the patient sued, claiming that the surgery had been unnecessary. Grossman was cited as a codefendant in the patient's lawsuit. An appeals court upheld summary judgment in Grossman's favor, holding that he had no duty to the patient because he had no direct contact with her and had no control over her treating physicians.

Ranier v. Grossman, Ct. of App. 2nd Dist., 31 Cal. App. 3rd 539, April 11, 1973.

Direct patient contact is not always necessary for establishing a duty, as the following court case illustrates.

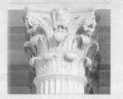

Court Case

Duty Established by Referral

A plastic surgeon examined a patient in a hospital emergency department. An X ray of the patient's knee revealed a possible malignant neoplasm, so the plastic surgeon referred the patient to an orthopedist but did not tell the patient why. The patient did not show up for any of the three appointments he scheduled with the orthopedist, and the orthopedist refused to reschedule him. The patient subsequently died of cancer, and his estate sued the two physicians. A lower court granted summary judgment to the orthopedist, but an appeals court reversed, holding that a doctor-patient relationship began when the orthopedist accepted the referral and scheduled the patient for an appointment. The court also said that "a letter to plaintiff advising him of his condition and to consult with another physician without delay might well have been sufficient" to discharge the duty to the patient.

Davis v. Weiskopf, Ill. App. 64 Ill. Dec. 131, 439 N.E.2nd 60, 108 Ill. App. 3rd 505.

Other Health Care Practitioners

As discussed in Glencoe's text *Medical Assisting: A Patient-Centered Approach to Administrative and Clinical Competencies,* by Prickett-Ramutkowski, Barrie, Keller, Dazarow, and Abel, medical assistants are expected to uphold legal concepts by:

- Practicing within the scope of their training and capabilities (relates to standard of care).
- Maintaining confidentiality.
- Preparing and maintaining health records.
- Documenting accurately.
- Using appropriate guidelines when releasing information.
- Following an employer's established policies dealing with the health care contract.
- Following legal guidelines and maintaining awareness of health care legislation and regulations.
- Maintaining and disposing of regulated substances in compliance with government guidelines.
- Following established risk-management and safety procedures.
- Recognizing professional credentialing criteria.
- Helping to develop and maintain personnel, policy, and procedure manuals.

Although these guidelines were written for medical assistants, they can also help other health care practitioners stay within the scope of their practices and operate within the law and the employing health care facility's policy.

Laws often dictate what a member of a health care profession can and cannot do on the job. In addition to the law, a health care practitioner should know what policies and procedures apply specifically to his or her place of employment. Policy and procedure manuals that clearly define a health care practitioner's responsibilities can serve as a valuable guide.

Check Your Progress

1. As employers, physicians have general liability for:

_____

_____

_____

Write "T" or "F" in the blank to the left of each numbered statement to indicate whether you think it is true or false.

_____ 2. *Standard of care* refers to the level of performance expected of a health care practitioner in carrying out his or her professional duties.

_____ 3. *Duty of care* is the obligation of health care workers to patients but never applies to nonpatients.

_____ 4. An obstetrician who helps deliver a baby to a woman who happens to be riding with him in a taxicab would be held to the reasonable-person standard.

_____ 5. Policies and procedures of the employing medical facility, as well as the law, should be considered when a health care practitioner performs his or her duties.

Privacy, Confidentiality, and Privileged Communication

confidentiality *The act of holding information in confidence, not to be released to unauthorized individuals.*

privileged communication *Information held confidential within a protected relationship.*

Not only do physicians and other health care professionals owe a duty of care to patients, but it is also their ethical and legal duty to safeguard a patient's privacy and maintain **confidentiality.** A breach of confidentiality is both unethical and illegal.

Privileged communication refers to information held confidential within a protected relationship. Attorney-client and physician-patient are examples of relationships in which the law, under certain circumstances, protects the holder of information from forced disclosure. Privileged communication statutes vary from state to state, but in most states patients may sue a physician for breach of confidence if the holder released protected information and damage to the patient resulted. In many states breach of confidence is grounds for revocation of a physician's license.

Since any medical facility presents numerous opportunities for a breach of confidentiality, health care workers must make every effort to safeguard each patient's privacy. The following suggestions for maintaining confidentiality in the medical facility can serve as a guide for all health care practitioners who may be asked to provide or release information about patients:

- Do not disclose any information about a patient to a third party without signed consent. This extends to insurance companies, attorneys, and curious neighbors, and it includes acknowledging whether or not the person in question is a patient.

- Do not decide confidentiality on the basis of whether or not you approve of or agree with the views or morals of the patient.

- Do not reveal financial information about a patient, since this is also confidential. For instance, be discreet when revealing a patient's account balance orally, so that others in the office waiting room do not overhear. Be discreet, also, when providing such information electronically, so that unauthorized persons do not see the information on a computer screen, fax machine, copier, printer, and so on.

- When talking on the telephone, do not use the caller's name if others in the room might overhear.

- Use caution in giving the results of medical tests to patients over the telephone to prevent others in the medical office from overhearing. Furthermore, when leaving a message on a home answering machine or at a patient's place of employment, simply ask the patient to return a call regarding a recent visit or appointment on a specific date. No mention should be made of the nature of the call. It is inadvisable to leave a message with a receptionist or coworker on an answering machine for the patient to call an oncologist, OB-GYN physician, and so forth. If test results are abnormal, usually the physician speaks directly to the patient and an appointment is made to discuss the results.

- Do not leave medical charts or insurance reports out where patients or medical facility visitors can see them.

- See that confidentiality protocol is duly noted in the medical facility's procedures manual, and make sure new employees learn it.

- If a patient is unwilling to release privileged information, the information should not be released. Exceptions include legally required disclosures, such as those ordered by subpoena; those dictated by statute to protect public health or welfare; or those considered necessary to protect the welfare of a patient or a third party.

- Follow all regulations and procedures for safeguarding the confidentiality of electronically created, stored, and transmitted records, including use of passwords, levels of access, and so on.

Confidentiality may be waived under certain circumstances, but such situations are not absolute, depending on state law, HIPAA provisions, and other factors such as the following:

- Sometimes when a third party requests a medical examination, such as for employment, and that party pays the physician's fee.

- Generally when a patient sues a physician for malpractice.

- When a waiver has been signed by the patient allowing the release of information (see Figure 4-1).

I authorize: Name of person or institution_____

                                              (Provider of information)

                Street address _____

                City, state, Zip Code _____

To release medical information to:

                Name of person or institution: _____

                                            (Recipient of information)

                Street address _____

                City, state, Zip Code _____

                Attention: _____

Nature of information to be disclosed:

                ☐ Clinical notes pertaining to evaluation and treatment

                ☐ Other, please specify _____

Purpose of disclosure:

                ☐ Continuing medical care

                ☐ Second opinion

                ☐ Other, please specify _____

This authorization will automatically expire one year from the date of signature, unless specified otherwise _____

This consent may be revoked at any time by sending written notice to the above-named provider of information. Any release of information made prior to the revocation of this compliant authorization is not a breach of confidentiality. Disclosed information may be reviewed by contacting the provider of information.

Patient's name_____

Signature of patient or legal guardian _____ Date _____

Complete address _____

Relationship, if not the patient _____ Patient's date of birth _____

SPECIFIC CONSENT FOR RELEASE OF INFORMATION
PROTECTED BY STATE OR FEDERAL LAW

Iowa law (and in some cases federal law) provides special confidentiality protection to information relating to substance abuse, mental health, and HIV-related testing. In order for information to be released on this subject matter, this specific authorization and the above authorization must be signed:

I authorize release of information relating to:

☐ Substance abuse (alcohol/drug abuse)
    Signature of patient or legal guardian

    _____ Date_____

☐ Mental health (includes psychological testing and mental health counseling)
    Signature of patient or legal guardian

    _____ Date_____

☐ HIV-related information (AIDS-related testing)
    Signature of patient or legal guardian

    _____ Date_____

Date information is sent _____ Sent by (name) _____

To the recipient of this information: This information has been disclosed to you from records protected by federal confidentiality rules. The federal rules prohibit you from making further disclosure without additional consent.

Figure 4-1
Consent to Release Information

6. Define *privileged communication.*

_____

_____

7. Explain why health care practitioners are obligated to protect confidentiality of health records.

_____

_____

_____

8. Before health records can be released to authorized sources, such as insurance companies, what must be obtained?

_____

_____

VOICE OF EXPERIENCE
CMA Instructor's Views on Confidentiality

Carol, a certified medical assistant (CMA) and registered health information technician (RHIT), is an instructor in the medical assisting program at a community college in the Northwest. She has been a medical clinic manager and is a consultant on reimbursement issues, such as coding and billing. Carol says one of her pet peeves is patient sign-in sheets in medical offices. "Patient names are there for everyone to see. I'd like to see that abolished. It may seem unimportant," says Carol, "but if another patient recognizes a name on the OB-GYN sign-in sheet, for example, inferences can be made."

"Also," adds Carol, "the receptionist and the person who makes appointments should be two different people." The appointment scheduler should be located in a more private part of the medical office than the busy waiting room, because that person asks for names and reasons for seeing the physician that might be overheard.

(*Note:* As HIPAA is fully implemented, such practices as those mentioned above will no longer be legal. As a health care practitioner who is responsible for patient appointments or waiting room procedures, be sure you function within the law.)

The following case, concerning privacy and the release of autopsy information, made headlines in 2001, after the death of well-known NASCAR driver Dale Earnhardt.

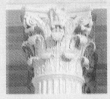

Newspaper Cannot Get Autopsy Photos

On February 18, 2001, while driving the last lap of the Daytona 500 race at the Daytona International Speedway, NASCAR driver Dale Earnhardt's car struck the wall, and he was killed instantly. An autopsy was performed the following day.

Since the *Orlando Sentinel* had been running a series of articles about NASCAR safety, the newspaper requested copies of Earnhardt's autopsy photos so a medical examiner they had hired could determine if wearing the HANS device for head stabilization might have saved the race car driver's life. Upon learning of the *Sentinel's* request, Dale Earnhardt's widow, Teresa, filed suit in Volusia County Circuit Court seeking an injunction to prevent the *Sentinel's* representative from examining the photos. Mrs. Earnhardt claimed releasing the photos would violate the Earnhardt family's privacy. The Circuit Court judge granted a temporary injunction, stating that the family's privacy interest outweighed the public interest in seeing the photographs.

Before the case was settled, the Florida legislature passed a law, known as the Earnhardt Family Protection Act, that allows autopsy photographs or recordings of the autopsy to be examined only by a surviving spouse, parent, or child. Anyone else must obtain a court order and examine the materials under the "direct supervision of the custodian." Exceptions were made for some service providers, such as the medical examiner and state or federal agencies performing official duties. The law restricted access to such information by journalists and others.

Mrs. Earnhardt settled her suit against the *Orlando Sentinel* on March 16, 2001. An independent medical expert could examine Earnhardt's autopsy photos, then the photos would be permanently sealed.

Several news organizations challenged the constitutionality of the Earnhardt Family Protection Act, but as of the end of 2001, the law had been upheld in Florida as constitutional.

Earnhardt v. Volusia County Office of the Medical Examiner, Case No. 2001-30373-C1C1 (Fla. Cir. Ct.).

YOU BE THE JUDGE

A physician told her group practice she was leaving the practice to move to another state. She asked other physicians in the group to continue to care for her patients. Her plans to move fell through, however, and she asked to resume her position. The practice had decided not to replace her, and her request was denied. In response, the physician contacted many of her former patients, asking them to write the practice and urge her colleagues to reinstate her. In your opinion, was it ethically appropriate for the physician to contact her former patients to ask them to intervene on her behalf? Explain your answer.

_____

_____

_____

_____

The Tort of Negligence

The unintentional tort of negligence is the basis for professional malpractice claims and is the most common liability in medicine. Because the term *malpractice* refers to just one area of medical liability and implies "bad" or dishonorable behavior, the term preferred by most health care practitioners is *medical professional liability.* When health care practitioners are sued for medical malpractice, the term generally means any deviation from the accepted medical standard of care that causes injury to a patient.

In a court case decided in 1965, for the first time a hospital was found guilty of negligence. Since then, under the theory of corporate liability, hospitals have been found to have an independent duty to patients, including a duty to grant privileges only to competent doctors, to supervise the overall medical treatment of patients, and to review the competence of staff physicians.

Court Case

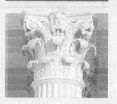

Landmark Case: Hospital Found Negligent

A patient was admitted to a small, southern Illinois hospital's emergency room with a broken leg. The treating doctor was not an orthopedic specialist and complications developed. The patient developed gangrene in the injured leg and it was amputated.

In a lawsuit the patient brought against the hospital, the hospital was required to pay damages when the court decided that the facility was negligent in permitting the treating doctor to do orthopedic work and in not requiring him to review his operative procedures to be sure they were current. The hospital was also found negligent in failing to exercise adequate supervision in the case and in not requiring consultation, especially after complications developed.

Darling v. Charleston Community Hospital, 211 N.E.2d 253 (Ill., 1965).

All medical professional liability claims are classified in one of three ways, based on the root word *feasance,* which means "the performance of an act."

malfeasance *The performance of a totally wrongful and unlawful act.*

Malfeasance is the performance of a totally wrongful and unlawful act. For example, in the absence of the employing physician, a medical assistant determines that a patient needs a prescription drug and dispenses the wrong drug from the physician's supply. Medical assistants are not licensed to practice medicine, and the wrong drug was dispensed, so the act was totally wrongful and unlawful and could be called malfeasance.

misfeasance *The performance of a lawful act in an illegal or improper manner.*

Misfeasance is the performance of a lawful act in an illegal or improper manner. Suppose a physician orders his or her nurse/employee to change a sterile dressing on a patient's burned hand. The nurse changes the dressing but does not use sterile technique, and the patient's burn becomes infected. The nurse is legally authorized to carry out the physician's instructions in dressing the patient's hand but violated proper procedure in carrying out the physician's order.

nonfeasance *The failure to act when one should.*

Nonfeasance is the failure to act when one should. For example, a newly certified emergency medical technician is first upon the scene of a traffic accident. An injured motorist stops breathing and appears to be in cardiac arrest. The EMT, though trained in cardiopulmonary resuscitation, "freezes" and does nothing. The patient dies. In failing to act, the EMT could be guilty of nonfeasance.

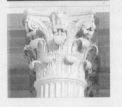

Court Case

Physician Operates on Wrong Side

A New York trial court ruled a surgeon was negligent in performing misplaced surgery on a prison inmate. Before making an incision, the surgeon saw a large left hernia bulge. However, he proceeded to perform a right inguinal repair because the only records available stated that there was a right hernia. The records were wrong.

The New York State Board for Professional Medical Conduct investigated and found that the surgeon did not properly examine the inmate, did not obtain an adequate medical history, and did not evaluate the inmate's medical condition before the operation. The inmate/patient sued the state. Although there was no testimony by a medical expert, the board's findings were introduced into evidence. The court found sufficient evidence to determine the surgeon's treatment constituted negligence, and his license was revoked.

Rivers v. State of New York, 537 N.Y.S.2d 968 (N.Y. Ct. of Claims, Jan. 25, 1989).

There are four elements that must be present in a given situation to prove a health care professional guilty of negligence. Sometimes called the "four Ds of negligence," these elements are:

- Duty—The person charged with negligence owed a duty of care to the accuser.

- Derelict—The health care provider breached the duty of care to the accuser.

- Direct cause—The breach of the duty of care to the accuser was a direct cause of the person's injury.

damages *Monetary awards sought by plaintiffs in lawsuits.*

- **Damages**—There is a legally recognizable injury to the accuser.

When a patient or other person (the plaintiff) sues a physician or other health care practitioner (the defendant) for negligence, the burden of proof is on the plaintiff. That is, it is up to the accuser's attorney to present evidence of the four Ds.

State statutes must be consulted for restrictions that apply to actions against health care providers. Some states limit damage awards or mandate procedural rules that must be followed in medical malpractice claims. In some states, for example, medical review panels must screen claims before they are brought to court. The panel examines the facts and then issues a finding of "malpractice" or "no malpractice." Such panels are generally comprised of physicians with expertise in the medical specialty in question and sometimes include a neutral attorney.

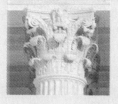

Negligence Charged in Penile Implant

A urologist performed penile implant surgery on a patient who had already attempted suicide in part due to his impotency. After surgery the patient suffered intense pain and urinary retention and was faced with the prospect of lifelong self-catheterization. Later corrective surgery left the patient permanently impotent.

After a failed suicide attempt, the patient was hospitalized and a urologist examined him. The urologist found that the wall of the patient's bladder was lacerated, causing urine to enter the surrounding body tissue and accumulate in the scrotum. Subsequently, the urologist performed three separate operations to correct problems caused by accumulation of scar tissue in the urethra.

In his malpractice action against the first urologist, the patient claimed the physician had breached the standard of care in failing to ascertain whether he was permanently, organically impotent before performing the penile implant. He argued that his impotency could have been cured without resorting to an implant. He also said the urologist's negligence had caused the bladder laceration, which he failed to diagnose.

An Ohio appellate court awarded the patient $300,000 for damages caused by the physician's negligence.

Bailey v. Emilio C. Chu, MD, Inc., 610 N.E.2d 531 (Ohio Ct. of App., Jan. 15, 1992).

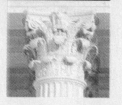

Court Increases Award to Patient

A patient entered the hospital to give birth to her second child. Before delivery she received an epidural block for anesthesia. The catheter used in the procedure was improperly inserted into the patient's back. When she awoke after surgery, her legs were numb and heavy. For the next few days while she was hospitalized, the patient had back pain and was sensitive to light. The catheter was removed two days after it had been inserted, and the patient was discharged from the hospital a few days later. Her condition worsened after discharge.

The patient saw her physician two days after discharge from the hospital and was diagnosed with an epidural abscess. Physicians performed a laminectomy and drained the abscess. At home the patient required intravenous antibiotics. She suffered bowel and bladder problems for several months and continued to have lumbar area pain and numbness and tingling in her right leg. The patient was eventually diagnosed with spinal meningitis, and she sued the hospital for the anesthesiologists' negligence.

At trial the patient was awarded $30,000. She appealed, claiming that the award was inadequate compensation for her damages. The appeals court agreed. The court held that there was no merit to the hospital's argument that the award was appropriate because the patient had failed to show the longevity of her injuries. On the contrary, the court said, there was evidence presented at trial to suggest that the patient would continue to suffer from back pain and numbness.

The court determined that the lowest permissible award for the patient was $125,000, and it increased the award to that amount.

Bush v. Arrow International, 646 So. 2d 1173 (La. Ct. of App., Nov. 23, 1994; rehearing denied Jan. 18, 1995).

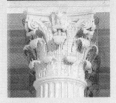
Check Your Progress

9. Name the four Ds of negligence.

   _____

   _____

   _____

   _____

10. In a lawsuit, the burden of proof is on which party?

    _____

11. State _____ must be consulted for restrictions that apply to actions against health care providers.

◆ ◆ ◆ ◆   ***Res Ipsa Loquitur***

res ipsa loquitur *"The thing speaks for itself"; also known as the doctrine of common knowledge. Under this doctrine no expert witnesses need be called.*

Under the doctrine of ***res ipsa loquitur,*** Latin for "the thing speaks for itself" (also known as the doctrine of common knowledge), expert witnesses need not be called to testify in a medical malpractice lawsuit. For *res ipsa loquitur* to apply, three conditions must exist:

1. The act of negligence must obviously be under the control of the defendant.

2. The patient must not have contributed to the accident.

3. It must be apparent that the patient would not have been injured if reasonable care had been used.

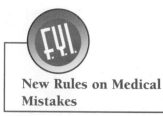
The Joint Commission on Accreditation of Healthcare Organizations evaluates approximately 80 percent of the hospitals in the United States for purposes of accreditation (2001 figure). The commission issued new rules for accreditation that took effect on July 1, 2001. Under the new standards, hospitals, doctors, and other medical professionals are required to tell patients when they have been harmed as a result of medical mistakes. Hospitals that fail to disclose such mistakes could lose their accreditation.

The new standards concerning disclosure were developed in response to a 1999 report issued by the National Academy of Sciences Institute of Medicine that revealed that medical mistakes kill as many as 98,000 individuals in the United States each year and cost billions of dollars.

Dr. Dennis O'Leary, president of the Joint Commission, emphasized that health care leaders "must radically change their thinking about medical mistakes. We need to create a culture . . . in which errors are openly discussed and studied."

Accordingly, the Veterans Administration and the National Aeronautics and Space Administration (NASA) were to implement a joint program called the Patient Safety Reporting System that would offer confidentiality and limited immunity from disciplinary action when mistakes were reported. The system would also disseminate the first nationwide medical alerts identifying patient safety hazards.

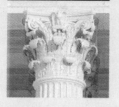

Court Case

Res Ipsa Loquitur Applied

A patient underwent surgery to correct hammertoes and awoke in the recovery room to find her front teeth missing. A podiatrist had performed the corrective surgery and general anesthesia had been administered by a board-certified anesthesiologist. An expert gave the opinion that the patient's injury was caused by use of excessive force by the anesthesiologist during the operation. A New York appellate court ruled:

- That the doctrine of *res ipsa loquitur* applied because, in the absence of negligence, a patient's teeth are not knocked out during foot surgery.
- That the injury was caused by an agency or instrumentality in the operating room, which was in the exclusive control of the podiatrist and the hospital.
- That the patient could not have contributed to the injury because she was anesthetized.

Kerber v. Saries, 542 N.Y.S.2d 94 (N.Y. Sup. Ct., App. Dov., June 2, 1989).

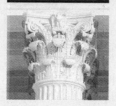

Court Case

Patient Sues Over Residual Surgical Drain

A Louisiana court awarded $20,000 to a patient who was infected after part of a surgical drain was left in his back.

An orthopedic surgeon performed back surgery on the patient to relieve his leg and back pain. After surgery a temporary drain was inserted in the patient's back to remove excess blood and fluid. The drain broke off when it was being removed, and the surgeon decided to leave the broken end inside the patient's back. The patient appeared to recover normally for two months but then began to suffer fever and pain. Finally, X rays revealed the piece of drain in the patient's back.

The patient sued the surgeon for malpractice, alleging that the surgeon had failed to comply with appropriate standards of care in removing the surgical drain. A jury agreed and awarded the patient $20,000, since no permanent impairment or disability resulted from the injury.

The surgeon appealed, arguing that he should have been allowed to present evidence of a manufacturing defect in the drain. The court ruled that evidence of a defect was irrelevant and said that the surgeon was at fault for his failure to use the appropriate standard of care.

Sebastien v. McKay, 649 So.2d 711 (La. Ct. of App., Nov. 23, 1994).

Cases that fall under the doctrine of *res ipsa loquitur* include:

- Unintentionally leaving foreign bodies, such as sponges or instruments, inside a patient's body during surgery.

- Accidentally burning or otherwise injuring a patient while he or she is anesthetized.

- Damaging healthy tissue during an operation.

- Causing an infection by the use of unsterilized instruments.

Check Your Progress

12. Expert witnesses usually testify to establish _____ .

13. *Res ipsa loquitur* means _____ .

14. Name three conditions that must be present for the doctrine of *res ipsa loquitur* to apply.

_____

_____

_____

Court Case

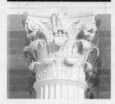

Wrongful Death Alleged

A patient was brought to a Texas hospital emergency room suffering from a gunshot wound to the chest. The nurse on duty telephoned the first surgeon on call, but he had an emergency at another hospital and could not respond. The nurse then paged the emergency physician who was second on call. He returned the call but did not want to come in, because he said he did not believe the first physician called actually had an emergency. The nurse finally convinced him to come. The patient was taken to surgery, but he died a short time later, before the emergency physician arrived.

The patient's family sued the hospital and its emergency nurses and physicians for wrongful death. Except for the second on-call physician, all of those named in the suit either settled with the family or were dropped from the complaint. The second on-call physician filed for summary judgment on grounds that he had no physician-patient relationship with the injured person and, therefore, had no duty of care. The trial court noted that the physician had never seen the patient and ruled in his favor. A Texas appellate court affirmed the summary judgment.

Ortiz v. Shah, 905 S.W.2d 609 (Texas Ct. of App., June 8, 1995; rehearing overruled Aug. 31, 1995).

◆ ◆ ◆ ◆ Damage Awards

When a defendant is found guilty of a tort—such as negligence, breach of contract, libel, or slander—the plaintiff is awarded compensation based on the extent of his or her injuries, loss of income, damage to reputation, or other harm that can be proved. This monetary compensation is called damages. Table 4-1 explains the various types of damages and how the court determines them.

Physicians and many other professional health care providers carry liability insurance, which pays damage awards in the event of a negligence or malpractice suit up to the limits of the policy. Some states have placed caps, or limits, on the amount of damages a plaintiff may be awarded in a medical malpractice action.

Some states have enacted **wrongful death statutes,** which allow a patient's beneficiaries to collect from a health care practitioner for loss to the estate of future earnings when a patient's death is judged to have been due to negligence of the health care practitioner. In most states, a cap has been placed on the amount of damages that can be recovered in a civil action for wrongful death.

The state may also prosecute a health care practitioner under criminal statutes for the wrongful death of a patient.

wrongful death statutes
State statutes that allow a person's beneficiaries to collect for loss to the estate of the deceased for future earnings when a death is judged to have been due to negligence.

Table 4-1   **DAMAGE AWARDS**

Types of Damages	Purpose	Considered by Court	Award
General Compensatory	To compensate for injuries or losses due to violation of patient's rights.	Physical disability? Loss of earnings? Mental anguish? Loss of service of spouse or child? Losses to date? Future losses?	Specified by court. Dollar value need not be proved; loss must be proved.
Special Compensatory	To compensate for losses not directly caused by the wrong.	Additional medical expenses?	Specified by court. Dollar value and loss must be proved.
Consequential	To compensate for losses caused indirectly by a product defect.	Loss covered by product warranty? Personal injury?	No limit on damages if personal injuries.
Punitive	To punish the offender.	How serious was the breach of conduct? How much can the defendant afford to pay?	In some cases, amount of damages is set by law.
Nominal	To recognize that rights of the patient were violated, though no actual loss was proved.	Legal rights of the patient violated? Actual loss proved?	Token award, usually $1.

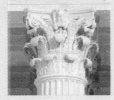

Doctor Sued for Wrongful Death Caused by Inadequate Hospital Discharge Instructions

A patient had chronic kidney failure that required continual dialysis treatment. In order to receive dialysis treatments, hemodialysis catheters, or access grafts, were surgically inserted in the patient's arms. When the access grafts caused problems, a vascular surgeon removed them. While the patient was hospitalized after the grafts in his arms were removed, he suffered two incidents during which he bled copiously from a surgery site in his left arm. Bleeding was stopped with pressure dressings, and the patient received a blood transfusion.

The patient remained hospitalized for observation for four days. He had no other bleeding episodes, received his dialysis treatment successfully, ate well, and had normal vital signs, so he was dismissed from the hospital. The physician noted in his discharge summary that the patient had been instructed on how to apply pressure if his arm should bleed and was told to call his physician if problems occurred.

On the evening of his return home, the patient had two bleeding incidents. Pressure was applied and the site was wrapped with gauze. No one called the physician to report the two bleeding incidents. The next day the patient was left alone while his wife took their daughter to school and filled a prescription. When she returned home about 30 minutes later, she found her husband dead, lying in a pool of blood.

The patient died from loss of blood caused by hemorrhaging from the incision in his left arm. His wife filed a wrongful death suit against the physician and his vascular surgery corporation. The trial judge found the physician had not erred in treating the patient's bleeding incidents in the hospital and had not discharged the patient too soon. The judge found, however, that the physician had issued inadequate discharge instructions to the patient and this constituted a breach of care. The discharge instructions were inadequate, according to the judge's ruling, in that the patient had not been warned about the seriousness of a potential bleeding episode and was not told to have someone at home with him at all times.

The patient was found to be 50 percent responsible for causing his own death, in that he failed to call the physician when he had two bleeding episodes after discharge from the hospital, as instructed.

An appeals court upheld the trial judge's ruling.

Samuel v. Baton Rouge General Medical Center, 2000 La.App. Lexis 321 (Ct. of App. of La., 1st Circ., Feb. 18, 2000).

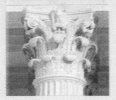

Hospital Sued for Wrongful Death

A 39-year-old Vietnam veteran was hospitalized in a Veteran's Administration hospital. The patient had posttraumatic stress syndrome, hypertension, liver damage, and a cholesterol level of 394. The VA hospital had tested his cholesterol five times but waited two years before starting treatment.

The patient had a heart attack and died, and his family filed a wrongful death claim, charging that the VA was negligent in treating his high cholesterol.

(continued)

The VA denied the claim. The patient's estate then filed a request for reconsideration, but the VA took no action. The estate filed suit in federal court for medical malpractice.

The trial court found that even though the patient was obese and hyperlipidemic, the VA failed to diagnose or treat him for these conditions initially. However, the trial court blamed the patient for any delay in treatment, due to his failure to take the tests in a fasting state. The court found in favor of the government.

The estate appealed and an appellate court found the fasting issue was misleading. Medical records did not show that any physician gave special consideration to the abnormal or critical cholesterol results. The court held that the VA did treat the patient's hypertension but failed to address his high cholesterol or obesity and thus failed to lessen the patient's risk of heart attack.

The trial court's judgment was vacated and the case remanded for further consideration.

Metzen vs. U.S., 19 F. ad 795 (C.A. 2., N.Y., March 23, 1994).

Elements of a Lawsuit

As indicated in Chapter 3, the type of court that hears a case depends on the offense or complaint. In civil malpractice or negligence cases, the party bringing the action (plaintiff) must prove the case by presenting evidence to a judge or jury that is more convincing than that of the opposing side (defendant).

◆ ◆ ◆ ◆ **Phases of a Lawsuit**

The typical malpractice or negligence lawsuit proceeds as follows:

1. A patient feels he or she has been injured.
2. The patient seeks the advice of an attorney.
3. If the attorney believes the case has merit, he or she then requests copies of the patient's health records. The attorney reviews the health records and the appropriate standard of care to ascertain merits of the case. In some states, before proceeding to a lawsuit, the attorney must obtain an expert witness report stating that the standard of care has been violated. An affidavit to that effect must then be submitted. An *affidavit* is a sworn statement in writing made under oath. It may also be a declaration before an authorized officer of the court.

Pleading Phase

summons *A written notification issued by the clerk of the court and delivered with a copy of the complaint to the defendant in a lawsuit, directing him or her to respond to the charges brought in a court of law.*

4. The plaintiff's (injured patient's) attorney files a complaint with the clerk of the court. In this document, the plaintiff states his or her version of the situation and the amount of money sought from the defendant (practitioner being sued) for the plaintiff's injury.
5. A **summons** is issued by the clerk of the court and is delivered with a copy of the complaint to the defendant, directing him or her to respond to the charges. If the defendant does not respond within the specified time limit, he or she can lose the case by default.

6. The defendant's attorney files an answer to the summons, and a copy of it is sent to the plaintiff. In this document the defendant presents his or her version of the case, either admitting or denying the charges. The defendant may also file a counterclaim or a cross-complaint.

7. If a cross-complaint is made, the plaintiff files a reply.

Interrogatory, or Pretrial Discovery, Phase

8. The court sets a trial date.

9. Pretrial motions may be made and decided. For example, the defendant may request that the lawsuit be dismissed, the plaintiff may amend the original complaint, or either side may request a change of venue (ask that the trial be held in another place).

10. Discovery procedures may be used to uncover evidence that will support the charges when the case comes to court. A court order called a **subpoena** may be issued commanding the presence of the physician or a medical office employee in court or requiring that a deposition be taken. A **deposition** is sworn testimony given and recorded outside the courtroom during the pretrial phase of a case. (See the section below entitled "Witness Testimony.")

An **interrogatory** may be requested instead of or in addition to a deposition. This is a written set of questions requiring written answers from a plaintiff or defendant under oath.

The subpoena commanding a witness to appear in court and to bring certain medical records is called a **subpoena *duces tecum.*** Failure to obey a subpoena may result in contempt-of-court charges. Contempt of court is willful disobedience to or open disrespect of a court, judge, or legislative body. It is punishable by fines or imprisonment.

11. A pretrial conference may be called by the judge scheduled to hear the case. During this conference the judge discusses the issues in the case with the opposing attorneys. This helps avoid surprises and delays after the trial starts and may lead to an out-of-court settlement. (*Note:* At any point after the complaint is filed before the case comes to trial, an out-of-court settlement may be reached.)

Trial Phase

12. The jury is selected (if one is to be used), and the trial begins.

13. Opening statements are made by the lawyers for the plaintiff and the defendant, summarizing what each will prove during the trial.

14. Witnesses are called to testify for both sides. They may be cross-examined by opposing attorneys.

15. Closing statements are made by each attorney. No new evidence may be presented during summation.

16. The judge gives instructions to the jury (if one was chosen), and the jury retires to deliberate.

17. The jury reaches a verdict.

18. The final judgment is handed down by the court. The judge bases his or her decision for judgment on the jury's verdict.

subpoena *A legal document requiring the recipient to appear as a witness in court or to give a deposition.*

deposition *Sworn testimony given and recorded outside the courtroom during the pretrial phase of a case.*

interrogatory *A written set of questions requiring written answers from a plaintiff or defendant under oath.*

subpoena *duces tecum* *A legal document requiring the recipient to bring certain written records to court to be used as evidence in a lawsuit.*

Appeals Phase

19. Posttrial motions may be filed.

20. An appeal may be made for the case to be reviewed by a higher court if the evidence indicates errors may have been made or if there was injustice or impropriety in the trial court proceedings. A judgment is final only when all options for appeal have been exercised.

Check Your Progress

15. Name the four phases of a typical medical professional liability lawsuit.

_____

_____

_____

_____

16. A subpoena *duces tecum* is issued during which trial phase? _____

17. The complaint is filed during which trial phase? _____

18. During which trial phase is the court's judgment handed down? _____

Witness Testimony

Nine out of ten lawsuits are settled out of court, but health care practitioners are often asked to give testimony. Testimony may be given in court on the witness stand, or it may be given in an attorney's conference room in a pretrial proceeding called a deposition. (See the earlier section entitled "Interrogatory, or Pretrial Discovery, Phase.")

Depositions are of two types: (1) discovery depositions and (2) depositions in lieu of trial.

Discovery depositions cover material that will most likely be examined again when the witness testifies in court. Since there will be an opportunity for the opposing attorney to question the witness a second time in court, the deposition need not cover every possible question.

Before both a deposition and in-court testimony, the witness is sworn to tell the truth and then is questioned by attorneys representing both sides. During courtroom testimony, however, a judge is present to rule on objections raised by the attorneys. When an objection is raised, the witness should stop speaking until the judge either sustains or overrules the objection. If the objection is sustained, the witness need not answer the question; if the objection is overruled, the witness must answer. If in doubt about whether an objection to a question was sustained or overruled, the witness may ask the judge whether a question should be answered. During a deposition, witnesses should take the attorney's advice regarding questions that should be answered.

Depositions in lieu of trial are used instead of the witness's in-person testimony in court. Since the opposing attorney has one opportunity to question the witness, questions are thorough, and the witness should carefully consider his or her answers.

Sometimes depositions in lieu of trial are videotaped, to be played in the courtroom during the trial. Witnesses whose depositions will be videotaped should be informed in advance, so they can dress as though they were appearing in court in person.

Witnesses may offer two kinds of **testimony:** fact and expert. *Fact testimony* may be offered by health care practitioners or laypersons and concerns only those facts the witness has observed. For example, regarding testimony in a medical malpractice case, medical assistants, LPNs/LVNs, and registered nurses may testify about how many times a patient saw the physician, the patient's appearance during a particular visit, or similar observations. If asked to give fact testimony, a health care practitioner's powers of observation and memory are more important than his or her professional qualifications.

Expert testimony is given by witnesses who have the education, skills, knowledge, and experience to be judged expert in a particular field relevant to the matter on trial. In medical negligence lawsuits, physicians are usually called as expert witnesses to testify to the standard of care regarding the matter in question. If the defendant/physician is a specialist, the expert witness generally practices or teaches in the same specialty. Acceptable expert witnesses are not coworkers, friends, or acquaintances of the defendant. It is ethical and acceptable for expert witnesses to set and accept a fee commensurate with time taken from regular employment and time spent preparing their expert testimony.

testimony *Statements sworn to under oath by witnesses testifying in court and giving depositions.*

◆ ◆ ◆ ◆ ## Courtroom Conduct

Most health care practitioners will never have to appear in court. If you should be asked to appear, however, the following suggestions may prove helpful:

- Attend court proceedings as required. If you were subpoenaed but fail to appear, you could be charged with contempt of court. (If either the plaintiff or defendant fails to appear, that person forfeits the case.)

- Find out in advance when and where you are to appear, and do not be late for scheduled hearings.

- Bring the required documents to court and present them only when requested to do so.

- Before testifying, refresh your memory concerning all the facts observed about the matter in question, such as dates, times, words spoken, and circumstances.

- Speak slowly, use layperson's terms instead of medical terms whenever possible, and do not lose your temper or attempt to be humorous.

- Answer all questions in a straightforward manner, even if the answers appear to help the opposing side.

- Answer only the question asked, no more and no less.

- Because you are testifying as to what you recall, be careful of broad generalizations, such as, "That is all that took place." A better answer might be, "As I recall, that is what took place."

- Your attorney may help you prepare your testimony, but do not discuss your testimony with other witnesses or others outside the courtroom. Answer truthfully if asked whether you discussed your testimony with counsel.

- Appear well groomed, and dress in clean, conservative clothing.

Alternative Dispute Resolution

alternative dispute resolution (ADR) *Methods of settling civil disputes between parties using neutral mediators or arbitrators without going to court.*

Alternative dispute resolution (ADR), also known as appropriate dispute resolution, consists of techniques for resolving civil disputes without going to court. As court calendars have become overcrowded in recent years, ADR has become increasingly popular. Several alternative methods of settling legal disputes are possible, including mediation, arbitration, and a combination of the two methods called med-arb.

Some states require mediation or arbitration for some civil cases, whereas in others these alternative dispute resolution methods are voluntary. Mediation is an ADR method in which a neutral third party listens to both sides of the argument and then helps resolve the dispute. The mediator does not have the authority to impose a solution on the parties involved.

Arbitration is a method of settling disputes in which the opposing parties agree to abide by the decision of an arbitrator. The arbitrator or arbitrators are selected directly by the disputing parties or are chosen in one of two ways:

- Under the terms of a written contract, an arbitrator is chosen by the court or by the American Arbitration Association.

- If no contract exists, each of the two involved parties selects an arbitrator and the two arbitrators select a third.

In an informal proceeding, each side presents evidence and witnesses. In the alternative dispute resolution method called med-arb, the mediator resolves the dispute if the two parties are unable to reach agreement after mediation.

Advocates of alternative dispute resolution claim that these methods are faster and less costly than court adjudication. Critics claim that medical malpractice cases are best decided when all the factual information is brought out, as in pretrial judicial discovery procedures. They also argue that selecting arbitrators acceptable to both parties can take weeks, months, and even years, and attorneys' fees and damage awards can be as costly as in court-tried cases. Figure 4-2 illustrates a sample arbitration agreement to be signed by the patient and physician involved in a dispute.

ARTICLE 1: It is understood that any dispute as to medical malpractice, that is as to whether any medical services rendered under this contract were unnecessary or unauthorized or were improperly, negligently, or incompetently rendered, will be determined by submission to arbitration as provided by California law, and not by a lawsuit or resort to court process except as California law provides for judicial review of arbitration proceedings. Both parties to this contract, by entering into it, are giving up their constitutional right to have such dispute decided in a court of law before a jury, and instead are accepting the use of arbitration.

ARTICLE 2: I understand and agree that this arbitration agreement binds me and anyone else who may have a claim arising out of or related to all treatment or services provided by the physician, including any spouse or heirs of the patient and any children, whether born or unborn at the time of the occurrence giving rise to any claim. This includes, but is not limited to, all claims for monetary damages exceeding the jurisdictional limit of the small claims court, including, without limitation, suits for loss of consortium, wrongful death, emotional distress or punitive damages. I further understand and agree that if I sign this agreement on behalf of some other person for whom I have responsibility, then, in addition to myself, such person(s) will also be bound, along with anyone else who may have a claim arising out of the treatment or services rendered to that person. I also understand and agree that this agreement relates to claims against the physician and any consenting substitute physician, as well as the physician's partners, associates, association, corporation or partnership, and the employees, agents, and estates of any of them. I also hereby consent to the intervention or joinder in the arbitration proceeding of all parties relevant to a full and complete settlement of any dispute arbitrated under this Agreement, as set forth in the CAHHS/CMA Medical Arbitration Rules.

ARTICLE 3: I understand and agree that I will be bound by this arbitration agreement and that this agreement will be valid and enforceable for any and all treatment provided by the physician in the future regardless of the length of time since my last visit to this physician, and regardless of the fact that the patient-physician relationship between myself and the physician may be interrupted for any reason and then recommenced.

ARTICLE 4: I UNDERSTAND THAT I DO NOT HAVE TO SIGN THIS AGREEMENT TO RECEIVE THE PHYSICIAN'S SERVICES, AND THAT IF I DO SIGN THE AGREEMENT AND CHANGE MY MIND WITHIN 30 DAYS OF TODAY, THEN I MAY CANCEL THIS AGREEMENT BY GIVING WRITTEN NOTICE TO THE UNDERSIGNED PHYSICIAN WITHIN THAT TIME STATING THAT I WANT TO WITHDRAW FROM THIS ARBITRATION AGREEMENT.

ARTICLE 5: On behalf of myself and all others bound by this agreement as set forth in Article 2, agreement is hereby given to be bound by the Medical Arbitration Rules of the California Association of Hospitals and Health Systems (CAHHS) and the California Medical Association (CMA), as they may be amended from time to time, which are hereby incorporated into this agreement. A copy of these Rules is included in the pamphlet in which this agreement is found. Additional copies of the Rules are available from the California Medical Association, P.O. Box 7690, San Francisco, Ca. 94120-7690, Attention: Arbitration Rules. I understand that disputes covered by this Agreement will be covered by California law applicable to actions against health care providers, including the Medical Injury Compensation Reform Act of 1975 (including any amendments thereto).

ARTICLE 6: OPTIONAL: RETROACTIVE EFFECT
If I intend this agreement to cover services rendered before the date it is signed (for example, emergency treatment), I have indicated the earlier date I intend this agreement to be effective from and initialed below.

Earlier effective date: _____ Patient's Initials: _____

ARTICLE 7: I have read and understood all the information in this pamphlet, including the explanation of the Patient-Physician Arbitration Agreement, this Agreement, and the Rules. I understand that in the case of any pregnant woman, the term "patient" as used herein means both the mother and the mother's expected child or children.

If any provision of this arbitration agreement is held invalid or unenforceable, the remaining provisions shall remain in full force and shall not be affected by the invalidity of any other provision.

NOTICE: BY SIGNING THIS CONTRACT YOU ARE AGREEING TO HAVE ANY ISSUE OF MEDICAL MALPRACTICE DECIDED BY NEUTRAL ARBITRATION AND YOU ARE GIVING UP YOUR RIGHT TO A JURY OR COURT TRIAL. SEE ARTICLE 1 OF THIS CONTRACT.

_____ Dated: _____, _____
(Patient, Parent, Guardian or Legally Authorized Representative of Patient)

If signed by other than patient, indicate relationship: _____

PHYSICIAN'S AGREEMENT TO ARBITRATE
In consideration of the foregoing execution of this Patient-Physician Arbitration Agreement, I likewise agree to be bound by the terms set forth in this agreement and in the rules specified in Article 5 above.

_____ Dated: _____, _____
(Physician or Duly-Authorized Representative)

_____   _____
Title — e.g., Partner, President, etc.   Print name of Physician, Medical Group, Partnership or Association
©California Medical Association, 1998

Figure 4-2
Sample Patient-Physician Arbitration Agreement
Published with permission of and by arrangement with the California Medical Association.

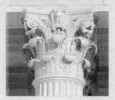

Physician Not Qualified as Expert Witness

A Florida appellate court ruled that a physician who had not practiced for more than ten years was not qualified to testify as an expert witness in a malpractice case.

The case in question involved a patient who sued her physician after a breast implant procedure. Before filing her claim, the patient engaged a physician to serve as an expert witness.

In accordance with Florida law, the expert witness submitted an affidavit to the trial court. The court held that the physician was not qualified to testify as an expert witness because he had not practiced medicine for a decade. His recent professional activity consisted of acting as an expert witness in similar cases. The trial court struck the affidavit, and since the statute of limitations had run out, the patient's action against the physician was dismissed.

An appellate court affirmed the trial court's action.

Winson v. Norman, 658 So.2d 625 (Fla. Dist. Ct. of App., July 19, 1995; rehearing denied Aug. 23, 1995).

Applying Knowledge

Answer the following questions in the spaces provided.

1. According to the reasonable-person standard, a person may be charged with negligence if someone is injured because of failure to perform an act that a reasonable person in similar circumstances would perform, or if an act is committed that

   _____

   _____ .

2. To whom is a duty of care owed? _____

3. Briefly explain and distinguish between the terms *standard of care* and *duty of care*.

   _____

   _____

4. What is the basis for most medical professional malpractice claims?

   _____

   _____

5. Explain the differences between the terms *malfeasance, misfeasance,* and *nonfeasance*.

   _____

   _____

   _____

   _____

   _____

   _____

6. List and describe the four Ds of negligence.

   _____

   _____

   _____

   _____

   _____

   _____

7. When a patient sues a physician for negligence, who has the burden of proof, the plaintiff or the defendant? _____

8. In a case in which a patient sues a physician, the patient is called the _____ and the physician is called the _____ .

Review and Case Studies

9. Why are expert witnesses allowed in a medical professional negligence lawsuit?

   _____

10. When is the doctrine of *res ipsa loquitur* applied? _____

11. Explain the status of expert witnesses in cases in which *res ipsa loquitur* is applied.

    _____

12. Monetary compensation awarded by a court of law is called _____ .

13. Why might a medical assistant/dental assistant/surgical assistant purchase a professional liability insurance policy separate from his or her employer's policy?

    _____

14. A court order for an individual to appear in court is called a(n) _____ and an order
    for bringing certain records is called _____ .
    An order to appear in court to defend yourself is a(n) _____ .

15. What is the difference between a deposition and an interrogatory?

    _____

    _____

    _____

16. Define the two types of depositions that might be taken prior to a medical malpractice lawsuit.

    _____

    _____

    _____

17. As a health care practitioner asked to testify, are you more likely to give factual or expert testimony?
    Why?

    _____

    _____

    _____

18. Define *alternative dispute resolution.* List two commonly used ADR methods.

    _____

    _____

    _____

19. As a health care practitioner, can you legally and ethically use any title you want? Explain your answer.

    _____

    _____

20. Define *res ipsa loquitur.*

    _____

    _____

21. Explain what legal action may be taken if you are subpoenaed to appear in court as a witness or to give a deposition and you fail to appear.

_____

_____

22. What is the result if you are the plaintiff or the defendant in a lawsuit and you fail to appear in court?

_____

_____

_____

Match each description that follows with the correct type of damages by writing the appropriate letter in the space provided.

_____**23.** Token damages, recognizing the wrong.

_____**24.** Specific losses not proven to be a direct cause of the wrong; dollar amount and loss must be proven.

_____**25.** Punishment.

_____**26.** No limit for damages involving personal injury caused by indirect product defect or warranty.

_____**27.** Damages awarded by court paying for violation of rights; dollar value need not be proved.

a. general compensatory

b. special compensatory

c. consequential

d. punitive

e. nominal

Match each of the following actions with the appropriate phase of a lawsuit by writing the appropriate letter in the space provided.

_____**28.** The jury reaches a verdict.

_____**29.** A complaint is filed.

_____**30.** A trial date is set.

_____**31.** A subpoena may be issued.

_____**32.** A jury is selected.

_____**33.** A summons is issued.

_____**34.** Pretrial motions are made or decided.

_____**35.** A deposition may be taken.

_____**36.** Witnesses are called to testify.

_____**37.** Opening and closing statements are made by the attorneys.

_____**38.** An answer to the summons is filed.

_____**39.** A pretrial conference is called by the judge.

_____**40.** Judgment is handed down by the court.

_____**41.** A plea is made for the case to be reviewed by a higher court.

a. pleadings phase

b. interrogatory, or pretrial discovery, phase

c. trial phase

d. appeals phase

Case Studies

Use your critical-thinking skills to answer the questions that follow each of the case studies.

A trained anesthesiologist ran out of oxygen before the operation was completed, causing the patient to suffer a fatal cardiac arrest.

42. **This case was adjudicated as a strong medical malpractice case and was won by the plaintiff. Referring to the four Ds of negligence, explain why.**

_____

_____

_____

_____

_____

During an endoscopic retrograde cholangiopancreatography (ERCP), an inexperienced nurse injected the dye too forcefully and caused the patient to develop pancreatitis and other debilitating injuries.

43. **The patient sued and won. Refer to the four Ds of negligence to explain the court's decision.**

_____

_____

_____

_____

_____

An on-call ophthalmologist, without seeing the patient, diagnosed his eye pain, sensitivity to light, and nausea as sinusitis. In fact, the patient had acute angle closure glaucoma and lost sight in the eye.

44. **When this case came to trial, the court found in favor of the patient/plaintiff. Explain the court's decision based on the four Ds of negligence.**

_____

_____

_____

_____

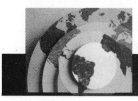

Complete the activities and answer the questions that follow.

45. Visit the Web site of the American Arbitration Association. Click on "Rules/Procedures," then "Model Standard of Conduct for Mediators." List three major points you find there for standards of conduct for mediators.

_____

_____

_____

_____

46. Find the Web site for the American Health Information Management Association (AHIMA). Do a site search for "patient confidentiality." Click on "Frequently Asked Questions." List a question asked about this issue and record the answer.

_____

_____

_____

_____

47. Visit the Web site for the Association for Responsible Medicine (ARM). What sources might be used by laypersons to check credentials and malpractice records of physicians?

_____

_____

_____

_____

5

DEFENSES TO LIABILITY SUITS

Objectives

After studying this chapter, you should be able to:

1. Relate how the guidelines for physicians' malpractice prevention apply to other health care practitioners.

2. Discuss the various defenses to professional liability suits.

3. Know where to find the statute of limitations for malpractice litigation in your state.

4. Debate the question of whether liability insurance is practical for the medical career you plan to practice.

5. Discuss two different types of medical liability insurance.

Key Terms

- affirmative defenses
- assumption of risk
- claims-made insurance
- comparative negligence
- contributory negligence
- denial
- emergency

- liability insurance
- occurrence insurance
- release of tortfeasor
- *res judicata*
- statute of limitations
- technical defenses

Preventing Liability Suits

Malpractice litigation not only adds to the cost of health care; it takes a psychological toll on both patients and health care practitioners. Both sides would probably agree that prevention is preferable to litigating a malpractice claim. Health care practitioners who use reasonable care in preventing professional liability claims are least likely to be faced with defending themselves against such claims. The following guidelines, adapted from "commandments" for malpractice prevention devised by the American Medical Association's Committee on Medicolegal Problems, can help medical practitioners avoid malpractice lawsuits.

◆ ◆ ◆ ◆ ## Standards of Care and Safety

The first responsibility of the health care practitioner is always to provide competent, courteous, and compassionate health care to patients. The following suggestions for providing effective health care can help you meet your professional responsibilities while at the same time avoiding liability that can lead to lawsuits:

- Know and follow standards of care and appropriate procedures for medical practitioners in similar practices and in similar communities. Avoid what you are not fully trained or equipped to handle.

- Know the requirements of good medical practice in caring for each patient.

- Maintain accurate and complete files relevant to the patient's condition, including X rays, test results, and progress notes.

- If your duties include taking telephone messages, relate them accurately. Offer to make appointments when appropriate. Remember that when health care practitioners other than physicians diagnose or prescribe, they may be charged with practicing medicine without a license.

- If you prepare or administer medications, check each drug three times: once when taking it from the supply cabinet, again when preparing the dosage, and a third time when returning the container to the shelf. All outdated medications should be discarded and promptly replaced. Prescription blanks should not be left on desktops or work areas.

- Avoid destructive and unethical criticism of the work of other physicians or other health care practitioners. Do not discuss with a patient his or her former physician. Listen carefully to each patient's complaints and remarks about dissatisfaction with treatment, and see that they reach the treating physician.

- Stay informed of general medical and scientific progress by reading professional journals, attending seminars and professional association meetings, and fulfilling continuing study requirements.

The following guidelines for employing physicians can help you evaluate the quality of care offered by your employing physician or medical facility and make appropriate suggestions for improving patient care and reducing liability risks in the workplace environment:

- Employing physicians should carefully select and supervise all employees and should be careful in delegating duties to them, expecting them to perform only those duties they may reasonably be expected to perform, based on their qualifications, credentials, training, and experience.

- Physicians should exhaust all reasonable methods of securing a diagnosis before embarking on a therapeutic course.

- Physicians should use conservative and the least dangerous methods of diagnosis and treatment whenever possible, rather than those that involve highly toxic agents or risky surgical procedures.

- Physicians should not diagnose or prescribe by telephone.

- Except in emergencies, male physicians should not examine female patients and female physicians should not examine male patients unless an assistant, a nurse, or a member of the patient's family is present. Ideally, a female medical assistant or female nurse should be present when a male physician examines a female patient. Likewise, when a female physician examines a male patient, a male medical assistant or male nurse should be present.

- Employing physicians should check equipment and facilities frequently for safety, including the reception area. All employees should know safe procedures for operating equipment and should remind employing physicians when repair or replacement of equipment is necessary for continued safe operation. Employees should be alert to all hazards in the medical office that might cause injury, such as slippery floors, electrical cords in unsafe places, tables with sharp edges, and so forth. The reception area at the health care facility should include a safe area for children, perhaps including such items as child-sized tables and chairs and picture books.

- When using toxic agents for diagnosis or treatment, physicians should know customary dosages or usage for such substances, any possible side effects or known toxic reactions, and the proper methods for treating reactions. Medical assistants and other medical office employees should ensure that when supplies are received, they are handled according to office policy and all relevant literature is readily accessible to physicians.

◆ ◆ ◆ ◆ **Communicating with Patients**

Patients who see the medical office as a friendly place are generally less likely to sue. You can help by:

- Developing good listening skills and nonverbal communication techniques so that patients feel the time spent with them is not rushed. For example, patients will see a health care practitioner as caring and interested if he or she sits rather than stands while interviewing or convers-

Why Do Patients Sue?

A survey by the Texas Medical Liability Trust asked six thousand physicians why they thought patients sue. They offered the following reasons:

- Unrealistic expectations. Because of the abundance of available medical information, patients may expect perfection. When the outcome of medical care is not perfect, patients may feel betrayed by the health care system.
- Poor rapport and poor communication. Few patients sue health care practitioners they like and trust. On the other hand, if a patient perceives health care providers as cold, uncaring, or rude, they may be more inclined to sue if something goes wrong.
- Greed. Although money is seldom the reason for medical malpractice lawsuits, in some cases it may be an influencing factor. Patients read about huge awards made by juries, and some may feel that a lawsuit is worth the potential reward.
- Lawyers and our litigious society. Since contingency arrangements are common in the United States and the loser of a lawsuit does not have to pay the winner's legal expenses, lawyers may be more apt to accept a medical malpractice suit.
- Poor quality of care. Poor quality *in fact* means that a patient is truly not receiving quality health care. Poor quality *in perception* means that the patient *believes* he or she is not receiving quality health care, even if that is untrue. Either situation can lead to a malpractice lawsuit.
- Poor outcome. If medical treatment is unsuccessful or adds to a patient's health problems and a plaintiff can provide evidence of the four Ds of negligence, an attorney will probably accept his or her medical malpractice lawsuit.
- Failure to keep the family informed. When physicians do not return telephone calls or are otherwise unavailable to a patient's family members and they perceive the unresponsive physicians as cold and uncaring, those family members may be more apt to sue if something goes wrong.

ing with the patient. Conversely, lack of eye contact and defensive body postures convey disinterest to a patient. In short, obey the Golden Rule when communicating with patients.

- Setting aside a certain time period during the day for returning patients' telephone calls, and advising patients accordingly. Medical facility staff members responsible for answering the telephone should learn to recognize when patients' reported symptoms require the physician's immediate attention and when patients should be advised to seek emergency care.

- Reminding physicians to explain illnesses and treatment options thoroughly, including risks and possible complications, in terms the patient can understand. Patients should be encouraged to ask questions and to participate in the decision-making process. The best way to keep patients' expectations in line is through education. When dealing with accidents and bad results, a straightforward approach is desirable.

- Checking to be sure that all patients or their authorized representatives sign informed-consent forms before they undergo medical and surgical procedures. Next-of-kin or designated representatives must also sign informed-consent forms to authorize autopsies.

- Avoiding statements that could be construed as an admission of fault on the physician's part. If a lawsuit is filed against a physician, his or her employees should say nothing to anyone except as required by the physician's attorney or the court. However, an employee may be held liable if he or she knowingly remains silent to protect a physician who has performed an illegal act.

- Using tact, good judgment, and professional ability in handling patients. Physicians should insist on a professional consultation if the patient is not doing well, if he or she is unhappy and complaining, or if the patient's family expresses dissatisfaction.

- Refraining from making overly optimistic statements about recovery or prognoses. Health care practitioners who are not physicians should not discuss patients' ailments with them, compare treatments, attempt to diagnose their condition, or make promises on the physician's behalf, such as, "The doctor will have you feeling better soon."

- Advising patients when their physicians intend to be gone and reminding physicians to recommend or make available qualified substitutes. The patient must not be abandoned. A copy of a letter of referral, notice of a physician's intended absence from practice, or letter of dismissal should be placed in the patient's record. Notices of a physician's intended absence should be posted in the office and sent with the monthly billing or be published in the local newspaper. The name and telephone number of the covering physician should be available for patients requesting care in the absence of their regular physician.

- Making every effort to reach an understanding about fees with the patient before treatment so that billing does not become a point of contention. When handling fees for the physician, employees should explain all charges to patients, detailing those that are not included in regular fees. They should also follow legal collection procedures.

♦ ♦ ♦ ♦   Documentation

Patient records are often used as evidence in professional medical liability cases, and improper documentation can lose a case (see Chapter 6). In some situations that may arise in medical practice, such as drug testing or the examination of a rape victim, evidence may need to be collected in a certain manner in order to be admissible in court. When in doubt about what documentation to make, contact legal authorities for advice.

Physicians should keep records that clearly show what treatment was done and when it was done. It is important that they be able to demonstrate that nothing was neglected and that the care given fully met the standards demanded by law. Physicians should also document all referrals to other physicians, withdrawals from a case, and cases in which patients refuse to follow their advice. Today's health care environment requires complete documentation of actions taken and, in many cases, actions not taken. Medical facility employees should pay particular attention to the following:

REFERRALS   Make sure the patient understands whether the referring physician's staff will make the appointment and notify the patient or whether the patient must call to set up the appointment. Make notations that the patient has been referred, and follow up with telephone calls to verify that an appointment was scheduled and kept. Note whether reports of the consultation were received in your office, and document all recommendations from the referring physician concerning further care of the patient.

MISSED APPOINTMENTS   At the end of the day, a designated person in the medical office should gather all patient records of those who missed or canceled appointments without rescheduling. Charts should be dated, stamped, and documented "no show" or "canceled, no reschedule," respectively. The treating physician should review these records and note whether follow-up is indicated. If follow-up occurs, it should be documented as completed.

DISMISSALS   To avoid charges of abandonment, the physician must formally withdraw from a case or formally dismiss the patient. Be sure a letter of withdrawal or dismissal has been filed in the patient's records.

ALL OTHER PATIENT CONTACT   Patients' records should include reports of all tests, procedures, and medications prescribed, including refills. Make sure all necessary informed-consent papers have been duly signed and filed in the patient's record. Keep a record of all telephone conversations with the patient. Remember that correct documentation requires the initials or signature of the person making a notation on the patient's medical record, as well as the date and time. Remember the rule, "If it wasn't documented, it wasn't done."

Types of Defenses

When, in spite of all best efforts to avoid litigation, a medical professional liability lawsuit is filed, the physician or other health care professional must defend himself or herself against the charges.

Denial

denial *A defense that claims innocence of the charges or that one or more of the four Ds of negligence are lacking.*

Denial of wrongdoing, or the assertion of innocence, may be used as a defense in professional liability suits. If some of the alleged facts are true, defendants may not claim innocence. Instead, they should claim that the charge or charges do not meet all of the elements of the theory of recovery. In other words, the charge may be missing one of the four Ds of negligence.

Affirmative Defenses

affirmative defenses *Defenses used by defendants in medical professional liability suits that allow the accused to present factual evidence that the patient's condition was caused by some factor other than the defendant's negligence.*

Affirmative defenses that may be used by the defendant in a medical professional liability suit allow the accused to present factual evidence that the patient's condition was caused by some factor other than the physician's negligence.

Contributory Negligence

contributory negligence *An affirmative defense that alleges that the plaintiff, through a lack of care, caused or contributed to his or her own injury.*

comparative negligence *An affirmative defense claimed by the defendant, alleging that the plaintiff contributed to the injury by a certain degree.*

Claimed by the defense, **contributory negligence** alleges that the patient or complaining party, through a "want of ordinary care," caused or contributed to his or her own injury. The physician may deny that he or she committed a negligent act and claim the patient was totally responsible for the damage or injury. Alternatively, the physician may admit negligence but claim that the patient was also somehow at fault and so contributed to the injury.

In some states, damages are apportioned according to the degree a plaintiff contributed to the injury. This is called **comparative negligence.** For instance, if the court decides a patient, through the consequences of his or her own negligence, contributed 20 percent toward the injury and the physician contributed 80 percent, the patient's damage award may be reduced by 20 percent.

Court Case

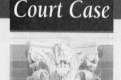

Patient Can Contribute to Negligence

A patient had a bilateral mastectomy, then filed medical negligence and informed consent lawsuits against two of her physicians. The plaintiff alleged that the physicians failed to adequately disclose her treatment options and the risks involved before performing surgery.

A jury found one physician negligent in obtaining the plaintiff's consent to surgery but also assigned 50 percent causal negligence each to that physician and to the plaintiff, thus cutting the plaintiff's jury award in half.

The plaintiff appealed the trial court's decision. The appellate court held that in most circumstances a patient cannot be contributorily negligent by consenting to treatment that a physician presents as a viable option. The appellate court restored the plaintiff's jury award to 100 percent.

On further appeal, the state Supreme Court held that a patient could be contributorily negligent by failing to provide a complete and accurate medical history but could not be contributorily negligent for failing to ascertain the truth or completeness of information presented by the physician. The patient also could not be contributorily negligent in following a viable treatment option presented by the physician. Based on this ruling, the court remanded to the trial court for a new trial because the standard contributory negligence jury instruction presented at the first trial did not include the above limitations on how a patient could be contributorily negligent in an informed consent action.

Brown v. Dibbell, 220 Wis.2d 200, 582 N.W.2d 134 (June 23, 1999).

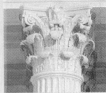
Contributory Negligence Proved

A patient sued her physician for prescribing a drug that allegedly caused brain damage. The patient took the drug for eight years without calling the prescribing physician's attention to the fact that she had suffered ill effects.

The court held that the physician had no way of knowing that the patient was suffering ill effects because she did not tell him, and that the patient should have told the physician of the problems when they arose. The physician was not liable because the patient did not exercise ordinary care for her own protection.

Tisdale v. Johnson, 339 S.E.2d 764 (Ga. App. 1986).

In hearing cases alleging contributory negligence, the court will consider the patient's ability to comprehend and carry out the physician's instructions. Minors, or adults who are unconscious, mentally impaired, insane, or otherwise incompetent, may be judged unable to have contributed to a negligent act.

Assumption of Risk

assumption of risk *A legal defense that holds that the defendant is not guilty of a negligent act because the plaintiff knew of and accepted beforehand any risks involved.*

Assumption of risk is a defense based on the contention that the patient knew of the inherent risks before treatment was performed and agreed to those risks. Informed consent (see Chapter 6) is vital to this defense, since the defendant must show that the patient was fully informed of the risks prior to treatment and that the risks inherent in the treatment were the cause of the patient's injury.

For example, in one lawsuit in which assumption of risk was used as a defense by the defendant, it was held that a physician was not liable for injuries suffered by a chronically ill woman when she fell in the examining room while attempting to undress without assistance. Because she had refused assistance, the woman had assumed the risk of injury.

In other cases it has been held that individuals submitting to X-ray treatment assume the risk of burns from a proper exposure to X rays but not the risk of negligence in applying it.

Emergency

emergency *A type of affirmative defense in which the person who comes to the aid of a victim in an emergency is not held liable under certain circumstances.*

If services were provided during an **emergency,** this may also be used as an affirmative defense. The health care practitioner who comes to the aid of a victim in an emergency would not be held liable under common law if the defense establishes that:

1. A true emergency situation existed and was not caused by the defendant.
2. The appropriate standard of care was met, given the emergency situation.

Health care professionals who provide assistance in emergencies may also be protected from liability under Good Samaritan Acts, which are discussed in Chapter 6.

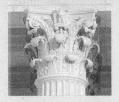

Court Case

Emergency Defense Established

The father of a minor plaintiff sought consequential damages in a malpractice suit against an anesthesiologist. The patient suffered cardiac arrest during a tonsillectomy. Resuscitation was performed and the patient's heartbeat was restored, but she was left with severe and extensive brain damage.

The defendants used an emergency defense. The plaintiff alleged that cardiac arrest is a complication that is a constant possibility in surgery and, therefore, not to be considered "an emergency within the meaning of the emergency doctrine."

A trial court found for the defendants. The court held that:

1. In an emergency a person does not have the time to think in the way that he or she would in ordinary circumstances.

2. When a layperson or a professional is confronted with an emergency, conduct is to be judged according to his or her skill, care, and due diligence with respect to the emergency.

Linhares v. Hall, 257 N.E.2d 429 (1970).

◆ ◆ ◆ ◆ ## Technical Defenses

technical defenses *Defenses used in a lawsuit that are based on legal technicalities.*

Technical defenses to liability suits hinge on legal technicalities rather than factual evidence.

Release of Tortfeasor

A tortfeasor is one who is guilty of committing a tort. Suppose a third party causes injury to a person, as in an automobile accident, and a physician treats the injured person. In most states the party who caused the accident (the tortfeasor) is liable both for the victim's injury and for any medical negligence by the physician who treats the injured victim. This is the basis for the **release of tortfeasor** defense.

release of tortfeasor *A technical defense that prohibits a lawsuit against the person who caused an injury (the tortfeasor) if he or she was expressly released from further liability in the settlement of a suit.*

If the injured party sues the tortfeasor, settles the case, and then releases the tortfeasor from further liability, the injured party cannot also sue the physician, unless the victim expressly reserved that right in the release. If the victim's settlement with the tortfeasor provided compensation for all medical expenses, the release of tortfeasor is usually an absolute defense.

Laws governing release of tortfeasor contain many modifiers, which must be applied in individual cases.

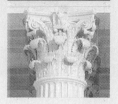

Release of Tortfeasor

A passenger in an automobile was injured in an accident. One leg was badly broken, and an osteopathic physician treated the patient, giving her a choice of procedures in treating her injury. The woman chose to have a closed reduction of her fracture. The result was that the leg was bowed and 1 inch shorter than the other leg. The patient sued the physician for negligence.

The physician claimed he could not be held liable since the woman had signed a release of tortfeasor when she made a $20,000 settlement with the driver of the automobile.

The court held that according to state law, the driver and the physician were joint tortfeasors. Nevertheless, the release of one party did not release third parties and was not a bar to malpractice action. However, the court found that the plaintiff could recover damages only for those injuries due to the physician's negligence and not for those sustained in the auto accident. The patient was awarded $50,000 for mental suffering.

Day v. Wynne, D.O., 702 F.2d 10 (1983).

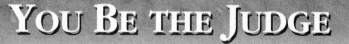

YOU BE THE JUDGE

A patient in her mid-twenties saw an ophthalmologist for a routine eye exam. Due to her young age a glaucoma test was not performed. She later was diagnosed with glaucoma and sued the ophthalmologist group, alleging negligence in failing to perform a glaucoma test.

The defense argued that the standard of care was to not administer the test to patients younger than 40 because the instance of glaucoma at younger ages was rare.

Which of the following statements do you think best describes the applicable standard of care in this case? Explain your choice.

The defense should prevail because the reasonable, customary, and prudent course of action followed by practitioners in the same or similar circumstances would be the same.

_____

_____

_____

The plaintiff should prevail because all patients should be protected against glaucoma, regardless of age.

_____

_____

_____

Res Judicata

Under the doctrine of *res judicata,* "The thing has been decided," a claim cannot be retried between the same parties if it has already been legally resolved. For example, if a patient sues a physician for negligence and loses, the patient cannot then sue the physician for breach of contract based on evidence presented in the trial for negligence. If a patient refuses to pay a physician's fees on the grounds that the physician was negligent and the physician sues for money owed and wins, the patient cannot then sue the physician for negligence. However, if the patient fails to respond to the suit (defaults) or does not allege negligence in his or her defense, then usually he or she may sue the physician for negligence. If a physician has been sued by a nonpaying patient for negligence and does not file a counterclaim for the fee while defending the suit, the patient cannot be sued later for unpaid bills.

Statute of Limitations

Since statutes of limitations vary with states, health care practitioners must be familiar with specific laws for their state. Statutory time limits apply to a number of legal actions, including collections, damages for child sexual abuse, retaining medical records, wrongful-death claims, medical malpractice, and many other causes of action. The **statute of limitations** for filing professional negligence suits varies with states but generally specifies one to six years, with two years being most common. In other words, patients may not file suit for negligence against physicians if the designated length of time has elapsed.

Establishing when the statue of limitations begins also varies with state law, but the most common occurrences for marking the beginning of the statutory period are:

- On the day the alleged negligent act was committed.

- When the injury resulting from the alleged negligence was actually discovered, or should have been discovered, by a reasonably alert patient.

- The day the physician-patient relationship ended or the day of the last medical treatment in a series.

In some states statutory periods may be modified for minors, for the legally insane, or for certain circumstances, such as imprisonment or when foreign objects were left in the body during surgery.

Since statutes of limitations vary greatly from one state to another, health care practitioners must be familiar with specific laws in their state. Specific statutory time limits may be found in the state code, available in most libraries.

Court Case

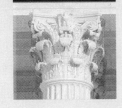

Action Dismissed Due to Statute of Limitations

A patient's family sued a physician in Texas for wrongful death for failure to diagnose the patient's cancer. The Supreme Court of Texas barred the action because the statute of limitations had run out.

The patient was first evaluated for anemia in 1986, but test results revealed a lesion in the stomach. A biopsy showed no sign of malignancy in the lesion. A

(continued)

second biopsy performed in 1987 was also negative for cancer, but upon further examination two weeks later, cells from the lesion were found to be consistent with carcinoma.

Follow-up exams and another biopsy performed a year later revealed cancer cells in the patient's stomach lesion, which by then had ulcerated. Surgery was recommended but was not performed when advanced cancer was found in the patient's lung and stomach. The patient died.

The appellate court ruled that the statute of limitations period began at the time of the second biopsy in 1987; therefore, the time limitation had run out.

Bala v. Maxwell, 909 S.W.2d 889 (Texas Sup. Ct., Nov. 2, 1995).

Check Your Progress

1. What is the difference between an affirmative defense and a technical defense?

_____

_____

_____

2. Identify the type of defense described in each of the following:

One in which the defendant claims innocence.

_____

One in which the accused is allowed to present factual evidence that the physician's negligence did not cause the patient's condition.

_____

One in which the defendant claims that the patient contributed to his or her own injury.

_____

One in which informed consent is a vital factor.

_____

One that hinges on legal technicalities rather than factual evidence.

_____

Professional Liability Insurance

liability insurance *Contract coverage for potential damages incurred as a result of a negligent act.*

Because costs for defending a medical professional liability lawsuit can be high, **liability insurance** may be purchased to cover the costs, up to the limits of the policy. For example, if a medical professional liability insurance policy covers an insured physician up to $10 million, in the event that he or she loses a malpractice suit and must pay damages, the insurance company will not pay more than that amount.

The cost of liability insurance premiums for physicians is based on the dollar amount covered by the policy and the physician's specialty. Insurance for physicians in the least risky insurance risk class (for example, family practitioners and specialists who do not perform surgery) is generally less costly than for those in specialties considered more risky (for example, orthopedic surgeons and obstetricians). States vary regarding which medical specialties carry the highest risk of liability and, therefore, are subject to the highest liability insurance premiums.

Some physicians drop liability insurance coverage when rates become too high. However, this can adversely affect a physician's practice, since most hospitals require proof of coverage up to a predetermined minimum amount in order to grant hospital privileges. In addition, managed-care organizations require physicians to provide proof of liability insurance coverage as a prerequisite for entering into a contractual agreement and as a component of their credentialing process.

There are two main types of medical professional liability insurance. **Claims-made insurance** covers the insured only for those claims made (not for any injury occurring) while the policy is in force. With this kind of insurance, the determining factor is when the claim is made, not when the injury occurs. For example, a policy in force during a previous year would cover only those claims made during that year.

Occurrence insurance (also known as claims-incurred insurance) covers the insured for any claims arising from an incident that occurred or is alleged to have occurred while the policy is in force, regardless of when the claim is made. For example, suppose an alleged incident of negligence by a physician occurred in September 2001, while the physician's occurrence insurance policy was in effect with XYZ Insurance Company. If the patient files a claim against the physician in January 2003, after the policy period has passed, the physician is covered under the terms of the occurrence insurance policy.

The physician should notify his or her insurance company immediately if advised of the possibility of a malpractice lawsuit. Insurance companies almost always provide legal representation for covered physicians, and some insurance contracts require that the insurance company's attorneys represent the insured physician.

Once a lawsuit seems imminent, neither the physician nor his or her employees should mention the suit on the telephone or in correspondence unless the insurance company's legal counsel approves such a reference.

claims-made insurance *A type of liability insurance that covers the insured only for those claims made (not for any injury occurring) while the policy is in force.*

occurrence insurance *A type of liability insurance that covers the insured for any claims arising from an incident that occurred, or is alleged to have occurred, during the time the policy is in force, regardless of when the claim is made.*

Court Case

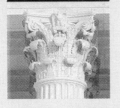

Insurer Obligated to Defend

According to the Rhode Island Supreme Court, a physician's professional liability insurer was obligated to defend an action against him for improperly disclosing a patient's blood-alcohol level.

The physician was on emergency room duty when he treated the patient for head and body injuries. He tested the patient's blood-alcohol level, and the results were later published in the local newspaper. The patient filed an action against the physician for invasion of privacy.

(continued)

The physician's professional liability carrier and his homeowner's insurance company both refused to defend the action. After the physician had successfully defended the action, he filed suit against both companies for expenses incurred in the lawsuit.

A trial court granted summary judgment in favor of both insurance companies, but the appellate court said the professional liability insurer was obligated to defend the physician, since the patient's allegations were sufficient to bring the claim within, or potentially within, the liability policy coverage.

Mellow v. Medical Malpractice Joint Underwriting Assn. of Rhode Island, 567 A.2d 367 (R.I. Sup. Ct., Dec. 21, 1989).

Check Your Progress

3. If a physician receives notice of a lawsuit, he or she should first notify

_____ .

4. Claims-made insurance pays for _____

_____ .

5. Occurrence insurance pays for _____

_____ .

VOICE OF EXPERIENCE
Dealing with Unhappy Patients

Rita, CMA, teaches medical assisting at a Midwestern community college and has worked for physicians in private practice. It is important to make patients feel comfortable and welcome when they visit a medical office, Rita tells her students, but sometimes this can be difficult. "I worked for an orthopedic surgeon once. He was always behind in seeing his appointments because his appointment schedule was frequently interrupted for surgery. Once a Hispanic man got really upset and accused me of discrimination because he had waited so long. I apologized for his long wait and explained that others had also been waiting quite a while. I asked him if he wanted to reschedule. He agreed to wait for the doctor, but he was still upset when he finally saw him, and he mentioned to the doctor that he was unhappy about the long wait."

Medical assistants in similar situations can help maintain rapport with patients by being honest, Rita continues, and by treating patients with respect and consideration at all times.

Applying Knowledge

Match each of the following statements with the correct term by writing the appropriate letter in the space provided.

_____ **1.** The defendant is allowed to introduce factual evidence.

_____ **2.** The defense hinges on legal technicalities.

_____ **3.** The defendant claims the plaintiff in some way caused his or her own injury.

_____ **4.** The plaintiff knew of the risks and agreed to them ahead of time.

_____ **5.** The claim has been previously tried and decided.

_____ **6.** A time limit for filing a suit has been established.

_____ **7.** The accused asserts his or her innocence.

_____ **8.** Damages and guilt are proportioned.

_____ **9.** A third party is responsible for the injury and has settled the case.

_____ **10.** Because of the urgent nature of care given and the judgment that an appropriate standard of care was used, no liability exists.

a. denial

b. affirmative defenses

c. contributory negligence

d. comparative negligence

e. assumption of risk

f. emergency

g. technical defenses

h. release of tortfeasor

i. statute of limitations

j. *res judicata*

Write "A" for affirmative or "T" for technical in the space provided to identify the type of defense described in each of the following phrases:

_____**11.** release of tortfeasor

_____**12.** contributory negligence

_____**13.** statute of limitations

_____**14.** comparative negligence

_____**15.** assumption of risk

_____**16.** *res judicata*

_____**17.** emergency

18. Name eight guidelines for physicians and other health care practitioners to follow that may help prevent malpractice lawsuits.

_____ _____

_____ _____

_____ _____

_____ _____

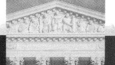

Case Studies

Use your critical-thinking skills to answer the questions that follow each case study.

Deb, a 17-year-old high school student, had a tonsillectomy. The general surgeon who performed the operation informed Deb and her family after the surgery that when her tonsils were excised, the uvula was also inadvertently removed. He said this should pose no problems.

As healing progressed, Deb had difficulty in swallowing and with food "going down the wrong way," but she attributed this to the normal postoperative condition and said nothing.

Two years later, Deb's symptoms were still present. She also had problems with emesis occasionally entering her nasal cavity. Deb wondered if she could recover damages from her physician for negligence.

19. **In your opinion, does Deb have a standing to sue? Explain your answer.**

    _____

    _____

    _____

20. **Could the statute of limitations prevent her from filing? How could she find out?**

    _____

    _____

    _____

21. **Do you think Deb would be successful in a suit? Why or why not?**

    _____

    _____

    _____

A urologist removed a cancerous prostate from a patient. During surgery the balloon that held a urinary catheter in place burst inside the patient's bladder. After the patient regained consciousness, the urologist told him about the incident. He said he had meticulously removed all fragments of the catheter balloon, but he cautioned the patient to report any untoward symptoms. The patient recovered without incident.

22. **In your opinion, does the patient have a standing to sue either the company that manufactured the urinary catheter or the urologist who operated on him? Why or why not?**

    _____

    _____

    _____

    _____

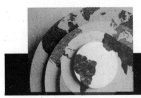

Internet Activities

Complete the activities and answer the questions that follow.

23. Visit the Web site for Healthcare Providers Service Organization (HPSO). Is liability insurance offered by HPSO for members of your profession? How many other professions may obtain liability insurance from HPSO?

_____

_____

_____

List those most likely to be employed in a medical office.

_____

_____

_____

How much is the current annual premium listed for the health care profession in which you plan to practice? In your opinion, is the expense justified?

_____

24. Search the Web site of the American Tort Reform Association (ATRA). Briefly summarize the association's membership composition and its position regarding tort reform in the United States.

_____

_____

_____

What measures do they advocate for tort reform?

_____

_____

What other organizations support liability reform?

_____

_____

6

MEDICAL RECORDS AND INFORMED CONSENT

Objectives

After studying this chapter, you should be able to:

1. Explain the purpose of medical records and the importance of proper documentation.

2. Discuss those entries necessary in a medical record for legal protection.

3. Demonstrate the procedure for making a correction in a medical record.

4. Identify ownership of medical records.

5. Tell how long medical records must be legally retained.

6. Describe the purpose of obtaining a patient's consent for release of medical information.

7. Explain the doctrine of informed consent.

8. State the purpose of Good Samaritan Acts.

9. State the purpose of the Uniform Anatomical Gift Act.

Key Terms

- **Confidentiality of Alcohol and Drug Abuse, Patient Records**

- **consent**

- **doctrine of informed consent**

- **doctrine of professional discretion**

- **fiduciary duty**

- **Good Samaritan Acts**

- **medical record**

- **National Organ Transplant Act**

- **Uniform Anatomical Gift Act**

Medical Records

A **medical record** is a collection of data recorded when a patient seeks medical treatment. Hospitals, surgical centers, clinics, physicians' offices, and other facilities providing health care services maintain patients' medical records. Medical records serve many purposes:

- They are required by licensing authorities and provide a format for tracking, documenting, and maintaining a patient's communication data, both inside and outside a health care facility.
- They provide documentation of a patient's continuing health care, from birth to death.
- They provide a foundation for managing a patient's health care.
- They serve as legal documents in lawsuits.
- They provide clinical data for education, research, statistical tracking, and assessing the quality of health care.

Entries

As a legal document, a patient's medical record may be subpoenaed (via subpoena *duces tecum*) as evidence in court. When conscientiously compiled, medical records may prevail over a patient's recollection of events during a trial. What is omitted from the record may be as important to the outcome of a lawsuit as what is included.

Records may be kept on paper, microfilm, or computer tapes or disks. For legal protection, as well as continuity of care, the following information must be recorded in a patient's record:

- The patient's full name; Social Security number; birth date; full address; home and work telephone numbers, if applicable; marital status; name and address of employer, if applicable.
- The patient's medical history.
- The dates and times of the patient's arrival for appointments.
- A complete description of the patient's symptoms and reason for making an appointment.
- The examination performed by the physician.
- The physician's assessment, diagnosis, recommendations, treatment prescribed, progress notes, and instructions given to the patient.
- X rays and all other test results.
- A notation for each time the patient telephoned the medical facility or was telephoned by the facility, listing date, reason for the call, and resolution.
- A notation of copies made of the medical record, including date copied and to whom the copy was sent.
- Notes documenting all prescriptions and refill authorizations.
- Documentation of informed consent, when necessary.

- Name of the guardian or legal representative to be contacted if the patient is unable to contract and give informed consent.

- Other documentation such as complete written descriptions, photographs, samples of body fluids, foreign objects, clothing, and so on. All items should be carefully labeled and preserved.

- Condition of the patient at the time of termination of treatment, when applicable, and reasons for termination, including documentation if the physician-patient contract was terminated before completion of treatment.

Entries in the medical record must be objective, concise, and clearly and legibly written. They should never include inappropriate personal judgments or observations, or attempts at humor.

◆ ◆ ◆ ◆

Photographs, Videotaping, and Other Methods of Patient Imaging

In today's health care environment, it has become increasingly common to record patients' images through the use of photography, videotaping, digital imaging, and other visual recordings. For example, surgeons may photograph, videotape, or otherwise record procedures used during an operation for purposes of education or review. Cosmetic surgeons and physicians who treat accident victims may want to document visually the patient's condition "before" and "after." Such images then become part of the patient's medical record, subject to the same requirement for written release as the rest of the record.

Photographing or otherwise recording a patient's image without proper consent may be interpreted in a court of law as invasion of privacy. Invasion of privacy charges are most often upheld in court if the patient's image was used for commercial purposes, but such claims have also been upheld under public disclosure of embarrassing private facts. For example, "before" and "after" photographs published by a cosmetic surgeon may cause embarrassment to the patient if he or she did not give consent for the photographs to be published.

If a health care facility routinely photographs patients to document care, a special consent form should be signed, stating that:

- The patient understands that photographs, videotapes, and digital or other images may be taken to document care.

- The patient understands that ownership rights to the images will be retained by the health care facility, but that he or she will be allowed to view them or to obtain copies.

- The images will be securely stored and kept for the time period prescribed by law or outlined in the health care facility's policy.

- Images of the patient will not be released or used outside the health care facility without written authorization from the patient or his or her legal representative.

If the images will be used for teaching or publicity, a separate consent form should be used.

Check Your Progress

1. Define *medical record.*

_____

_____

2. List five purposes served by a patient's medical record.

_____

_____

_____

_____

_____

◆ ◆ ◆ ◆ Corrections

Errors made when making an entry in a medical record or errors discovered later can be corrected, but corrections must be made in a certain manner, so that if the medical records are ever used in a medical professional liability lawsuit, it will not appear that they were falsified. Follow these guidelines when correcting errors in a client's medical record:

- Draw a line through the error so that it is still legible. Do not black out the information or use correction fluid to cover it up.

- Write or type in the correct information above or below the original line or in the margin. If necessary, you may attach another sheet of paper or another document with the correction on it. In this case, note in the record "See attached document A" to indicate where the corrected information can be found.

- Note near the correction why it was made (for example, "error, wrong date," or "error interrupted by a phone call"). You can place this note in the margin or, again, add an attachment. Do not make a change in the record without noting the reason for it.

- Enter the date and time, and initial the correction.

- If possible, ask another staff member or the physician to witness and initial the correction to the record when you make it.

Ownership

Patients' medical records are considered the property of the owners of the facility where they were created. For example, a physician in private practice owns his or her records; records in a clinic are property of the clinic. Hospital records are the property of the admitting hospital. The facility where the medical records were created owns the documents, but the patient owns the information they contain. Upon signing a release, patients may usually obtain access to or copies of their medical records, depending on state law. However, under the **doctrine of professional discretion,** courts have held that in some cases patients treated for mental or emotional conditions may be harmed by seeing their own records. To avoid misunderstandings, records are best reviewed in the presence of a health care professional.

When a physician examines a patient for a job-related physical, scheduled and paid for by the patient's employer or prospective employer, those records are the property of the employer, not the patient. The patient must obtain permission from the employer to release to another party information contained in the records.

Retention and Storage

As a protection in the event of litigation, records should be kept until the applicable statute of limitations period has elapsed, which generally ranges from two to seven years. In some cases this involves keeping the medical records for minor patients for a specified length of time after they reach legal age. Some states have enacted statutes for the retention of medical records. However, most physicians retain records indefinitely because, in addition to their value as documentation in medical professional liability suits and for tax purposes, the patient's medical history may be vital in future treatment.

Confidentiality

Because health care practitioners have a duty to protect the privacy of the patient, medical records should not be released to a third party without written permission, signed by the patient or the patient's legal representative. Only the information requested should be released.

Requests for release of records may ask for records concerning a specific date or time span. Records may also be requested for a specific diagnosis, symptom, or body system, or for results of certain diagnostic tests. Never send unsolicited records. Carefully review the signed release form to ensure that the correct records are sent.

When medical records are requested for use in a lawsuit, a signed consent for the release of the records must be obtained from the patient, unless a court subpoenas the records. In this case, the patient should be notified in writing that the records have been subpoenaed and released.

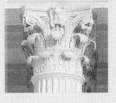

Court Case

Wrong HIV Test Result Leads to Suit

A food service employee of a Veteran's Canteen Service in Puerto Rico consented to a voluntary blood test for HIV. The test results revealed he had been exposed to the virus. The treating VA physician told the employee's supervisor he was unfit to work in food handling and the man was dismissed.

Several months later it was discovered that the man was not HIV positive, and he brought suit against the government for medical malpractice. The employee claimed that the hospital and the physician were negligent in handling the test results. He also claimed that the physician improperly disclosed test results to the personnel supervisor, thus breaching the confidentiality of the physician-patient relationship.

The trial court found that, because the employee was diagnosed as having pneumocystis carini pneumonia, a condition often occurring in persons with AIDS, the laboratory results seemed consistent. The court said that although the patient did not suffer from AIDS, the physician was not negligent because his diagnosis was within the range of accepted medical practice.

On the issue of physician-patient confidentiality, the court concluded that no breach of confidentiality had occurred because the memo the physician sent to the VA personnel supervisor stated only that the employee was unfit to work in food handling. No confidential information relating to the employee's condition was divulged.

Sierra Perez v. United States, 779 E.Supp. 637 (D.C. Puerto Rico, Oct. 25, 1991).

◆ ◆ ◆ ◆ **Technological Threats to Confidentiality**

Modern health care facilities rely on technology for creating, maintaining, and transporting patients' medical information. The implementation of HIPAA imposes penalties for breaches of confidentiality regarding medical records that identify patients by name. The following guidelines can help ensure that confidentiality is not breached when using copiers, fax machines, computers, and printers.

Copiers

- Do not leave confidential papers anywhere on the copier where others can read the information.

- Do not discard copies in a shared trash container; shred them.

- If a paper jam occurs, be sure to remove from the machine the copy or partial copy that caused the jam.

Fax Machines

- Always verify the telephone number of the receiving location before faxing confidential material.

- Never fax confidential material to an unauthorized person.

- Do not fax confidential material if others in the room can observe the material.

- Do not leave confidential material unattended on a fax machine.

- Do not discard fax copies in a shared trash container; shred them.

- Use a fax cover sheet that states, "Confidential: To addressee only. Please return if received in error."

Computers

- Locate the monitor in an area where others cannot see the screen.

- Do not leave a monitor unattended while confidential material is displayed on the screen.

- Because it is difficult to ensure the privacy of e-mail messages, sending confidential patient information via e-mail is not recommended.

Printers

- Do not print confidential material on a printer shared by other departments or in an area where others can read the material.

- Do not leave a printer unattended while printing confidential material.

- Before leaving the printing area, check to be sure all computer disks containing confidential material and all printed material have been collected.

- Do not direct print jobs to the wrong location.

- Do not discard printouts in a shared trash container; shred them.

Court Case

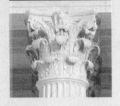

fiduciary duty *A physician's obligation to his or her patient, based on trust and confidence.*

Not Guilty of Breach of Confidentiality

A physician cannot be sued for breach of confidentiality when required to produce a patient's medical records for use in court testimony.

A patient (Cruz) sued a physician (Agelides) for breach of fiduciary duty. (**Fiduciary duty** is a physician's duty to his or her patient, based on trust and confidence.) In a previous malpractice action brought by Cruz against another physician, Agelides had given a sworn pretrial affidavit and video deposition in favor of the defending physician. The court held Agelides was immune from any civil liability action as a result of his testimony as a witness in the previous trial.

Cruz v. Agelides, 574 So.2d 278 (Fla. App. 3 Dist. 1991).

---

3. Define *fiduciary duty.*

_____

_____

4. Who owns a patient's medical records?

_____

_____

5. Define *doctrine of professional discretion.*

_____

_____

◆ ◆ ◆ ◆   **Release of Information**

Medical information about a patient is often released for the following purposes:

INSURANCE CLAIMS   The medical office supplies specific requested information but does not usually send the patient's entire medical record. An authorization to release information, signed by the patient, is required before records may be released.

TRANSFER TO ANOTHER PHYSICIAN   The physician may photocopy and send all records or may send a summary. The patient must sign an authorization to release records.

USE IN A COURT OF LAW   When a subpoena *duces tecum* is issued for certain records (the subpoena commanding a witness to appear in court and to bring certain medical records), the patient's written consent to release the records is waived.

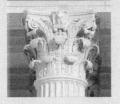

Court Case

Psychiatrist's Records Examined

In June 1991 a woman was injured in a car accident. She sued the driver of the other vehicle, claiming that after the crash she was unable to work due to continuous "severe and great pain of body and mind."

Before the trial the plaintiff was examined by an orthopedic surgeon who said she suffered from a "major psychosocial dysfunction" and that her physical injuries were not substantiated by clinical findings.

(continued)

The defendant petitioned the trial court for records of the psychiatrist who had treated the woman before and after the crash. The trial court reviewed the records, judged them to be privileged, and granted the woman a protective order.

The defendant appealed, but the protective order was upheld. The appellate court said that even when the nature of a patient's psychiatric care has been put at issue in a civil or criminal proceeding, psychiatrist-patient communications must remain privileged. The court also ruled, however, that information in the psychiatrist's records that was not a part of these communications was not privileged. Therefore, the trial court was ordered to again review the psychiatrist's records, in conformance with the appellate court's opinion.

Plunkett v. Ginsburg, 456 S.E.2d 595 (Ga. Ct. of App., Feb. 17, 1995; reconsideration denied March 29, 1995).

When complying with a subpoena to produce specified medical records in court, it is usually the responsibility of the medical office employee in charge of medical records to:

- Check the subpoena to be sure the name and phone number of the issuing attorney and the court docket number of the case are listed.

- If a carbon copy of the subpoena is received, verify that it is the same as the original in every way.

- Verify that the patient named was a patient of the physician named.

- Verify the trial date and time as listed on the subpoena.

- Notify the physician that a subpoena was received, and then notify the physician's insurance company or attorney, if so directed.

- Check all subpoenaed records to be sure they are complete, but never alter them in any way.

- Document the number of pages in the record and itemize its contents.

- Store the record in a locked safe until trial time.

- Make a photocopy of the original to be submitted, if permitted by state law and the court.

- Offer sworn testimony regarding the record, if so instructed by the court.

Confidentiality of Alcohol and Drug Abuse, Patient Records *A federal statute that protects patients with histories of substance abuse regarding the release of information about treatment.*

Some state laws specifically address the release of confidential medical information, especially as it pertains to treatment for mental or emotional health problems, HIV testing, and substance abuse. In addition, the federal statute **Confidentiality of Alcohol and Drug Abuse, Patient Records** protects patients with histories of substance abuse regarding the release of information about treatment. Under no circumstances should information of this type be released without specific, written permission from the patient to do so. The patient also has the right to rescind (cancel) a consent to release information, in which case the information should not be released.

The following rules for authorizations for the release of medical records can serve as a general guide for medical assistants and other medical office employees.

- Authorizations should be in writing.

- Authorizations should include the patient's name, address, and date of birth.

- The patient should sign authorizations, unless he or she is not a legal, competent adult. In that case, parents or guardians should sign authorizations.

- Only the information specifically requested should be released.

- The patient has the right to rescind a **consent** to release information, in which case information should not be released.

consent *Permission from a patient, either expressed or implied, for something to be done by another.*

Requests for information coming into the medical office from insurance companies, physicians, or other sources should:

- Be witnessed and dated and include the complete name, address, and signature of the party requesting the information, as well as that of the party asked to release the information.

- Include a specific description of the information that is needed.

- List the purpose for which the data will be used and the date on which the consent expires.

Check Your Progress

6. Name three reasons a medical office might be requested to release a patient's medical records.

_____

_____

_____

7. In which of the three situations named in question 6 might a patient's written consent to release records be waived?

_____

_____

8. What is needed before the medical office can send a patient's medical record to the insurer?

_____

_____

Consent

As already stated, consent means that the patient has given permission, either expressed (orally or in writing) or implied, for the physician to examine him or her, to perform tests that aid in diagnosis, or to treat for a medical condition. When the patient makes an appointment for an examination, implied consent for the physician to perform the exam has been given. Likewise, when he or she cooperates with various diagnostic testing procedures, implied consent for the tests has been given.

◆ ◆ ◆ ◆ ## Informed Consent

For surgery and for some other procedures, such as a test for HIV, implied consent is not enough. In these cases it is important to ask the patient to sign a consent form, thereby establishing informed consent (see Figure 6-1).

doctrine of informed consent
The legal basis for informed consent, usually outlined in a state's medical practice acts.

The **doctrine of informed consent** is the legal basis for informed consent and is usually outlined in a state's medical practice acts. Informed consent implies that the patient understands:

- Proposed modes of treatment.
- Why the treatment is necessary.
- Risks involved in the proposed treatment.
- Available alternative modes of treatment.
- Risks of alternative modes of treatment.
- Risks involved if treatment is refused.

Informed consent involves the patient's right to receive all information relative to his or her condition and then to make a decision regarding treatment based on that knowledge. Informed consent also proves that the patient was not coerced into treatment.

Adults of sound mind are usually able to give informed consent. Individuals who cannot give informed consent include the following:

MINORS, PERSONS UNDER THE AGE OF MAJORITY   Exceptions include:
- Emancipated minors—those who are living away from home and are responsible for their own support.
- Married minors.
- Mature minors—those who, through the doctrine of mature minors, have been granted the right to seek birth control or care during pregnancy, treatment for reportable communicable diseases, or treatment for drug- or alcohol-related problems without first obtaining parental consent.

THE MENTALLY INCOMPETENT   Individuals judged by the court to be insane, senile, mentally retarded, or under the influence of drugs or alcohol cannot give informed consent. In these cases a competent person may be designated by the court to act as the patient's agent.

THOSE WHO SPEAK ONLY A FOREIGN LANGUAGE   When patients do not speak or understand English, interpreters may be necessary to inform the patient and obtain his or her consent for treatment.

Other problems in obtaining informed consent may arise, as in situations such as when foster children need medical attention or a spouse seeks sterilization or an abortion. In each case health practitioners must determine who is legally able to give informed consent for treatment. When in doubt, seek legal advice.

Patient education can be vital to the issue of informed consent. Stocking the medical office with brochures about various medical problems is not sufficient if the physician does not review the material with the patient. Patients who sue have successfully claimed lack of informed

AUTHORIZATION FOR
DISCLOSURE OF THE RESULTS OF THE
HIV ANTIBODY BLOOD TEST

A. AUTHORIZATION

I herby authorize Hamilton County Public Hospital to furnish to

_____

(Name of person or entity who is to receive results)

the results of my blood test for antibodies to HIV.

B. USES

The Receiver may use the information for the following purpose(s):

_____

_____

C. RESTRICTIONS

This authorization is being given with the understanding that the Receiver will be informed in writing by the Hospital that state law protects the confidentiality of this information and prohibits any further disclosure of the information without my specific, written consent, or as otherwise permitted by law. The Receiver will be informed that a general authorization for the release of medical or other information is not sufficient for this purpose.

D. DURATION

This authorization shall become effective immediately and shall remain in effect indefinitely or until _____ , whichever is shorter.

(Date)

_____   _____

Date   Patient's signature

                                     _____

                                     Print name of patient

Figure 6-1
A Sample Consent Form

consent because they did not read the consent form they signed or did not read brochures handed to them. Health care personnel should be sure patients understand all forms and all treatment or surgery to be performed before signing.

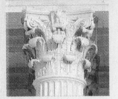
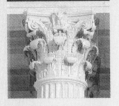

9. Who may give informed consent?

_____

10. Who may not give informed consent?

_____

_____

Court Case

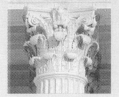

Patient Not Competent to Sign Forms

The U.S. Supreme Court overruled two lower federal courts, stating that a Florida mental patient had a cause of action. The patient claimed that he was admitted to a state mental health treatment facility as a voluntary patient, based on forms he signed when he was heavily medicated, disoriented, and suffering from a psychotic disorder. He had been found wandering along a highway, appearing to be injured and disoriented. He was taken to a private mental health facility. While he was hallucinating, confused, and psychotic, he signed forms for admission.

The U.S. Supreme Court held that allegations that employees of the state hospital admitted him as a voluntary patient without taking steps to ascertain whether he was mentally competent to sign the admission forms stated a cause of action.

Zinermon v. Burch, 110 S.Ct. 975 (U.S. Sup. Ct., Feb. 27, 1990).

◆ ◆ ◆ ◆ ## When Consent Is Unnecessary

In emergency situations, when the patient is in immediate danger, the physician is not expected to obtain consent before proceeding with treatment.

All 50 states have passed a **Good Samaritan Act.** This protects physicians and, in some states, other health care practitioners and laypersons from charges of negligence or abandonment if they stop to help the victim of an accident or other emergency, provided they:

Good Samaritan Acts *State laws protecting physicians and sometimes other health care practitioners and laypersons from charges of negligence or abandonment if they stop to help the victim of an accident or other emergency.*

• Give such care in good faith.

• Act within the scope of their training and knowledge.

• Use due care under the circumstances.

• Do not bill for their services. (If a physician treats a patient as a "Good Samaritan" and later bills the patient for services, he or she may be held as having established a physician-patient relationship and may not have the immunity from civil damages that a Good Samaritan law would otherwise provide.)

Sally, Michael, and Teresa handle requests for release of patients' medical records for a Midwestern hospital. They stress that they can release records only with signed authorization from the patient or upon subpoena, and that photocopies are then released, but never original medical records. When someone visits the hospital to pick up copies of a patient's records, that person is asked to show identification.

"If a request for release of records doesn't feel right, check it out," advises Michael. For example, when a husband brings an authorization form for release of medical records that he says was signed by his wife, the person in charge may want to check the signature against the signature on hospital admission forms, because in divorce or custody cases a spouse may want medical records to prove that a husband or wife is an unfit parent. "It's most important to use common sense," Michael emphasizes.

Never release medical records simply because you are intimidated by the person requesting them, stresses Teresa. "The most officious person I've dealt with was an FBI agent who told me, 'I want this record. If you don't give it to me, I'll get it myself.' I said, 'Go for it.' Later the agent called and apologized to me."

"Military investigative officers can also be difficult," adds Sally. "Once a military person on leave was injured in a car wreck and was treated here. Alcohol was involved, and later military investigators wanted the patient's medical records. They couldn't locate his wife for authorization, and they called us several times, each time with a different story. All three of us said the same thing, 'We cannot release a patient's records without authorization.' "

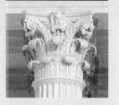

Court Case

Good Samaritan Act a Defense

When a woman in labor was admitted to the hospital, her regular attending physician was not available. Another physician was called to deliver the patient's baby. During the delivery the physician learned the fetus was in distress, and he performed a mid-forceps delivery. The baby suffered from quadriplegia and cerebral palsy from birth, and the mother sued the physician who delivered the child.

The court ruled that the physician was immune from liability under the Good Samaritan Act, saying that the law applies if the doctor does not have notice of the patient's illness or injury, provides emergency care, and does not charge a fee.

Roberts v. Myers, 569 N.E.2d 135 (Ill. App. 1 Dist. 1991).

Uniform Anatomical Gift Act

Uniform Anatomical Gift Act
A national statute allowing individuals to donate their bodies or body parts, after death, for use in transplant surgery, tissue banks, or medical research or education.

In 1968 the **Uniform Anatomical Gift Act** was approved by the National Conference of Commissioners on Uniform State Laws for the purpose of allowing individuals to donate their bodies or body parts, after death, for use in transplant surgery, tissue banks, or medical research or education. The act made certain provisions uniform throughout all states within the United States. Major provisions include:

- Any person 18 years of age or older who is of sound mind may make a gift of his or her body, or certain bodily organs, to be used in medical research or for transplantation or storage in a tissue bank.

- Donations made through a legal will are not to be held up by probate.

- Except in autopsies, the donor's rights override those of others.

- Survivors may speak for the deceased if arrangements were not made prior to his or her death (provided the deceased did not express an objection to donation before his or her death).

- Physicians who rely on donation documents for the acceptance of bodies or organs are immune from civil or criminal prosecution. However, if the physician (or hospital) knows the deceased was opposed to donation or if, in the absence of prior arrangements, survivors express an objection, then the donation should be refused.

- Hospitals, surgeons, physicians, accredited medical or dental schools, colleges and universities, and tissue banks or storage facilities may accept anatomical gifts for research, advancement of medical or dental science, therapy, or transplantation.

- Time of death of the donor must be established by a physician who is not involved in transplanting the donor's designated organs, and the donor's attending physician cannot be a member of the transplant team.

- Donors may revoke the gift, and gifts may be rejected.

Some states provide for prospective donors to indicate their wish to donate on the back of their driver's licenses. Alternatively, donors may carry signed and witnessed Uniform Donor Cards (see Figure 6-2).

◆ ◆ ◆ ◆ Frequently Asked Questions About Organ Donation

Because there are more people waiting for organ transplants than there are organs available, individuals are encouraged to indicate their willingness to become donors. One way to increase the number of possible organ donors is to make sure that potential donors understand the process. Here are a few of the most commonly asked questions about organ donation, followed by summarized answers from the experts:

Q: What organs and tissues can be transplanted?
A: Organs that can be transplanted include heart, kidney, pancreas, lung, stomach, and small and large intestines. Other tissues often transplanted include bone, corneas, skin, heart valves, veins, cartilage, and other connective tissues.

Figure 6-2
A Sample Uniform Donor Card

UNIFORM DONOR CARD

Of _____
Print or type name of donor

in the hope that I may help others, I hereby make this anatomical gift, if medically acceptable, to take effect upon my death. The words and marks below indicate my desires.

I give: (a) ☐ any needed organs or parts
      (b) ☐ only the following organs or parts

_____
Specify the organ(s) or part(s)

for the purposes of transplantation, therapy, medical research or education:
      (c) ☐ my body for anatomical study if needed.

Limitations or special wishes, if any: _____
_____

Front of card

Signed by the donor and the following two witnesses in the presence of each other:

Signature of Donor _____

Date of Birth of Donor _____

Date Signed _____

City and State _____

Witness _____

Witness _____

THIS IS A LEGAL DOCUMENT UNDER THE UNIFORM ANATOMICAL GIFT ACT OR SIMILAR LAWS.

Back of card

Q: Is the donor or the donor's family responsible for paying for transplantation of donated organs?
A: No. Costs are borne by the recipient or his or her insurance plan, when applicable.

Q: If a prospective, designated donor is injured in an accident, will the attending doctors allow that person to die in order to harvest donated organs?
A: Absolutely not. A willingness to donate organs in no way compromises the medical care provided to accident victims. The organ procurement organization (OPO) is notified that organs are available only after a patient is declared dead, and the transplant team is not notified until surviving family members have consented to donation.

Q: How old or young can a donor be?
A: Donors range from newborns to about the age of 70.

Q: If a person donates an organ, may the recipient or the recipient's family learn the donor's identity and contact the donor or his or her family?
A: A donor's name is released to recipients only if the recipient asks for the information and the donor's family agrees.

Q: Are organs transplanted only after a prospective donor has died?
A: Not necessarily. Voluntary transplants from living donors to living recipients may also take place. For example, kidneys, lungs, skin, and other tissues are successfully transplanted from compatible living donors to recipients.

Q: If I, as a willing organ donor, sign the back of my driver's license indicating that I am a donor, then I die, can my relatives legally "undo" my wishes?
A: No. A signed declaration on the back of a driver's license still is legally effective to authorize donation in virtually every state in the United States. Moreover, the relevant laws specify that the consent of the donor's relatives is not needed in such circumstances. However, prospective organ donors should also make their wishes known to family members while they are able, because in spite of having signed a card, if relatives protest the donation, fear of bad publicity regarding organ donation will likely prevent the donation from occurring.

The National Organ Transplant Act

National Organ Transplant Act *Passed in 1984, a statute that provides grants to qualified organ procurement organizations and established an Organ Procurement and Transplantation Network.*

Passed in 1984, the **National Organ Transplant Act** addresses the severe shortage of organs available for transplantation. It provides funds for (1) grants to qualified organ procurement organizations (OPOs) and (2) the establishment of an Organ Procurement and Transplantation Network (OPTN) to assist OPOs in the distribution of unused organs outside their geographical area. The existing United Network for Organ Sharing (UNOS), a registry for kidney transplant patients, is designated as the OPTN.

YOU BE THE JUDGE

A patient who had lived in several states and had sought medical attention in those states requested that copies of records from the last three states be forwarded to him so he would have access to his most recent treatments when he saw a physician in yet another state. The patient was able to access his medical records in two of the states but was denied access by the third state.

How is this possible, if patients own the information in their medical records?

_____

_____

Can this patient sue to obtain personal copies of the records in the refusing state?

_____

Can you obtain a copy of your medical records in the state where you live? Where can you find this information?

_____

_____

Applying Knowledge

Answer the following questions in the spaces provided.

1. List seven items that must be recorded in a patient's chart for each visit to the physician's office.

   _____

   _____

   _____

   _____

   _____

   _____

   _____

2. After an entry in the medical record has been written and an error is discovered, what procedure should be followed to correct the error?

   _____

   _____

   _____

   _____

   _____

3. Dr. Wellness works as an employee of Anytown Medical Clinic. Who owns the records of his patients?

   _____

4. Dr. Wellness also sees patients at Anytown General Hospital, where he maintains records of hospital stays, procedures, and emergency room visits. To whom do these records belong?

   _____

5. Jan B. sees Dr. Wellness on occasion for routine illnesses and physicals. She will soon be moving and wishes to transfer these records to her new physician, Dr. Good.

   Who has ownership of the records before Jan moves? _____

   Who has ownership of the records after Jan moves? _____

   What procedure should be followed for the records to be transferred to Jan's new physician?

   _____

   _____

   _____

6. What is the statute of limitations in your state for filing a medical malpractice suit?

_____

_____

7. List all items that should be noted when releasing medical information to a third party.

_____

_____

8. List two precautions regarding maintaining confidentiality of patients' records when copying, faxing, printing, sending by e-mail, or entering information in computers.

_____

_____

9. Give two examples of persons who would need an agent to give informed consent for them.

_____

_____

10. For informed consent to be complete, what six items need to be explained to a patient?

_____

_____

_____

_____

_____

_____

11. State and federal laws protect patients with a medical history of drug or alcohol abuse, treatment for mental or emotional problems, or HIV/AIDS from release of confidential information about this history. What does the law require?

_____

_____

_____

_____

12. Medical records are often subpoenaed in court, because a patient's medical record is what kind of document?

_____

13. In a court of law, which testimony will prevail, a patient's recollection of events or the written documentation in a medical record? Explain your answer.

_____

_____

14. Can physicians, nurses, and other health care practitioners write any comment they choose in a patient's medical record? Why or why not?

_____

_____

Review and Case Studies

Match the following statements with the correct terms by writing the appropriate letter in the space provided.

_____15. Addresses the severe shortage of organs available for transplantation.

_____16. Protects a patient from being coerced into treatment.

_____17. Protects health care providers from lawsuits when providing care at an accident or emergency.

_____18. Allows individuals to donate their bodies or parts of their bodies for transplants or scientific use.

_____19. Allows physicians to decide whether or not to show medical records to patients treated for mental or emotional disorders.

_____20. A federal statute that protects the confidentiality of medical records of patients with histories of substance abuse.

a. Good Samaritan Act

b. National Organ Transplant Act

c. Uniform Anatomical Gift Act

d. doctrine of informed consent

e. Confidentiality of Alcohol and Drug Abuse, Patient Records

f. doctrine of professional discretion

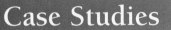

Case Studies

Use your critical-thinking skills to answer the questions that follow each of the case studies.

When Ruth applied for health insurance, she listed a colonoscopy examination as part of her medical history. The insurance company asked for more information. Ruth requested, in writing, that the clinic where she was examined send just the colonoscopy records to her insurance company. The clinic sent all of Ruth's medical records for the past five years, which included the diagnoses of fibrocystic breast disease and obesity, in addition to the requested information on her colonoscopy. As a result, the insurance company issued Ruth a policy but attached riders stipulating that they would not pay for any illnesses arising from the fibrocystic breast disease or obesity.

Ruth complained to the clinic administrator, explaining that she had requested that only those records concerning her colonoscopy be forwarded to the insurance company. The administrator apologized and assured Ruth that the clinic's policy concerning release of medical records would be reviewed. He also told Ruth that should she ever incur medical expenses for those conditions excepted in her insurance policy, she should contact him.

21. **Did the clinic err in sending all of Ruth's medical records to the insurance company? Why or why not?**

   _____

   _____

22. **In your opinion, did Ruth have a legal cause for action against the clinic? Explain.**

   _____

   _____

   _____

23. **What would you do, in the clinic administrator's place, to rectify the situation and make sure that similar problems do not arise in the future?**

   _____

   _____

   _____

A patient asked her dermatologist for the name of an internist. She visited the recommended internist several times and then learned that, without informing her, he had sent the dermatologist two detailed reports on her condition and family medical history. Since her gastrointestinal condition had nothing to do with her dermatological complaint, she believed the internist sent the records to show his appreciation for the referral. She told the internist that she felt her privacy had been violated.

24. **Do you agree with the patient? Why or why not?**

   _____

   _____

   _____

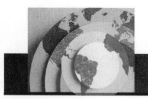

Internet Activities

Complete the activities and answer the questions that follow.

25. Visit the Web site for the United Network of Organ Sharing. How does the organization explain its mission?

   _____

   _____

   Find the statistics for the numbers of patients currently waiting for kidney transplants and heart transplants. Record those numbers here. How many patients die each day for lack of a donated organ?

   _____

   Find the donor and recipient stories and record relevant facts for one such story here:

   _____

   _____

   _____

   _____

   _____

   _____

26. Visit the Web site for an organization called Transweb. What are the organization's goals?

   _____

   _____

   Take the quiz on organ transplants. List the questions you missed, summarizing the correct answer or answers.

   _____

   _____

   _____

   _____

27. Visit the Web site of the American Health Information Management Association. Through the link to Lexis-Nexis, scan recent articles about health information confidentiality. Summarize the most recent attempts of the U.S. Congress to protect patients' privacy rights. Do health care practitioners, managed care plans, insurance companies, and health information managers agree that federal legislation is necessary to protect patient privacy?

   _____

   _____

   _____

   _____

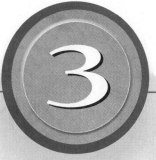

PART

PROFESSIONAL, SOCIAL, AND INTERPERSONAL HEALTH CARE ISSUES

CHAPTER

7

PHYSICIANS' PUBLIC DUTIES AND RESPONSIBILITIES

Objectives

After studying this chapter, you should be able to:

1. List at least four vital events for which statistics are collected by the government.
2. Discuss the procedures for filing birth and death certificates.
3. Explain the purpose of public health statutes.
4. Tell when a medical examiner or coroner is required to sign a death certificate.
5. Cite examples of reportable diseases and explain how they are reported.
6. Identify three types of reportable injuries.
7. Discuss federal drug regulations.
8. State the purpose of the Controlled Substances Act.

Key Terms

- administer
- Amendments to the Older Americans Act
- autopsy
- Child Abuse Prevention and Treatment Act
- Controlled Substances Act
- coroner
- dispense

- Drug Enforcement Agency (DEA)
- Food and Drug Administration (FDA)
- forensics
- medical examiner
- National Childhood Vaccine Injury Act
- prescribe
- vital statistics

Vital Statistics

vital statistics *Numbers collected for the population of live births, deaths, fetal deaths, marriages, divorces, induced terminations of pregnancy, and any change in civil status that occurs during an individual's lifetime.*

In order to assess population trends and needs, state and federal governments collect **vital statistics.** Vital events for which statistics are collected include live births, deaths, fetal deaths, marriages, divorces, induced terminations of pregnancy, and any change in civil status that occurs during an individual's lifetime. Health care practitioners help in gathering this information and in filling out forms for filing with the appropriate state and federal agencies.

The information provided through the reporting of vital statistics is useful to educational institutions, governmental agencies, research scientists, private industry, and many other organizations and individuals. For example, the recording of vital statistics allows for tracking population composition and growth, measuring educational standards, and monitoring communicable diseases and other community and environmental health problems. Health care practitioners play an important role in collecting and recording valuable health data required by law and should know the correct methods and procedures for reporting public health information.

Many states use U.S. Standard Certificates of Birth and Death to report births and deaths. Birth and death certificates are permanent legal records. The following guidelines can help ensure that information is recorded correctly:

- Type or legibly print all entries. In some states, only black ink may be used.

- Leave no entries blank. Each state has specific requirements for recording information.

- Avoid corrections and erasures.

- Where requested, provide signatures. Do not use rubber stamps or initials in place of signatures.

- Verify the spelling of names.

- Avoid abbreviations, except those recommended in instructions for specific items.

- File only originals with state registrars.

- Refer any problems to the appropriate state officials.

◆ ◆ ◆ ◆ **Births**

All live births must be reported to the state registrar. Figure 7-1 illustrates a sample birth certificate. In some states separate birth and death certificates must be filed for stillbirths, whereas in others there are special forms for stillbirths that include both birth and death information. Generally, birth and death certificates are not required for fetal deaths in which the fetus has not passed the twentieth week of gestation.

Hospitals file birth certificates for babies born to mothers who have been admitted as patients. The attending physician must verify all medical information. For nonhospital births, the person in attendance is responsible for filing the birth certificate.

DO NOT WRITE IN MARGIN RESERVED FOR ODH DATA CODING

Reg. Dist. No. _____

Primary Reg. Dist. No. _____

Registrar's No. _____

Ohio Department of Health
VITAL STATISTICS
CERTIFICATE OF LIVE BIRTH
TYPE OR PRINT IN PERMANENT *BLACK* INK

Birth No. 134 —

a. _____
b. _____
c. _____

CHILD

1. CHILD - NAME   *First*   *Middle*   *Last* | 2. SEX | 3a. DATE OF BIRTH *(Month, Day, Year)* | 3b. TIME OF BIRTH   M
➤

d. _____
e. _____
f. _____
g. _____
h. _____

4a. FACILITY NAME - *(If not institution, give street and number)* | 4b. CITY, VILLAGE OR LOCATION OF BIRTH | 4c. COUNTY OF BIRTH
➤

5. PLACE OF BIRTH
☐ Hospital ☐ Freestanding Birthing Center ☐ Clinic/Doctor's Office ☐ Residence ☐ Other (Specify)_____

6. REGISTRAR'S SIGNATURE | 7. DATE FILED BY REGISTRAR *(Month, Day, Year)*

ATTENDANT

8a. I certify that the above named child was born alive at the place and time and on the date stated above.
SIGNATURE ➤ | 8b. DATE SIGNED | 8c. ATTENDANT ☐ M.D. ☐ D.O. ☐ C.N.M. ☐ OTHER MIDWIFE ☐ OTHER (Specify)

8d. ATTENDANT - NAME   *(Type or Print)* | 8e. MAILING ADDRESS   *(Street or R.F.D. No., City or Village, State, Zip)*
➤

MOTHER

9a. MOTHER'S NAME   *(First, Middle, Last)* | 9b. MAIDEN NAME | 10a. DATE OF BIRTH *(Month, Day, Year)* | 10b. AGE
➤

11. BIRTHPLACE   *(State or Foreign Country)* | 12a. RESIDENCE - STATE | 12. COUNTY | 12c. CITY, TOWN, OR LOCATION

12d. STREET AND NUMBER | 12e. INSIDE CITY LIMITS? ☐ Yes ☐ No | 13. MOTHER'S MAILING ADDRESS   *(If same as residence, enter zip code only)*
➤

FATHER

14. FATHER'S NAME   *(First, Middle, Last)* | 15a. DATE OF BIRTH *(Month, Day, Year)* | 15b. AGE | 16. BIRTHPLACE   *(State or Foreign Country)*

INFORMANT

17. I certify that the personal information provided on this certificate is correct to the best of my knowledge and belief. (ENTER INFORMANT'S NAME OR WHEN REQUIRED BY LAW, PARENTS' SIGNATURES.)

INFORMATION FOR MEDICAL AND HEALTH USE ONLY

MOTHER

18. OF HISPANIC ORIGIN? (Specify No or Yes - if yes, specify Cuban, Mexican, Puerto Rican, etc.) | 19. RACE American Indian, Black, White, etc. (Specify below) | 20. EDUCATION (Specify only highest grade completed) Elementary / Secondary (0 - 12) College (1 - 4 OR 5+) | 21.OCCUPATION AND BUSINESS/INDUSTRY *(Worked during last year)* Occupation   Business/Industry

18a. ☐ NO ☐ YES   Specify: | 19a. | 20a. | 21a. | 21b.

FATHER

18b. ☐ NO ☐ YES   Specify: | 19b. | 20b. | 21c. | 21d.

i. _____
j. _____
k. _____
l. _____
m. _____
n. _____
o. _____
p. _____
q. _____
r. _____
s. _____
t. _____
u. _____
v. _____
w. _____
x. _____
y. _____
z. _____
aa. _____
bb. _____
cc. _____
dd. _____
ee. _____
ff. _____
gg. _____
hh. _____
ii. _____
jj. _____
kk. _____
ll. _____
mm. _____

22. PREGNANCY HISTORY (Complete each section) | 23. MOTHER MARRIED? (At birth, conception, or any time between) (Yes or No) | 24. DATE LAST NORMAL MENSES BEGAN (Month, Day, Year)

LIVE BIRTHS (Do not include this child) | OTHER TERMINATIONS (Spontaneous and induced at any time after conception) | 26a. TOTAL PRENATAL VISITS (If none, so state)

22a. NOW LIVING NUMBER _____ ☐ NONE | 22b. NOW DEAD NUMBER _____ ☐ NONE | 22d. NUMBER _____ ☐ NONE | 25. MONTH OF PREGNANCY PRENATAL CARE BEGAN First, Second, Third, etc. (Specify) | 26b. CITY | 26c. COUNTY

27. BIRTH WEIGHT IN GRAMS | 28. CLINICAL ESTIMATE OF GESTATION *(Weeks)*

22c. DATE OF LAST BIRTH (Month, Year) | 22e. DATE OF LAST OTHER TERMINATION (Month, Year) | 29a. PLURALITY - Single, Twin, Triplet, etc. (Specify) | 29b. IF NOT SINGLE BIRTH - Born First, Second, Third, etc. (Specify)

30. APGAR SCORE | 31a. MOTHER TRANSFERRED PRIOR TO DELIVERY? ☐ No ☐ Yes If yes, enter name of facility and city transferred **FROM**

30a. 1 MINUTE | 30b. 5 MINUTES | 31b. FACILITY NAME | 31c. CITY

31d. INFANT TRANSFERRED? ☐ No ☐ Yes If yes, enter name of facility and city transferred **TO.**
31e. FACILITY NAME | 31f. CITY

MULTIPLE BIRTHS Enter State File Number for Mate(s) LIVE BIRTH(S)

FETAL DEATH(S)

32a. MEDICAL RISK FACTORS FOR THIS PREGNANCY (Check all that apply)
Anemia (Hct. < 30/Hgb. < 10) ....01 ☐
Cardiac disease ....02 ☐
Acute or chronic lung disease ....03 ☐
Diabetes ....04 ☐
Genital herpes ....05 ☐
Hydramnios/Oligohydramnios ....06 ☐
Hemoglobinopathy ....07 ☐
Hypertension, chronic ....08 ☐
Hypertension, pregnancy-associated ....09 ☐
Eclampsia ....10 ☐
Incompetent cervix ....11 ☐
Previous infant 4000 + grams ....12 ☐
Previous preterm or small-for-gestational-age infant 13 ☐
Renal disease ....14 ☐
Rh sensitization ....15 ☐
Uterine bleeding ....16 ☐
None ....00 ☐
Other (Specify)_____ ....17 ☐

32b. OTHER RISK FACTORS FOR THIS PREGNANCY (Complete all items)
Tobacco use during pregnancy ....Yes ☐ No ☐
Average number cigarettes per day _____
Alcohol use during pregnancy ....Yes ☐ No ☐
Average number drinks per week _____
Weight gained during pregnancy _____ lbs.
Pre-Pregnancy weight _____ lbs.

33. OBSTETRIC PROCEDURES (Check all that apply)
Amniocentesis ....01 ☐
Electronic fetal monitoring ....02 ☐
Induction of labor ....03 ☐
Stimulation of labor ....04 ☐
Tocolysis ....05 ☐
Ultrasound ....06 ☐
None ....00 ☐
Other (Specify)_____ ....07 ☐

34. COMPLICATIONS OF LABOR AND/OR DELIVERY (Check all that apply)
Febrile (>100° F. or 38° C.) ....01 ☐
Meconium, moderate/heavy ....02 ☐
Premature rupture of membrane (>12 hours) ....03 ☐
Abruptio placenta ....04 ☐
Placenta previa ....05 ☐
Other excessive bleeding ....06 ☐
Seizures during labor ....07 ☐
Precipitous labor (< 3 hours) ....08 ☐
Prolonged labor (> 20 hours) ....09 ☐
Dysfunctional labor ....10 ☐
Breech/Malpresentation ....11 ☐
Cephalopelvic disproportion ....12 ☐
Cord prolapse ....13 ☐
Anesthetic complications ....14 ☐
Fetal distress ....15 ☐
None ....00 ☐
Other (Specify)_____ ....16 ☐

35. METHOD OF DELIVERY (Check all that apply)
Vaginal ....01 ☐
Vaginal birth after previous C-section ....02 ☐
Primary C-section ....03 ☐
Repeat C-section ....04 ☐
Forceps ....05 ☐
Vacuum ....06 ☐

36. ABNORMAL CONDITIONS OF THE NEWBORN (Check all that apply)
Anemia (Hct. < 39/Hgb. < 13) ....01 ☐
Birth injury ....02 ☐
Fetal alcohol syndrome ....03 ☐
Hyaline membrane disease/RDS ....04 ☐
Meconium aspiration syndrome ....05 ☐
Assisted ventilation < 30 min ....06 ☐
Assisted ventilation ≥ 30 min ....07 ☐
Seizures ....08 ☐
None ....00 ☐
Other (Specify)_____ ....09 ☐

37. CONGENITAL ANOMALIES OF CHILD (Check all that apply)
Anencephalus ....01 ☐
Spina bifida/Meningocele ....02 ☐
Hydrocephalus ....03 ☐
Microcephalus ....04 ☐
Other central nervous system anomalies (Specify)_____ ....05 ☐
Heart malformations ....06 ☐
Other circulatory / respiratory anomalies (Specify)_____ ....07 ☐
Rectal atresia / stenosis ....08 ☐
Tracheo-esophageal fistula / Esophageal atresia .09 ☐
Omphalocele / Gastroschisis ....10 ☐
Other gastrointestinal anomalies (Specify)_____ ....11 ☐
Malformed genitalia ....12 ☐
Renal agenesis ....13 ☐
Other urogenital anomalies (Specify)_____ ....14 ☐
Cleft lip / palate ....15 ☐
Polydactyly / Syndactyly / Adactyly ....16 ☐
Club foot ....17 ☐
Diaphragmatic hernia ....18 ☐
Other musculoskeletal / integumental anomalies (Specify)_____ ....19 ☐
Down's syndrome ....20 ☐
Other chromosomal anomalies (Specify)_____ ....21 ☐
None ....00 ☐
Other (Specify)_____ ....22 ☐

37a. PARENT(S) REQUEST ISSUANCE OF A SOCIAL SECURITY NUMBER FOR THIS CHILD
☐

38. NAME OF PROPHYLACTIC USED IN EYES OF CHILD | 39. DATE OF APPROVED TEST FOR SYPHILIS, IF NONE, STATE REASON | 40. DATE OF APPROVED TEST FOR GONORRHEA, IF NONE, STATE REASON

HEA 2703 5112.06 (REV. 7/92)

Figure 7-1
A Sample Birth Certificate

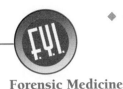
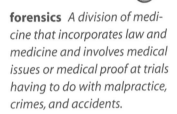
forensics *A division of medicine that incorporates law and medicine and involves medical issues or medical proof at trials having to do with malpractice, crimes, and accidents.*

autopsy *A postmortem examination to determine the cause of death or to obtain physiological evidence, as in the case of a suspicious death.*

coroner *A public official who investigates and holds inquests over those who die from unknown or violent causes; he or she may or may not be a physician, depending on state law.*

medical examiner *A physician who investigates suspicious or unexplained deaths.*

Deaths

After a person is pronounced dead, the attending physician must complete the medical portion of the certificate of death, which generally includes the following information:

- Disease, injury, or complication that caused the death, and how long the decedent was treated for this condition before death occurred.

- Date and time of death.

- Place of death.

- If decedent was female, presence or absence of pregnancy.

- Whether or not an autopsy was performed. An **autopsy** is a postmortem examination to determine the cause of death or to obtain physiological evidence, as in the case of a suspicious death.

In most states it is against the law for an attending physician to sign a death certificate if the death was:

- Possibly due to criminal causes.

- Not attended to by a physician within a specified length of time before death.

- Due to causes undetermined by the physician.

- Violent or otherwise suspicious.

If any of these situations exist, the coroner or medical examiner (see below) must sign the death certificate.

After authorization has been obtained from the next of kin or from a legally responsible party, the body can be removed to a funeral home. In many states the death certificate must be signed within 24 to 72 hours. The *mortician* or *undertaker* (person trained to attend to the dead) files the death certificate with the state. (See Figure 7-2 on p. 158 for a sample death certificate.)

If the deceased has not been under a physician's care at the time of death, the appropriate county health officer—usually the coroner or medical examiner—is responsible for completing the death certificate. A **coroner** is a public official who investigates and holds inquests over those who die from unknown or violent causes. He or she may or may not be a physician, depending on state law.

The purpose of a coroner's inquest is to gather evidence that may be used by the police in the investigation of a violent or suspicious death. It is not a trial, but it is a criminal proceeding, in the nature of a preliminary investigation.

Some states employ medical examiners instead of coroners. A **medical examiner** is a physician, frequently a pathologist, who investigates suspicious or unexplained deaths in a community. As a physician, the medical examiner can order and perform autopsies.

Ohio Department of Health
VITAL STATISTICS
CERTIFICATE OF DEATH

DO NOT WRITE IN MARGIN RESERVED FOR ODH DATA CODING

Reg. Dist. No. _____

Primary Reg. Dist. No. _____

State File No. _____

Registrar's No. _____

a. _____
b. _____
c. _____
d. _____
e. _____

DECEDENT

1. DECEDENT'S NAME *(First, Middle, LAST)*	2. SEX	3. DATE OF DEATH *(Month, Day, Year)*

4. SOCIAL SECURITY NUMBER	5a. AGE - Last Birthday *(Years)*	5b. UNDER 1 YEAR		5c. UNDER 1 DAY		6. DATE OF BIRTH *(Month, Day, Year)*	7. BIRTHPLACE *(City and State or Foreign Country)*
		Months	Days	Hours	Minutes		

8. WAS DECEDENT EVER IN U.S. ARMED FORCES? ☐ Yes ☐ No

9a. PLACE OF DEATH *(Check only one)*
HOSPITAL: ☐ Inpatient ☐ ER/Outpatient ☐ DOA
OTHER ☐ Nursing Home ☐ Residence ☐ Other *(Specify)*

9b. FACILITY NAME *(If not institution, give street and number)*	9c. CITY, VILLAGE, TWP., OR LOCATION OF DEATH	9d. COUNTY OF DEATH

IF DEATH OCCURRED IN INSTITUTION, GIVE RESIDENCE BEFORE ADMISSION →

10. MARITAL STATUS - Married, Never Married, Widowed, Divorced *(Specify)*	11. SURVIVING SPOUSE *(If wife give maiden name)*	12a. DECEDENTS USUAL OCCUPATION *(Give kind of work done during most of working life. Don't use retired.)*	12b. KIND OF BUSINESS/INDUSTRY

13a. RESIDENCE - STATE	13b. COUNTY	13c. CITY, TOWN, TWP., OR LOCATION	13d. STREET AND NUMBER

13e. INSIDE CITY LIMITS? *(Yes or No)*	13f. ZIP CODE	14. WAS DECEDENT OF HISPANIC ORIGIN? *(Specify No or Yes - If yes, specify Cuban, Mexican, Puerto Rican, etc.)* ☐ No ☐ Yes Specify:	15. RACE - American Indian, Black White, etc. *(Specify)*	16. DECEDENT'S EDUCATION *(Specify only highest grade completed)* Elementary/Secondary (0-12) | College (1-4 or 5+)

PARENTS

17. FATHER'S NAME *(First, Middle, Last)*	18. MOTHER'S NAME *(First, Middle, Maiden Surname)*

INFORMANT

19a. INFORMANT'S NAME *(Type/Print)*	19b. MAILING ADDRESS *(Street and Number or Rural Route Number, City or Town, State, Zip Code)*

DISPOSITION

20a. METHOD OF DISPOSITION ☐ Burial ☐ Cremation ☐ Removal from State ☐ Donation ☐ Other *(Specify)*	20b. PLACE OF DISPOSITION *(Name of cemetery, crematory, or other place)*	20c. LOCATION - City or Town, State

20d. DATE OF DISPOSITION	21a. NAME OF EMBALMER	21b. LICENSE NUMBER

22a. SIGNATURE OF FUNERAL DIRECTOR OR OTHER PERSON ►	22b. LICENSE NUMBER *(of Licensee)*	23. NAME AND ADDRESS OF FACILITY

REGISTRAR

24. REGISTRAR'S SIGNATURE ►	25. DATE FILED *(Month, Day, Year)*

f. _____
g. _____
h. _____
i. _____

26a. SIGNATURE OF PERSON ISSUING PERMIT ►	26b. DIST. No.	27. DATE PERMIT ISSUED

CERTIFIER

28a. CERTIFIER *(Check only one)*

☐ CERTIFYING PHYSICIAN
To the best of my knowledge, death occurred at the time, date, and place, and due to the cause(s) and manner as stated.

☐ CORONER
On the basis of examination and/or investigation, in my opinion, death occurred at the time, date, and place, and due to the cause(s) and manner as stated

28b. TIME OF DEATH M	28c. DATE PRONOUNCED DEAD *(Month, Day, Year)*	28d. WAS CASE REFERRED TO CORONER? ☐ Yes ☐ No

j. _____
k. _____

28e. SIGNATURE AND TITLE OF CERTIFIER ►	28f. LICENSE NUMBER	28g. DATE SIGNED *(Month, Day, Year)*

l. _____
m. _____
n. _____
o. _____
p. _____
q. _____
r. _____
s. _____
t. _____
u. _____

29. NAME AND ADDRESS OF PERSON WHO COMPLETED CAUSE OF DEATH *(Type/Print)*

CAUSE OF DEATH

SEE INSTRUCTIONS ON OTHER SIDE

30. PART I. Enter the diseases, injuries, or complications that caused the death Do not enter the mode of dying, such as cardiac or respiratory arrest, shock, or heart failure. List only one cause on each line. TYPE OR PRINT IN PERMANENT INK | Approximate Interval Between Onset and Death

IMMEDIATE CAUSE (Final disease or condition resulting in death) → a. _____
DUE TO (OR AS A CONSEQUENCE OF):

Sequentially list conditions, if any, leading to immediate cause. Enter UNDERLYING CAUSE (Disease or injury that initiated events resulting in death) LAST
b. _____
DUE TO (OR AS A CONSEQUENCE OF):

c. _____
DUE TO (OR AS A CONSEQUENCE OF):

d. _____

PART II. Other *significant* *conditions* contributing to death but not resulting in the underlying cause given in Part I.	31a. WAS AN AUTOPSY PERFORMED? ☐ Yes ☐ No	31b. WERE AUTOPSY FINDINGS AVAILABLE PRIOR TO COMPLETION OF CAUSE OF DEATH? ☐ Yes ☐ No

32. MANNER OF DEATH ☐ Natural ☐ Pending Investigation ☐ Accident ☐ Suicide ☐ Could not be Determined ☐ Homicide	33a. DATE OF INJURY *(Month, Day, Year)*	33b. TIME OF INJURY M	33c. INJURY AT WORK? ☐ Yes ☐ No	33d. DESCRIBE HOW INJURY OCCURRED
	33e. PLACE OF INJURY - At home, farm, street, factory, office building, etc. *(Specify)*			33f. LOCATION *(Street and Number or Rural Route Number, City or Town, State)*

HEA 2717 5152.06 Rev. 2/89

Figure 7-2
A Sample Death Certificate

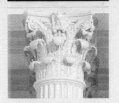

Newspaper Allowed to Inspect Death Records

A New Jersey appellate court ruled that a newspaper could inspect the death records of the state registrar of vital statistics.

A newspaper reporter received information from a hospital nurse that a baby had died due to lack of staff to watch monitors but that the parents had been told the baby died of toxemia. The nurse refused to name the infant but promised to verify the name if the reporter obtained it. The newspaper filed suit under the right-to-know law to examine the death records.

The appellate court ruled:

1. That death certificates are public records, available for inspection by any citizen, and could be copied under the supervision of a representative of the registrar.

2. That the newspaper had a right to inspect randomly the records during regular business hours, in the presence of a representative of the registrar.

3. That the registrar could charge a reasonable fee.

Home News Publishing Co. v. State of New Jersey, Dept. of Health, 570 A.2d 1267 (N.J. Sup. Ct., App. Div., March 1, 1990).

Check Your Progress

1. Define *vital statistics.*

_____

_____

2. Define *autopsy.*

_____

_____

3. Define *coroner.*

_____

_____

4. Define *medical examiner.*

_____

_____

5. Define *forensics.*

_____

_____

6. Where are birth certificates and death certificates filed?

_____

_____

7. Birth certificates must be filed for _____ .

_____

Requirements vary with states for _____ .

_____

8. Name three circumstances in which an attending physician may not legally complete a death certificate.

_____

_____

_____

Public Health Statutes

In all states, to help guarantee the health and well-being of citizens, physicians or other health care practitioners must report births, deaths, certain communicable diseases, specific injuries, and child and drug abuse to the appropriate local, state, and federal authorities. Public health statutes vary with states concerning the reporting of fetal deaths and stillbirths, time limits for filing reports, and the manner in which information must be recorded. However, all provide for:

- Guarding against unsanitary conditions in public facilities.

- Inspecting establishments where food and drink are processed and sold.

- Exterminating pests and vermin that can spread disease.

- Checking water quality.

- Setting up measures of control for certain diseases.

- Requiring physicians, school nurses, and other health care workers to file certain reports for the protection of citizens.

◆ ◆ ◆ ◆ **Communicable and Other Notifiable Diseases**

Under each state's public health statutes, physicians, other health care practitioners, and anyone who has knowledge of a case must report to county or state health agencies the occurrence of certain diseases that, if left unchecked, could threaten the health and well-being of the population.

The list of reportable diseases is long and varies with the state. Requirements for reporting, such as time lapses and whether to report by telephone or mail, also vary, so medical office personnel should be familiar with the specific requirements for reporting communicable diseases in their county and state of employment. Requirements for reporting and forms for reporting by mail are available from county and state health departments. The communicable diseases most likely to have mandated reporting by state statutes are diphtheria, cholera, meningococcal meningitis, plague, smallpox, tuberculosis, anthrax, AIDS, brucellosis, infectious and serum hepatitis, leprosy, malaria, rubeola, poliomyelitis, psittacosis, rheumatic fever, rubella, typhoid fever, trichinosis, and tetanus. Other diseases that may have mandated reporting if a higher than normal incidence occurs are influenza and streptococcal and staphylococcal infections.

VOICE OF EXPERIENCE

The Importance of Confidentiality

Mary, R.N., B.S.N., is a community health nurse working for a county health department in a rural area of a Northwestern state. She says that tact, understanding, and diplomacy are necessary when contacting individuals who may have been exposed to a sexually transmitted disease. "When a patient sees a physician who diagnoses an STD, the physician discusses test results with the patient, then reports the case to the health department. If the patient lives in the area we serve, then we visit that person and try to determine recent sexual partners. We emphasize that information will be kept confidential and hope that the person will feel a sense of responsibility so that their sexual partners can see a physician. Most do, but some are reluctant for one reason or another.

"We then contact all the named sexual partners of the person diagnosed with an STD and encourage them to see a physician or visit a clinic for examination, even if they have no symptoms," Mary continues. "Of course, we also ask them for names of their sexual partners, so they can also be contacted. Unfortunately, lists can be long and some individuals may not even recall everyone with whom they have been intimate. It's a difficult task, because it's embarrassing and upsetting for everyone involved, but it's also necessary, to see that people who have been exposed [to STDs] get treatment."

[*Note:* Contact procedures differ with states. In some states, for instance, "community disease specialists," who may or may not be nurses or other health care practitioners, contact individuals diagnosed with STDs.]

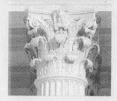
Physician's Duty to Notify the Public Is Questioned

A patient of a Delaware physician suffered an epileptic seizure while driving and hit another vehicle. The patient survived, but passengers in her car were killed, as well as passengers and the driver of the other vehicle.

Representatives of the estates of the deceased individuals in the car that was hit sued the patient's physician for his alleged negligence in treating her for epilepsy and for his failure to take steps to protect the public from the danger of the patient's driving. (The physician had treated the patient for several years and was aware of a previous car accident that had resulted from a seizure while driving.)

At trial, both sides filed for summary judgment, but the court did not rule in favor of either party. It held that the physician's failure to follow state law requiring him to notify the department of motor vehicles of the patient's condition did not constitute a breach of duty to the public. The purpose of the state law was to enforce licensing procedures relating to the operation of motor vehicles, the court explained, not to establish a physician's duty to protect the public.

Under common law, the plaintiffs could have claimed that the physician had a duty to the deceased, stemming from his treatment of the driver who had allegedly caused the accident. The court referred the case back to the trial court for a jury to determine.

Harden v. Allstate Insurance Co., 883 F.Supp. 963 (D.C., De., May 2, 1995).

Certain sexually transmitted diseases (STDs), also called venereal diseases, must be reported whenever diagnosed. Reportable STDs differ with states but generally include gonorrhea, syphilis, chlamydia (lymphogranuloma venereum), chancroid, and granuloma inguinale (genital warts). Public health practitioners use reported cases to find and treat others who may have been infected through sexual contact with the named individual.

Reporting requirements for communicable diseases are usually more stringent for patients who are employed in restaurants, cafeterias, day care centers, schools, health care facilities, and other places where contagion can be rampant.

Through extensive vaccination programs, many communicable diseases that decimated world populations in the past have largely been eradicated. In the United States, for example, smallpox has virtually disappeared and very few cases of poliomyelitis, typhoid fever, or diphtheria are reported annually.

In some states certain noncommunicable diseases must also be reported, to allow public health officials to track causes and treatment or to otherwise protect the public's health and safety. These diseases include cancer (to determine environmental causes); congenital metabolic disorders in newborns, such as phenylketonuria, congenital hypothyroidism, and galactosemia (to allow for prompt treatment); epilepsy and some other diseases that cause lapse of consciousness (to determine eligibility to drive a vehicle); and pesticide poisoning.

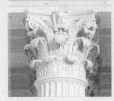

State Law Mandates Notification of Sexual Partners by HIV Carrier

Michigan passed a state law requiring individuals who know they are HIV-infected to notify their sexual partners before sexual activity. A defendant was convicted of having sexual contact as defined under the act without notifying her partner of her HIV status. She was sentenced to 2 years 8 months to 4 years in prison on each of three counts.

The defendant appealed, claiming that the statute is unconstitutionally broad because it applies both to consensual and nonconsensual sexual acts, and because it does not require intent. The appeals court addressed the issue of intent by comparing killing someone with a car while driving drunk to the defendant's having sexual contact with someone without telling them of her HIV status. The comparison made was that the statute against driving while intoxicated does not require an intent to kill but recognizes that there is intent in the reckless action of driving drunk. The court found that the intent in the HIV notification statute is satisfied by the reckless action of having sexual contact without warning one's partner about exposure to HIV. The court held that the statute was constitutional and that punishment in this case was appropriate under the law.

People v. Jensen, 231 Mich.App. 439, 586 N.W.2d 748 (Mich.App., Aug. 28, 1998). (Appeal denied, *People v. Jensen*, 595 N.W.2d 850 (Mich. May 25, 1999).

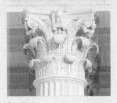

Physician's Duty to Protect Others From Contaminated Tissue Samples Determined by Court

A surgeon operating on a patient infected with HIV and tuberculosis drew a sample of pus into a syringe, then put the syringe, with the needle still attached, into a sample container and sent it to the lab. The surgeon's action violated proper standards for handling such samples.

A lab technician received the sample and stuck herself while trying to recap the needle, an action that violated hospital infection control procedures. The technician was accidentally infected with HIV and tuberculosis as a result of the injury. She sued the surgeon, who claimed that he owed no duty to the technician, that the sample was improperly packaged by a hospital nurse, and that plaintiff's injury resulted from her own negligence.

The court disagreed with the physician's assertion of no duty, finding that although a physician may not owe a duty to the general public, there is a duty to persons who would reasonably be expected to come into contact with such contaminated samples. The court also held that whether or not the nurse was under the physician's control in the operating room was an issue to be decided by a jury, as was the issue of the physician's negligence, if any, as the proximate cause of the plaintiff's injury.

Doe v. Smith, N.Y.S.2d, 2000 West Law 557362 (N.Y.S. 2000).

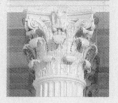
Case Establishes Right of State to Quarantine

A California man was diagnosed with pulmonary tuberculosis, a reportable, communicable disease. A state health officer served the man with a quarantine order and he was admitted to a hospital. The patient deserted the hospital one month later, but he still had tuberculosis. The man was subsequently arrested, tried, and convicted of violating the Health and Safety Code of California. He was sentenced to 180 days in jail, but the sentence was suspended and he was placed on 3-year probation. The health officer again served the man with an order of isolation and he was returned to the hospital, this time to the security section. The county public health officer then served the man with successive orders of isolation for periods of 6 months each.

The man asked for a writ of habeas corpus, claiming that the Health and Safety Code of California was unconstitutional, and therefore the health officer had no legal authority to issue consecutive certificates of quarantine and isolation.

The court held that it is the "duty of the state to protect the public from the danger of tuberculosis," therefore the Health and Safety Code of California was not unconstitutional. The court also held that, "The health officer may make an isolation or quarantine order whenever he shall determine in a particular case that quarantine or isolation is necessary for the protection of the public health." The petition for a writ of habeas corpus was denied.

In re. Halko, 246 Cal. App. 2d 553, 54 Cal. Rptr. 661 (Cal. App. Dist. 2, Nov. 18, 1966).

◆ ◆ ◆ ◆ ### The National Childhood Vaccine Injury Act of 1986

Parents usually begin programs of vaccination against certain communicable diseases for their children when they are infants. When children reach school age, most states ask for proof of vaccination for children entering the public school system for the first time. Since a small percentage of vaccinated children suffer adverse effects from the vaccine **administered,** parents or guardians are informed of risks associated with each vaccine and must sign consent forms allowing health care practitioners to administer the vaccine (see Figure 7-3).

The **National Childhood Vaccine Injury Act** of 1986 created the National Vaccine Injury Compensation Program (VICP). The VICP is a no-fault system designed to compensate individuals, or families of individuals, who have been injured by childhood vaccines. The program serves as an alternative to suing vaccine manufacturers and providers. Vaccines covered by the original act include diphtheria, tetanus, pertussis, measles, mumps, rubella, and polio. Vaccines added to the program from 1997 to 1999 include hepatitis B, haemophilus influenza type b, varicella, rotavirus, and pneumococcal conjugate vaccines. A rule was published in 1997 that provides for the automatic addition of future vaccines recommended by the Centers for Disease Control and Prevention (CDC) for routine administration to children.

The National Childhood Vaccine Injury Act also initiated programs to educate the public about vaccine benefits and risks. The act requires physicians and other health care providers administering vaccines to report adverse events following vaccination and to keep permanent

administer *To instill a drug into the body of a patient.*

National Childhood Vaccine Injury Act *A federal law passed in 1986 that created a no-fault compensation program for citizens injured or killed by vaccines, as an alternative to suing vaccine manufacturers and providers.*

Patient Name _____

Address _____

Birth Date _____

Patient's Name _____

Phone Number _____ Physician _____

Clinic Name/Address

Health care providers, health care facilities, federal or state agencies, welfare agencies, schools or family day care facilities may have access to this information. Immunization records remain confidential, and any person who fails to protect the confidentiality of this information is guilty of a Class 1 misdemeanor.

REFUSAL TO RELEASE INFORMATION: I have read or had explained to me the immunization information system. I understand the benefits of allowing my child's immunization record to be shared with other primary care providers and public health officials. However, I choose NOT to have my child's immunization record shared with other providers.

Signature (parent or legal guardian if minor): _____ Date: _____

Reviewed with parent by (initials): _____ Date: _____

Vaccine	Date Given	Vaccine Mfg.	Vaccine Lot No.	Site Given	*Initials	Parent/Guardian Sig.@
DT DTP DTaP 1						
DT DTP DTaP 2						
DT DTP DTaP 3						
DT DTP DTaP 4						
DT DTP DTaP 5						
MMR 1						
MMR 2						
*Hep B-P 1						
Hep B-P 2						
Hep B-P 3						
*Hep B-H 1						
Hep B-H 2						
Hep B-H 3						
OPV EIPV 1						
OPV EIPV 2						
OPV EIPV 3						
OPV EIPV 4						
OPV EIPV 5						

*Initials   Initials indicate VIS were provided & vaccine administered.

Signature of Vaccine Administrator

_____

@ I have been provided a copy of, and have read or have had explained to me, information about the diseases and the vaccines listed above. I have had a chance to ask questions that were answered to my satisfaction. I believe I understand the benefits and risks of the vaccines cited and ask that the vaccine(s) listed above be given to me or the person named above (for whom I am authorized to make this request).

Figure 7-3
Sample Vaccination Consent Form

records on vaccines administered and health problems occurring after vaccination. Vaccine administrators are required to document in the patient's permanent medical record:

- The date the vaccine was administered.

- The vaccine manufacturer.

- The vaccine lot number.

- The name, address, and title of the health care provider who administered the vaccine.

The Vaccine Adverse Events Reporting System (VAERS), operated by the Food and Drug Administration and the Centers for Disease Control and Prevention, should be notified of any adverse event by completing a VAERS reporting form. Health care providers must report the following events:

- Any event listed in the Vaccine Injury Table, available at the Health Resources and Services Administration Web site and from the Health Resources and Services Administration Bureau of Health Professions, 5600 Fishers Lane, Rockville, Maryland 20857.

- Any contraindicating event listed in the manufacturer's package insert.

◆ ◆ ◆ ◆ **Reportable Injuries**

In all states, physicians must immediately report to law enforcement officials medical treatment of patients with injuries resulting from an act of violence, such as assault, rape, or domestic violence, so that authorities can investigate the incident.

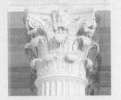

Court Case

No Liability for Report of Child Abuse

A Texas appellate court ruled a physician was immune from liability for reporting a case of child sexual abuse.

The physician examined a child brought in by a social worker. The physician's written report depicted a chronically abused child. The child was abnormally small for her age, was filthy, had lice, and showed signs of recent beatings and vaginal and rectal sexual assault.

A friend of the mother later pleaded *nolo contendere* to a felony charge of injuring a child. He filed suit against the physician for negligence and intentional, malicious, and bad-faith diagnosing and reporting of sexual abuse.

The court affirmed that the physician had probable cause to report the incident and was entitled to statutory immunity.

Dominguez v. Kelly, 786 S.W.2d 749 (Tex. Ct. of App., Jan. 10, 1990; rehearing overruled, March 14, 1990).

Child Abuse

Child Abuse Prevention and Treatment Act *A federal law passed in 1974 requiring physicians to report cases of child abuse and to try to prevent future cases.*

To help prevent violence against children, in 1974 Congress passed the **Child Abuse Prevention and Treatment Act,** mandating the reporting of cases of child abuse. All states have enacted legislation making child abuse a crime and requiring the reporting of child abuse and neglect by teachers, physicians, and other licensed health care practitioners. The report must immediately be made to the proper authorities—either in person or by telephone—and a written report is generally required within a specified time frame, such as 72 hours. Any individual reporting suspected child abuse is granted absolute immunity from criminal and civil liability resulting from the reported incident. Depending on state law, failure to report suspected cases of child abuse may be a misdemeanor.

Spousal Abuse

Unlike cases of child abuse, a state's laws may not specifically require a physician to report spousal abuse. Legal remedies available to battered spouses vary from state to state, but all states have laws protecting victims of domestic abuse. Advocacy programs can explain legal options to victims and can help them cope with the legal system. Courts may issue protective, or restraining orders, or they may issue injunctions that direct the batterer to stop abusing the victim. In some states police may be required to arrest batterers under certain conditions. Depending on laws within the jurisdiction, batterers may be criminally prosecuted for assault, battery, harassment, intimidation, or attempted murder.

Elder Abuse

Amendments to the Older Americans Act *A 1987 federal act that defines elder abuse, neglect, and exploitation but does not deal with enforcement.*

The Older Americans Act was signed into law by President Lyndon B. Johnson in 1965. The act created the Administration on Aging and outlined ten objectives aimed at preserving the rights and dignity of older citizens. The 1987 **Amendments to the Older Americans Act** define elder abuse, neglect, and exploitation but do not deal with enforcement. The year 2000 Amendments to the Older Americans Act include a five-year reauthorization for funding, maintain the original ten objectives, and add the National Family Caregiver Support Program for addressing the needs of caregivers to the elderly.

All 50 states and the District of Columbia have enacted legislation instituting reporting systems to identify domestic and institutional elder abuse, neglect, and exploitation. In most states reporting suspected elder abuse is mandatory for certain professionals, including physicians. (If not mandated by state law, reporting may be voluntary.) Physical, sexual, and financial abuses of the elderly are considered crimes in all states. Some forms of emotional abuse and types of neglect may be considered crimes in some states.

In addition to the above laws, some states have statutes protecting vulnerable adults, such as mentally ill and mentally challenged individuals. Some states also have statutes dealing with the prevention of fetal abuse stemming from sniffing paint and other chemicals, taking drugs, or drinking alcohol while pregnant.

◆ ◆ ◆ ◆ Identifying Abuse

Health care practitioners should be alert for signs of physical abuse, both for purposes of mandatory reporting and for possible intervention on behalf of the victim. It is imperative, however, that medical personnel not jump to conclusions and make unsubstantiated abuse reports.

Physical signs of abuse may include but are not limited to:

- Unexplained fractures.

- Repeated injuries, especially those in unusual places or those shaped like objects such as electrical cords, hair brushes, belt buckles, and so forth.

- Burns with unusual shapes, such as circles that may have been caused by a cigarette or those shaped like objects such as an iron.

- Friction burns apparently caused by a rope or cord.

- Bite marks.

- Signs of malnutrition or dehydration, such as extreme weight loss, dry skin, or red-rimmed, sunken eyes.

- Torn or bloody underwear.

- Pain or bruising in the genital area.

- Unexplained venereal disease or other genital infections.

Behavioral signs of abuse may include:

- Illogical or unreasonable explanations for injuries.

- Frequently changing physicians or missing medical appointments.

- Attempts to hide injuries with heavy makeup or sunglasses.

- Frequent anxiety, depression, or loss of emotional control.

- Changes in appetite.

- Problems at school or on the job.

Observation of individuals who accompany the patient may also identify a potential abuser. One might suspect abuse, for example, if in the presence of additional evidence an alleged victim of abuse is accompanied by someone who smells of alcohol, exhibits pensive or obsessive behavior, seems unusually or inappropriately emotional, or shows aggressive or otherwise suspicious body language toward the patient.

When a health care practitioner suspects abuse, care and tact must be used in eliciting information from patients. Direct, open-ended questions such as, "Has someone harmed you?" may encourage a patient to relate what has caused his or her injuries.

Health care practitioners should emphasize to the patient that information offered will be kept confidential, as required by physician-patient confidentiality, except in those cases in which the law mandates reporting abuse. Reporting requirements for abuse should be explained during the patient's first visit. Some sources recommend having patients sign a statement indicating that they understand the reporting requirements and agree with them.

Forcing the issue to encourage an adult to leave a batterer is not always the immediate answer. Similarly, providing hot line numbers, information on safe houses, or handouts about abuse may not be helpful if the batterer is waiting in the reception area for the patient or may later find the material and be further enraged. Instead, many medical facilities have bulletins posted in restrooms telling patients where to call for help. If tear strips with the telephone number are provided, a victim can tear off the small, easily concealed strip for future reference.

◆ ◆ ◆ ◆ Drug Regulations

Food and Drug Administration (FDA) *A federal agency within the Department of Health and Human Services that oversees drug quality and standardization and must approve drugs before they are released for public use.*

Drug Enforcement Agency (DEA) *A branch of the U.S. Department of Justice that regulates the sale and use of drugs.*

Controlled Substances Act *The federal law giving authority to the Drug Enforcement Agency to regulate the sale and use of drugs.*

prescribe *To issue a medical prescription for a patient.*

dispense *To deliver controlled substances in some type of bottle, box, or other container to a patient.*

The federal government has jurisdiction over the manufacture and distribution of drugs in the United States. The **Food and Drug Administration (FDA),** an agency within the Department of Health and Human Services, tests and approves drugs before releasing them for public use. This agency also oversees drug quality and standardization.

Both federal and state governments regulate the sale and use of certain drugs. At the federal level, the **Drug Enforcement Agency (DEA),** a branch of the Department of Justice, regulates the sale and use of drugs by the authority granted in the Comprehensive Drug Abuse Prevention and Control Act of 1970, commonly called the **Controlled Substances Act.**

General regulations mandated by the Controlled Substances Act require physicians who purchase, **prescribe, dispense,** administer, or in any way handle controlled drugs to:

- Register with the Drug Enforcement Administration through a division office. (A list of division offices is available online at the DEA Web site.) The physician will receive a registration number that must appear on all prescriptions for controlled substances and must be renewed periodically for a specified fee. Each DEA number is issued for a specific physician in a specific location. That location is the only one at which the physician may store controlled substances, including salespeople's samples. If a physician practices in more than one state, he or she needs a DEA number for each state. The physician must notify the appropriate state authorities and the DEA whenever he or she moves from a registered location.

- Keep records concerning the administering or dispensing of a controlled drug on file for two years. Such records must include the patient's full name and address, the reason for use of the drug, the date of the order, the name of the drug, the dosage form and quantity of the drug, and whether the drug was administered or dispensed.

- Note on a patient's chart when controlled substances are administered or dispensed.

- Make a written inventory of drug supplies every two years, and keep such records an additional two years.

- Keep drugs in a locked cabinet or safe, and report any thefts immediately to the nearest DEA office and the local police.

9. What two federal agencies control the manufacture and standardization of drugs and their sale and use?

   _____

   _____

Use these three terms correctly in the sentences that follow: prescribe, dispense, administer.

10. Dr. Wellness will _____ the drug to his patient, Mrs. Doe, when he starts an intravenous injection.

11. Under the law, medical assistants may not _____ drugs for patients but may _____ or _____ them under a physician's direct order.

12. When a pharmacist fills a patient's prescription, he or she then _____ the drug to the patient.

YOU BE THE JUDGE

In Mississippi in the year 2000, a mix-up in a hospital nursery resulted in a newborn baby being breast-fed by a woman who was not his mother. Hospital nurses discovered the error within a few hours and informed the baby's mother. The mother sued the hospital for the identity of the woman who had mistakenly nursed the baby and for access to the woman's medical records to detect any health threats to the baby, since breast milk can transmit communicable diseases such as HIV. The hospital refused to release the information. A trial court entered a discovery order for the information, then stayed it so the state appeals and Supreme Court could review the case.

The hospital asked the patient, who was a third party to the litigation, what she wanted to do. The patient said she was willing to give the plaintiff access to certain medical information, including her HIV test, but was unwilling to be identified or to give the plaintiff full access to her medical records.

In your opinion, what is most important in this situation, the privacy of the woman who mistakenly breast-fed someone else's baby or the health risk to the infant, who was in poor health? Explain your answer.

_____

_____

_____

Instead of bringing a legal suit against the hospital, would there have been alternative ways of handling the disclosure issue? Explain.

_____

_____

The Controlled Substances Act regulates drugs under the following five schedules, based on their potential for abuse and their medical usefulness.

- Schedule 1—Drugs with no proven or acceptable medical use and a high abuse potential. These include heroin, marijuana, peyote, mescaline, LSD, THC, and others. They are used for research only.

- Schedule 2—Narcotic drugs with a high potential for abuse but with currently accepted medical use in treatment (opiates, cocaine, methadone, meperidine).

    Schedule 2N—Nonnarcotic drugs with a high potential for abuse, such as amphetamines, phenmetrazine, methylphenidate, and short-acting barbiturates.

- Schedule 3—Narcotics in combination with other nonnarcotic drugs, such as codeine combined with acetaminophen or aspirin, phenacetin, and caffeine.

    Schedule 3N—Nonnarcotic central nervous system (CNS) depressants such as glutethimide, methyprylon, and barbiturates not listed in other schedules. Also included are anorectant agents (suppositories) that are not part of other schedules.

- Schedule 4—Narcotics in combination with other nonnarcotic drugs, antidiarrheals, mild CNS depressants, mild CNS stimulants, and tranquilizers. Also included are drugs such as chloral hydrate, meprobamate, phenobarbital, diphenoxylate with atropine sulfate, chlordiazepoxide, diazepam, diethylpropion, and phentermine.

- Schedule 5—Drugs containing small amounts of narcotics. Included are cough medications with codeine and drugs used for diarrhea, such as Lomotil and Donnagel.

Drugs included in Schedules 2 and 2N require a properly executed, manually signed prescription. (The N designation in 2N and 3N drugs stands for *nonnarcotic*.) No refills are permitted on these prescriptions. All other scheduled drugs (Schedules 3-5) may be prescribed on written or oral orders.

Whenever prescriptions are written for controlled substances, a copy should be filed in the patient's record. When a physician discontinues practice, he or she must return the registration certificate and any unused order forms (preferably marked "void") to the DEA. When it is necessary to dispose of controlled drugs, the physician or employee charged with disposal should contact the nearest field office of the DEA and the responsible state agency for disposal information.

State laws governing controlled substances may be as strict as or stricter than federal laws. Physicians may be required to register with the appropriate state agency as well as the DEA and must follow all state and federal requirements in prescribing, dispensing, and administering controlled substances. Whenever state and federal regulations differ, the more stringent regulation must be followed. For example, if federal law requires that records be held for two years and state law specifies five years, the state law takes precedence.

Because violation of a law dealing with a state- and/or federal-controlled substance is a criminal offense and can result in fines, jail sentences, and loss of license to practice medicine, physicians and medical facility employees should be familiar with all state and federal narcotics laws.

The role of the medical assistant concerning compliance with DEA regulations is to remind the physician of license renewal dates, keep accurate records for scheduled drugs, maintain an accurate inventory and inventory records, and assure the security of scheduled drugs kept in the office. This is accomplished by:

- Checking to be sure that all controlled substances are kept in a locked cabinet or safe.

- Reminding the physician to keep his or her "black bag" in a safe place.

- Keeping all prescription blanks, especially those used for narcotics, under lock and key.

- Ordering prescription blanks that are serially numbered or otherwise printed to help detect alterations and theft.

- Reporting to the physician any behavior by patients that would suggest an attempt to secure addictive drugs.

- Checking patients' records to verify all prescriptions that may be questioned by a pharmacist.

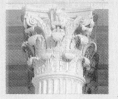

Court Case

Physician Convicted of Controlled Substance Violations

A California appellate court upheld the conviction of a physician for unlawfully prescribing controlled substances.

A patient had seen the physician for pain after back surgery. The patient's mother told the physician that her son took large amounts of codeine and Doriden and shared his pills with friends. The patient admitted that he had been treated for drug abuse twice before and had been caught burglarizing a pharmacy.

The physician wrote prescriptions for 100 tablets of Tylenol with codeine and 50 tablets of Doriden, and the pharmacist reported the prescriptions to the state's Bureau of Narcotic Enforcement. Two undercover agents subsequently visited the physician and were given prescriptions for Tylenol with codeine without undergoing a physical examination.

The physician was convicted on five counts of unlawful prescription of controlled substances. His sole defense was that he practiced medicine in good faith when he wrote the prescriptions. The appellate court upheld convictions on three counts and reversed convictions on two counts.

People of the State of California v. Lonergan, 267 Ca. Rptr. 887 (Cal. Ct. of App., March 26, 1990).

Applying Knowledge

Answer the following questions in the spaces provided.

1. Four vital statistics that the government collects are _____ , _____ , _____ , and _____ .

   Of these, the physician should be concerned with documenting _____ and _____ .

2. List eight federal recommendations to be followed in completing birth and death certificates.

   _____

   _____

   _____

   _____

   _____

   _____

   _____

   _____

   _____

3. After a person is pronounced dead, the attending physician must complete the medical portion of the death certificate. What information does this generally include?

   _____

   _____

   _____

   _____

4. Explain the difference between a coroner and a medical examiner.

   _____

   _____

   _____

   _____

5. List four situations in which a death certificate must be completed by a medical examiner or coroner.

   _____

   _____

   _____

   _____

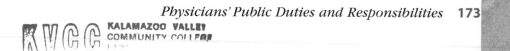

Review and Case Studies

6. What is the purpose of a coroner's inquest?

_____

_____

_____

_____

7. List five physical and five behavioral clues that may indicate that a patient has been a victim of abuse.

_____   _____

_____   _____

_____   _____

_____   _____

_____   _____

8. Give five examples of noncommunicable diseases for which reporting may be mandated in certain states.

_____   _____

_____   _____

_____

9. The _____ is responsible for testing and approving drugs for public use, whereas the _____ regulates the sale and use of drugs.

10. There are _____ schedules of controlled drugs. Schedule _____ drugs are the most addictive and have the most stringent controls. Schedule _____ drugs have the least potential for abuse of all the schedules for controlled substances.

11. Does your community have a coroner or a medical examiner? Is this an elective or an appointive office? Where will you find this information?

_____

_____

_____

12. What are the reportable diseases mandated by law in your state? Where will you find this information?

_____

_____

_____

_____

13. What regulations apply in your state to the reporting of HIV and AIDS cases? Is identity of the patient protected by law? Where will you find this information?

_____

_____

14. Are public health statutes in all states the same? Why or why not?

_____

_____

15. Who may legally file birth certificates for newborns?

_____

_____

16. Should a physician report to the state a greater than normal influenza outbreak in his or her community? Why or why not?

_____

_____

17. Which physicians must register with the federal Drug Enforcement Administration?

_____

_____

18. Referring to the drug schedules, name the categories of drugs that have the highest potential for abuse.

_____

19. If physicians may not prescribe Schedule 1 drugs for patients, what is the value of those drugs?

_____

20. Which federal agency tests and approves drugs before releasing them for public use and oversees drug quality and standardization?

_____

21. In the medical office, who is generally responsible for keeping accurate records concerning prescribing and dispensing drugs?

_____

Match each of the following descriptions with the correct term by writing the appropriate letter in the space provided.

_____ **22.** Tests and approves drugs for public use.

_____ **23.** Also known as the Comprehensive Drug Abuse Prevention and Control Act of 1970.

_____ **24.** As a branch of the Department of Justice, regulates the sale and use of drugs.

_____ **25.** Requires reports of communicable diseases and certain injuries, as mandated by state laws.

_____ **26.** Mandates reporting of child abuse.

_____ **27.** Created a no-fault compensation program for citizens injured or killed by vaccines, as an alternative to suing vaccine manufacturers and providers.

a. Drug Enforcement Agency (DEA)

b. National Childhood Vaccine Injury Act of 1986

c. Food and Drug Administration (FDA)

d. Controlled Substances Act

e. Child Abuse Prevention and Treatment Act of 1974

f. public health statutes

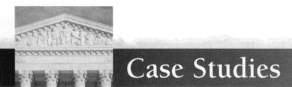

Case Studies

Use your critical-thinking skills to answer the questions that follow the case study.

Barbara, a medical assistant, noticed that her aunt, who suffered chronic pain from a neck injury, carried two bottles of Percodan in her purse. "Two doctors write prescriptions for me," Barbara's aunt confided, "but neither knows about the other. That's the only way I can get enough medication to control my pain."

28. In Barbara's place, would you report your aunt's deception to the physicians named on her prescriptions? Explain your answer.

   _____

   _____

29. What would you tell your aunt?

   _____

   _____

30. How can physicians guard against such abuses by patients?

   _____

   _____

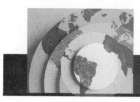

Complete the activities and answer the questions that follow.

31. Visit the Web site for federal statistics. According to the most recent statistics available at the site, what is the current birth rate in the United States?

_____

_____

What is the death rate? What is the leading cause of death in the United States?

_____

_____

32. Visit the Web site for the National Center for Health Statistics. List the current initiatives for the service.

_____

_____

_____

_____

_____

How might this site prove useful in the performance of your duties as a health care practitioner?

_____

_____

33. Visit the Web site for the National Vaccine Information Center. Who must report adverse vaccine reactions?

_____

_____

Where can forms and additional information be obtained?

_____

_____

8 WORKPLACE LEGALITIES

Objectives

After studying this chapter, you should be able to:

1. Recall at least three federal laws that protect employees from discrimination in the workplace.
2. Identify sexual harassment as a form of sexual discrimination.
3. Discuss major federal employment laws.
4. Identify four areas for which standards are mandated by the Occupational Safety and Health Administration (OSHA) for work done in a clinical setting.
5. Discuss the role of health care practitioners in following OSHA standards in the medical office.
6. Comply with the Centers for Disease Control and Prevention's (CDC's) guidelines for universal precautions.
7. Define the role of the Clinical Laboratory Improvement Amendments of 1988 (CLIA) in quality laboratory testing.
8. State the purpose of workers' compensation laws.
9. Explain legal concerns during the employment interview process.
10. Cite the information employers must record for each employee, as dictated by federal and state regulations.

Key Terms

- affirmative action
- Bloodborne Pathogen Standard
- Chemical Hygiene Plan
- Clinical Laboratory Improvement Amendments (CLIA)
- discrimination
- employment-at-will
- General Duty Clause
- Hazard Communication Standard (HCS)
- just cause
- Medical Waste Tracking Act
- Occupational Safety and Health Administration (OSHA)
- public policy
- right-to-know laws
- surety bond
- workers' compensation
- wrongful discharge

How the Law Affects the Workplace

This chapter provides an overview of workplace law, but it does not cover every employment statute and situation. For more detail, consult U.S. and state codes or an attorney specializing in employment law.

Many federal and state laws govern the workplace. Federal laws may apply only to those businesses with a certain number of employees (such as 15, 20, or 50) who work for a minimum number of weeks during the year. State laws may apply to those areas not covered by federal law, or they may extend or overlap existing federal law.

employment-at-will *A concept of employment whereby either the employer or the employee can end the employment at any time, for any reason.*

Traditionally, employment followed the principle of **employment-at-will.** This meant that employees could be refused employment and could be disciplined or fired for any or no reason. In fact, either the employer or the employee could end the employment at any time. Now employment-at-will is affected not only by federal and state statutes, executive orders, and case law but also by contracts between a worker and an employer, collective bargaining agreements between companies and unions, and civil service rules for government workers.

◆ ◆ ◆ ◆ **Hiring and Firing**

Employees generally cannot sue their employers simply because they have been fired, but an employer cannot fire an employee for an illegal reason. When no law exists that prohibits a specific reason for firing an employee, the discharged worker may have cause for litigation under precedent for

wrongful discharge *A concept established by precedent that says an employer risks litigation if he or she does not have just cause for firing an employee.*

just cause *An employer's legal reason for firing an employee.*

public policy *The common law concept of wrongful discharge.*

wrongful discharge. Generally, in such cases the employer must have documentation that shows **just cause** (a legal reason) for dismissing the employee. Promises made to the employee orally, in a written contract, or in a company handbook may be used as evidence should a suit involving wrongful discharge be filed against his or her employer.

State courts vary in their willingness to accept the common law concept of wrongful discharge, but most recognize **public policy,** or "common good," reasons for lawsuits brought by fired employees, such as refusing to commit an illegal act, whistleblowing, performing a legal duty, or exercising a private right.

Court Case

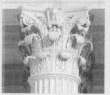

Fired Employee Sues and Wins

A discharged X-ray technician brought suit for breach of employment contract. Her complaint alleged that termination of employment-at-will was in retaliation for her refusal to perform catheterizations, which were illegal for her to perform, since she was not trained to do the procedure.

After the technician's dismissal, the New Jersey Board of Medical Examiners concluded that such an act performed by her would violate the state's medical practice act. The New Jersey Board of Nursing issued a cease-and-desist order to the defendants to stop ordering unqualified personnel to perform catheterizations.

The court ruled that public policy was an issue, since the public has a "foremost interest" in the administration of medical care. The technician won her suit.

O'Sullivan v. Mallon, 390 Atl.2d 149 (1987).

1. Define *employment-at-will.*

_____

_____

2. Define *wrongful discharge.*

_____

_____

3. Define *just cause.*

_____

_____

4. Define *public policy.*

_____

_____

◆ ◆ ◆ ◆ ## Discrimination

discrimination *Prejudiced or prejudicial outlook, action, or treatment.*

Discrimination in the workplace, or treating employees differently in hiring, firing, work assignments, or other aspects of employment because of personal traits or practices, is illegal. Federal laws prohibit employers from firing or otherwise discriminating against employees for any of the following reasons:

- Belonging to a particular race or religion, being one sex or another, or having a particular age or disability.

- Joining a union or engaging in political activity.

- Purposes of preventing the collection of retirement benefits.

- Reporting company safety violations.

- Exercising the right to free speech.

- Refusing to take drug or lie detector tests (with some exceptions).

Most states have passed laws that add to the federal list of prohibited discriminatory employment practices.

Sexual discrimination, or treating employees differently because of gender or sexual preference, has frequently made the news in recent years. Title VII of the Civil Rights Act makes sexual discrimination of any kind illegal. Sexual harassment is considered a form of sexual discrimination. In 1980 the Equal Employment Opportunity Commission (EEOC) defined sexual harassment as follows:

> Unwelcome sexual advances, requests for sexual favors, and other verbal or physical conduct of a sexual nature constitute sexual harassment when (1) submission to such conduct is made either explicitly or implicitly a term or condition of an individual's employment; (2) submission to or rejection of such conduct by an individual is used as a basis for employment decisions affecting such individual; or

(3) such conduct has the purpose or effect of unreasonably interfering with an individual's work performance or creating an intimidating, hostile, or offensive working environment.

Parts 1 and 2 of this definition prohibit what is known as *quid pro quo* (from Latin, meaning "something for something") sexual harassment. Part 3 prohibits conduct that interferes with an employee's work performance or creates a hostile working environment.

Court decisions have affirmed that sexual harassment of employees, either male or female, is cause for legal action. Employers may be found liable even though an employee actually committed the offense. For example, if the offending employee is a supervisor, the employer is usually automatically held liable. If a nonsupervisory employee sexually harasses another worker, the employer is held liable only if he or she knew or should have known about the offense and did nothing to stop it.

Court Case

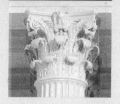

Landmark Case: A Sexual Harassment Case

A bank employee worked for Meritor Savings for more than four years. During that time she claimed that her supervisor continued to make sexual propositions. She finally complied, fearing for her job. She also claimed that her supervisor publicly fondled her and forcibly raped her. When she was fired after an indefinite sick leave, she sued for sexual harassment.

A trial court ruled for the bank, finding no *quid pro quo* discrimination, but the employee appealed, and the appellate court found in her favor. The bank appealed, but the U.S. Supreme Court upheld the appellate court's decision in the plaintiff's favor. In a precedent-setting pronouncement, the Court said, "a plaintiff may establish a violation of Title VII by proving that discrimination based on sex has created a hostile or abusive work environment. . . ." The Court remanded the case to the district court for further proceedings.

Meritor Savings Bank, FSB v. Vinson, 106 S.C. 2399, 91 L.Ed.2d 49, 447 U.S. 57 (U.S. Sup. Ct., 1986).

Check Your Progress

Write "T" or "F" in the space provided to indicate whether you think each statement that follows is true or false.

_____ 5. Sexual harassment in the workplace is cause for legal action.

_____ 6. Sexual harassment may involve any of the following types of interaction: male-female, male-male, female-female, or female-male.

_____ 7. A specific federal law called the Sexual Harassment Act prohibits sexual harassment in the workplace.

_____ 8. *Quid pro quo* refers to the demand for sexual favors in exchange for employment benefits.

_____ 9. Sexual harassment refers only to unwanted physical advances or explicit sexual propositions, not to the creation of an uncomfortable working environment.

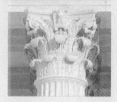
Labor and Employment Laws

The following federal laws cover discrimination in hiring and firing, workers' wages and hours, worker safety, and other workplace issues.

◆ ◆ ◆ ◆ Employment Discrimination Laws

WAGNER ACT OF 1935   This act makes it illegal to discriminate in hiring or firing because of union membership or organizational activities.

TITLE VII OF THE CIVIL RIGHTS ACT OF 1964   This act applies to businesses with 15 or more employees working at least 20 weeks of the year. The law prevents employers from discriminating in hiring or firing on the basis of race, color, religion, sex, or national origin. Some states have laws that also prohibit discrimination based on marital status, parenthood, mental health, mental retardation, sexual orientation, personal appearance, or political affiliation.

affirmative action *Programs that use goals and quotas to provide preferential treatment for minority persons determined to have been underutilized in the past.*

Title VII also specifically prevents federal judges from using **affirmative action** plans—programs intended to remedy the effects of past discrimination—just to correct an imbalance between the percentage of minority persons working for a specific employer and the percentage of qualified minority members in the workplace. Federal judges can order affirmative action plans only when they decide an employer has intentionally discriminated against a minority group.

Title VII created the U.S. Equal Employment Opportunity Commission (EEOC). The EEOC enforces Title VII provisions, the Age Discrimination in Employment Act, the Equal Pay Act, and Section 501 of the Rehabilitation Act. EEOC field offices handle charges or complaints of employment discrimination.

AGE DISCRIMINATION IN EMPLOYMENT ACT   This act applies to businesses with 20 or more employees working at least 20 weeks of the year. It prohibits discrimination in hiring or firing based on age, for persons aged 40 or older.

REHABILITATION ACT OF 1973   This act applies to employers with federal contracts of $2500 or more. It prohibits discrimination in employment practices based on physical disabilities or mental health. It also requires federal contractors to implement affirmative action plans in hiring and promoting disabled employees.

1976 PREGNANCY DISCRIMINATION ACT   This is an amendment to Title VII of the Civil Rights Act that makes it illegal to fire an employee based on pregnancy, childbirth, or related medical conditions.

AMERICANS WITH DISABILITIES ACT OF 1990   This act applies to all employers with 15 or more employees working at least 20 weeks during the year. Titles I and III of the act ban discrimination against disabled persons in the workplace, mandate equal access for the disabled to certain public facilities, and require all commercial firms to make existing facilities and grounds more accessible to the disabled.

Wage and Hour Laws

1935 SOCIAL SECURITY ACT   Funded by the Federal Insurance Contribution Act (FICA), the act now encompasses old-age survivors' insurance (OASI), public disability insurance, unemployment insurance (through the Federal Unemployment Tax Act), and the hospital insurance program (Medicare).

1938 FAIR LABOR STANDARDS ACT   This act prohibits child labor and the firing of employees for exercising their rights under the act's wage and hour standards. It also provides for overtime pay and a minimum wage.

EQUAL PAY ACT OF 1963   As an amendment to the Fair Labor Standards Act, this act requires equal pay for men and women doing equal work.

EMPLOYEE RETIREMENT INCOME SECURITY ACT OF 1974 (ERISA)
This act regulates private pension funds and employer benefit programs. As part of its provisions, employers cannot prevent employees from collecting retirement benefits from plans covered by the act.

Workplace Safety Laws

OCCUPATIONAL SAFETY AND HEALTH ACT OF 1970   This act ensures the safety of workers and prohibits firing an employee for reporting workplace safety hazards or violations.

Other Terms of Employment

FAMILY LEAVE ACT OF 1991   This act applies to employers with 50 or more employees. It mandates allowing employees to take unpaid leave time for maternity, for adoption, or for caring for ill family members.

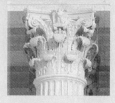
Check Your Progress

10. What federal act makes it illegal for employers to discriminate against employees or potential employees on the basis of race, color, religion, sex, or national origin?

    _____

11. Which act protects the rights of pregnant employees?

    _____

12. Social Security benefits are disbursed under the authority of which act?

    _____

Employee Safety and Welfare

Certain federal and state laws provide specifically for employee safety and welfare. Major areas include workplace safety regulations, including medical hazard regulations, job-related injuries and illnesses, and unemployment or reemployment.

◆ ◆ ◆ ◆ **Occupational Safety and Health Administration (OSHA)**

In the 1960s job-related disabilities and injuries caused more lost workdays in U.S. companies than did strikes. As a result of increasing concern over

Occupational Safety and Health Administration (OSHA) *Established by the Occupational Safety and Health Act of 1970, the act enforces compulsory standards for health and safety in the workplace.*

such statistics, in 1970 Congress passed the Occupational Safety and Health Act. The act established the **Occupational Safety and Health Administration (OSHA),** charged with writing and enforcing compulsory standards for health and safety in the workplace.

With few exceptions, the act covers all employers and employees. Standards cover four areas of employment—general industry, maritime, construction, and agriculture—and include regulations for the physical workplace, machinery and equipment, materials, power sources, processing, protective clothing, first aid, and administrative requirements.

All employers must know the standards that apply to their business. The *Federal Register,* a U.S. government publication that contains all administrative laws, is the primary source of information for OSHA standards.

Under the authority of the U.S. Secretary of Labor, OSHA inspectors may conduct workplace inspections unannounced, issue citations to employers for violations of the act, and in some cases levy fines. The priority of workplace inspections is as follows:

1. Imminent danger situations.

2. Catastrophes, fatalities, and accidents resulting in hospitalization of five or more employees.

3. Valid employee complaints about unsafe or unhealthful working conditions.

4. Specific high-hazard industries, occupations, or substances that are a threat to employees' health.

5. Follow-ups to see whether conditions previously cited have been corrected.

Fines are imposed as penalties for violations. Employers and employees may appeal under some circumstances.

Under OSHA standards both employers and employees have certain rights and responsibilities. Employers must provide a hazard-free workplace and comply with all applicable OSHA standards. Employers must also inform all employees about OSHA safety and health requirements, keep certain records, and compile and post an annual summary of work-related injuries and illnesses. It is the employer's responsibility to ensure that employees wear safety equipment when necessary, to provide safety training, and to discipline employees for violation of safety rules. The law prohibits employers from retaliating in any way against employees who file complaints under the act.

For their part, employees must comply with all applicable OSHA standards, report hazardous conditions, follow all safety and health rules established by the employer, and use protective equipment when necessary.

right-to-know laws *State laws that allow employees access to information about toxic or hazardous substances, employer duties, employee rights, and other workplace health and safety issues.*

Many states have employee **right-to-know laws,** which allow employees access to information about toxic or hazardous substances, employer duties, employee rights, and other health and safety issues.

Federal OSHA authority extends to all private sector employers with one or more employees, as well as to federal civilian employees. In addition, many states administer their own occupational safety and health programs through plans approved under section 18(b) of the federal OSHA act.

OSHA Health Standards

OSHA has created federal laws to protect health care workers from health hazards on the job. Because of the nature of their work, health care practitioners may accidentally become infected with dangerous or even fatal disease viruses. Exposure to toxic substances is another occupational hazard for medical facility workers.

Medical Hazard Regulations

The **Hazard Communication Standard (HCS)** is an OSHA standard that is intended to increase health care practitioners' awareness of risk, improve work practices and appropriate use of personal protective equipment, and reduce injuries and illnesses.

Under the HCS medical offices must have a written hazard communication program. A list of all office hazards must be compiled, posted on bulletin boards, and placed in a hazard communication manual. The list must include hazardous chemicals, hazardous equipment, and hazardous wastes. Hazards often found in the medical office include disinfectant sprays and lab reagents, electrical and mechanical equipment, and blood and body fluids.

Employers must obtain a Material Safety Data Sheet (MSDS) for each hazardous chemical in use in the office. These sheets should be kept on file, and new ones should be posted where employees can readily see them. Manufacturers must supply MSDSs when requested. Each hazardous product in use must have a hazard label, which is a condensed version of the MSDS.

Employees must determine what hazardous chemicals are used, initial and date new MSDSs as they are read, and initial and date records of safety training. Health care practitioners should see that a hazard communication manual is kept up to date and is accessible to all coworkers.

Under the **General Duty Clause** of the HCS, any equipment that may pose a health risk is included as a hazard. This clause covers all areas for which OSHA has not developed specific standards and holds the employer ultimately responsible for the safety of employees: "Each employer shall furnish a place of employment which is free from recognized hazards that are causing or are likely to cause death or serious physical harm to his/her employees."

Chemical Hygiene Plan

The Standard for Occupational Exposures to Hazardous Chemicals in Laboratories, or the **Chemical Hygiene Plan,** further clarifies the proper handling of hazardous chemicals in medical laboratories.

Occupational Exposure to Bloodborne Pathogen Standard

The Occupational Exposure to Bloodborne Pathogen Standard is an OSHA regulation passed in 1991. The standard is designed to protect workers in health care and related occupations from the risk of exposure to blood-borne *pathogens* (disease-causing organisms) such as the human immunodeficiency virus (HIV), which causes AIDS, and the hepatitis B virus (HBV). The standard requires posting safety guidelines, reporting exposure

Hazard Communication Standard (HCS) *An OSHA standard intended to increase health care practitioners' awareness of risks, improve work practices and appropriate use of personal protective equipment, and reduce injuries and illnesses in the workplace.*

General Duty Clause *A section of the Hazard Communication Standard stating that any equipment that may pose a health risk must be specified as a hazard.*

Chemical Hygiene Plan *The Standard for Occupational Exposures to Hazardous Chemicals in Laboratories, which clarifies the handling of hazardous chemicals in medical laboratories.*

incidents, and formulating a written exposure control plan that outlines the protective measures an employer will take to eliminate or minimize employee exposure to blood and other body fluids. The plan must be available to OSHA inspectors and to employees.

As mandated by the Needlestick Safety and Prevention Act, passed by Congress in 2000, the **Bloodborne Pathogen Standard** was revised in 2001 to include new provisions requiring employers to maintain a sharps injury log and to involve nonmanagerial employees in selecting safer medical devices.

Bloodborne Pathogen Standard *The authority by which OSHA can levy fines, based on guidelines of the Centers for Disease Control and Prevention.*

Medical Waste Tracking Act

By authority of the **Medical Waste Tracking Act,** OSHA may inspect hazardous medical wastes and will cite offices for unsafe or unhealthy practices regarding these wastes. Hazardous medical wastes include blood products, body fluids, tissues, cultures, vaccines (live and weakened), sharps, table paper (with body fluids on them), gloves, speculums, cotton swabs, and inoculating loops.

A puncture-proof, approved sharps container must be provided for the disposal of sharp objects. Chemicals should be discarded in a glass or metal container. Flushable chemicals can be washed down the drain with large quantities of water. Other hazardous medical wastes must be contained in plastic, leakproof biohazard bags. Incineration is often used to dispose of medical wastes. Reputable, licensed waste handlers should be used to handle this material.

Medical Waste Tracking Act *The federal law that authorizes OSHA to inspect hazardous medical wastes and to cite offices for unsafe or unhealthy practices regarding these wastes.*

Training and Accident Report Documentation

Under OSHA standards each employer must have a written training program detailing how employees will be provided with information and training regarding hazards in the workplace. Training should include information about hazards in the work area, the location of the list of hazards and MSDSs, explanations of MSDSs and the hazardous chemical labeling system, and any measures that employees can take to protect themselves against these hazards. Training logs should be kept, and employees who complete training should sign and date the log.

Accidents occurring in the office must be reported. Reports should include:

- Employer's name and address.

- Employee's name, address, and phone number.

- Specific information about the accident—that is, when, where, what, and how it occurred.

- Nature of the injury.

- Follow-up information such as medical treatment or hospitalization.

Each employer who is subject to OSHA record-keeping requirements must maintain a log of all occupational injuries and illnesses. Logs must be kept for five years following the end of the calendar year to which they relate and must be available for inspection by representatives of the U.S. Department of Labor, the U.S. Department of Health and Human Services, and state officials.

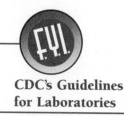

OSHA standards for health care settings may be obtained from the U.S. Department of Labor, Occupational Safety and Health Administration, Directorate of Health Standards Programs, 200 Constitution Ave., N.W., Washington, D.C. 20210 or from state or regional OSHA offices.

Centers for Disease Control and Prevention (CDC) Guidelines

CDC guidelines divide tasks for health care practitioners into two groups. Category I tasks include those that involve potential contact of mucous membranes or skin with blood, body fluids, or tissue. This category also includes potential for spills or splashes. Gloves, eye masks, gowns, and other protective equipment are required for these tasks. Such tasks include capillary puncture, phlebotomy, pelvic exams, minor suturing, and throat culture.

Category II tasks do not involve direct contact with blood, body fluids, or tissue. Because unplanned exposure may occur, however, protective equipment should be worn by health care practitioners who perform these tasks, which include urinalysis, fecal occult blood, X rays, ultrasound, ECG, injections, and the examination of sweat, tears, saliva, and nasal secretions.

The CDC maintains an online database of universal precautions guidelines that includes more specific information on a variety of disease and exposure topics.

Clinical Laboratory Improvement Amendments (CLIA) of 1988

The **Clinical Laboratory Improvement Amendments (CLIA)** of 1988 replaced 1967 laboratory testing legislation that established standards for Medicare and Medicaid. The 1988 amendments established minimum quality standards for all laboratory testing. The regulations define a laboratory as any facility that performs laboratory testing on specimens derived from humans for diagnosing, preventing, or treating disease, or for assessing health. The law requires that laboratories obtain certification, pay applicable fees, and follow regulations concerning testing, personnel, inspections, test management, quality control, and quality assurance.

The Centers for Medicare and Medicaid Services (CMS), formerly the Health Care Finance Administration (HCFA), enforces CLIA regulations. After laboratories register, they are inspected by the CMS. If approved, the laboratories are then issued a certificate and assessed appropriate fees.

Workers' Compensation ◆ ◆ ◆ ◆

Federal and state **workers' compensation** laws establish procedures for compensating workers who are injured on the job. The employer pays the cost of the insurance premium for the employee. These laws allow the injured worker to file a claim for compensation with the state or the federal government instead of suing. However, the laws require workers to accept workers' compensation as the exclusive remedy for on-the-job injuries. Federal laws cover workers in Washington, D.C.; coal miners;

YOU BE THE JUDGE

The relationship between cleanliness and disease has been established, over time, within the medical community. Despite the conclusive evidence that "germs" cause disease and clean hands help stop the spread of germs, a recent study suggests that many doctors and other health care practitioners are not as careful as they should be to wash hands between patient contacts. In one intensive care unit surveyed, only about 17 percent of physicians complied with the recommended regimen, which includes lathering hands with germicidal soap, rinsing twice for at least 30 seconds, then drying thoroughly.

Studies have revealed that 20,000 people die each year in the United States as the result of infections contracted in hospitals. Hand-washing alone won't solve the problem, but hand-to-hand and glove-to-glove contact between health care provider and patient is still a major route of disease transmission.

Some hospitals and other medical facilities are suggesting that patients remind doctors, nurses, and other health care practitioners to wash their hands before beginning an examination or treatment.

In your opinion, is this a reasonable approach to the problem? Explain your answer.

_____

_____

_____

What other methods might be used in addition to or instead of patient involvement to encourage proper hygiene among health care practitioners?

_____

_____

Do you believe hygiene is a moral obligation for health care practitioners? Explain your answer.

_____

_____

_____

Clinical Laboratory Improvement Amendments (CLIA)
Federal statutes passed in 1988 that established minimum quality standards for all laboratory testing.
workers' compensation *A form of insurance established by federal and state statutes that provides reimbursement for workers who are injured on the job.*

maritime workers; and federal employees. State laws cover workers not protected under federal statutes.

Workers who are injured on the job or who contract an occupational disease may apply for five types of state compensation benefits:

- Medical treatment, including hospital, medical and surgical services, medications, and prosthetic devices.

- Temporary disability indemnity, in the form of weekly cash payments made directly to the injured or ill employee.

- Permanent disability indemnity, which can be a lump sum award or a weekly or monthly cash payment.

- Death benefits for survivors, which consist of cash payments to dependents of employees killed on the job.

- Rehabilitation benefits, which are paid for medical or vocational rehabilitation.

Employees who are injured on the job or become ill due to work-related causes must immediately report the injury or illness to a supervisor. An injury report and claim for compensation are then filed with the appropriate state workers' compensation agency. Forms from the attending or designated workers' compensation physician who examines and treats the employee must also be filed with the appropriate agency as proof of the employee's injury or illness.

A medical facility employee may be responsible for filing the physician's report with the state workers' compensation agency. Requirements concerning waiting periods and other filing specifics vary with each state. When a claim is filed, all questions must be answered in full and as thoroughly as possible.

Court Case

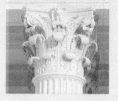

Negligence Tried Under Workers' Compensation

An employee who was seven months pregnant was suffering from severe abdominal pain and consulted the company's nurse. The nurse told her she had gas pains and should rest. When the employee's pain did not subside, the nurse took her to the company dispensary in a wheelchair. The employee asked to see a physician, but the nurse assured her that she did not need one. A coworker called the employee's husband, who persuaded the nurse to call an ambulance.

About 50 minutes after she first felt sick, the employee arrived at the hospital. There it was discovered that her uterus had ruptured. The baby was delivered by cesarean section and had brain damage and other medical problems. The infant died at the age of 28 months. The employee, her husband, and the deceased infant brought an action against the employer. They claimed that the nurse had negligently treated the employee's pregnancy complications, resulting in the infant's brain damage and eventual death.

The employee's claims for damages were brought under California's workers' compensation law. The employer said the claims were barred by the exclusive-remedy provisions of the law, and a trial court granted the employer's motion for summary judgment.

On appeal, however, the appellate court said the injury to the employee was caused by improper treatment at an employer-provided clinic and was within the compensation law. The court further held that the injury to the infant was a collateral consequence of the treatment of the employee. Since the infant's injuries were the direct result of the work-related negligence toward the employee, they were within the conditions of compensation of the workers' compensation law. Therefore, any mental distress suffered by the parents derived from the same source.

Bell v. Macy's California, 261 Cal. Rptr. 447 (Cal. Ct. of App., Aug. 11, 1989).

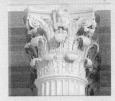

Nurse Who Developed MS Not Disabled Under ADA

A nurse who worked in a hospital's burn unit was also an AirMed Flight Nurse. After three years on the job, she was diagnosed with multiple sclerosis (MS). The nurse was hospitalized for five days, then was cleared to return to work. However, the nurse's supervisor was concerned that she could no longer perform her duties as a flight nurse. The supervisor and the director of the AirMed Department compiled a list of job qualifications and presented it to the nurse's doctor, who then stated that he could not provide her with a work release.

Due to the AirMed director's concerns about patient safety should the nurse suffer episodes because of her MS, the nurse was not allowed to return to duty as a flight nurse, but she did return to duty in the hospital's burn unit. She subsequently quit her job, then filed a complaint against the hospital alleging that she was disabled and that the hospital had violated the Americans with Disabilities Act by dismissing her from her AirMed duties.

A district court found that the nurse was not disabled within the meaning of the ADA and her case was dismissed. An appeals court confirmed the district court's ruling. The court held, in part, "Because [the nurse's] hospitalization and MS symptoms affected her for only a brief period of time and do not presently impact her ability to perform the job, [she] did not suffer an impairment that substantially limits a major life activity under the ADA."

Sorensen v. University of Utah Hospital, 194 F.3d 1084 (10th Cir.) (Oct. 14, 1999).

♦ ♦ ♦ ♦   **Unemployment Insurance**

Unemployment insurance (sometimes called reemployment insurance) funds are managed jointly by state and federal governments. Under the Federal Unemployment Tax Act (FUTA), employers contribute to a fund that is paid out to eligible unemployed workers. Each state also provides unemployment insurance, and credit is given employers against the FUTA tax for amounts paid to the state unemployment fund. The total cost is borne by the employer in all but a few states.

Out-of-work employees should contact a state unemployment office to determine whether they qualify for unemployment benefits. Ex-employees are denied unemployment compensation for three main reasons: (1) they quit their jobs without cause, (2) they were fired for misconduct, or (3) they are unemployed because of a labor dispute. Independent contractors and self-employed individuals usually do not qualify for unemployment compensation.

Individuals may file for unemployment benefits at state unemployment offices. Claimants need:

• Social Security card.

• W-2 statements for the past one to two years.

• Other wage records for the past 18 months.

• Employers' names and addresses for the past 18-month employment period.

• Statement of reasons for leaving the job.

• Employer's unemployment insurance account number, if available.

13. List three OSHA standards that deal specifically with health care workers' safety.

_____

_____

_____

14. Distinguish between workers' compensation and unemployment insurance.

_____

_____

_____

Hiring and the New Employee

When interviewing for a position or when asked to interview a job applicant, the health care practitioner must know legal boundaries.

◆ ◆ ◆ ◆ **Interviews**

Because of federal and state laws against discrimination in hiring, inquiries cannot be made concerning an applicant's:

- Race or color.
- Religion or creed.
- Gender.
- Family.
- Marital status.
- Method of birth control.
- Age, birth date, or birthplace.
- Disability.
- Arrest record (with some exceptions in many states).
- Residency duration.
- National origin. (However, the Immigration Reform and Control Act of 1986 requires new employees to complete an I-9 form, intended to prevent the employment of illegal aliens.)
- General military experience or discharge.
- Membership in organizations.

Questions concerning one's Social Security number, qualifications (including license or certificate), and job experience are proper, and they should be answered as thoroughly and truthfully as possible. As part of the hiring process, applicants may be asked to take a physical examination.

During a job interview, applicants may refuse to answer a question that is clearly improper or not job-related, but this could cost them the job. The question, "May I ask how this relates to the position?" is generally more acceptable than a blunt, "That question is illegal, and I don't have to answer it." Furthermore, the mere asking of an improper preemployment interview question does not in itself give an applicant grounds for a legal challenge if he or she is not hired.

The following guidelines can help employees who are responsible for conducting preemployment interviews:

- Make a list of questions that relate specifically to the job description of the position to be filled, and stick to them.

- Do not rush the interview, nor let it drag on beyond reasonable time limits.

- General questions that may prove helpful include these: What are your qualifications for this position? Why are you leaving your present position? Why do you want this job? What salary do you expect? When can you begin work? What are your professional strengths? What are your professional goals?

- Remain objective and listen well.

- End the interview on a positive note. Indicate when a decision will be made, and follow through on your promise to inform the applicant of your decision, one way or the other.

Check Your Progress

15. Place a check mark beside any questions that are considered to be illegal if asked in a preemployment interview.

_____ Why are you leaving your present position?

_____ Do you belong to a church?

_____ What do you hope to achieve over the next five years?

_____ How many children do you have, and how old are they?

_____ Who will watch your children while you work?

_____ Why do you want to work for us?

_____ How many years' experience do you have as a medical assistant?

_____ What nationality are you?

Lab Supervisor Emphasizes Importance of Documentation

As the supervisor of a state medical laboratory in the Midwest, Marie has been responsible for hiring employees to fill 11 positions and for firing employees whose work is unsatisfactory.

Because Marie's lab does microbiology tests for the state, including bacteriology, parasitology, serology, virology, and immunology, she is keenly aware of the importance of accuracy in test results.

"We have a litigious public," Marie remarks, "and we can be sued if a laboratory test is not right. We are dependent on machines for test results, but we [the lab director and lab supervisor] are responsible for the errors of laboratory employees. The federal guidelines for a technical supervisor say that that person is responsible for every test result signed out."

Marie recalls a false positive test result that was extremely troublesome because it could have caused injury to a patient. "[The patient] was pregnant and was given a certain medication as the result of a reported test result of 'positive' for a sexually transmitted disease. The result reported should have been 'negative.' The drug was not contraindicated for a pregnant woman, but she should not have had to take it. Plus, she had the emotional distress of receiving a false positive STD test result." The error was reported to the woman's treating physician, and Marie was never informed of any ill effects.

The laboratory employee who committed the error had a two-year work history of certain behavior problems, such as failing to show up for work and alcohol and drug problems that led to counseling. Marie had carefully documented the employee's behavior. She had also documented that she consistently checked and rechecked this person's work, often finding errors, and had met with the employee weekly to discuss progress and expectations. When the STD test result was reported in error, she felt the employee responsible could no longer be trusted, and that she had ample grounds for dismissal.

The employee was fired. Because of Marie's careful documentation, the employee had scant grounds for protesting the action and did not. "Good documentation is essential for those responsible for hiring and firing employees," Marie reiterates.

◆ ◆ ◆ ◆ **Bonding**

surety bond *A type of insurance that allows employers, if covered, to collect up to the specified amount of the bond if an employee embezzles or otherwise absconds with business funds.*

In some medical offices and other workplace locations where employees are responsible for collecting fees and handling financial matters, prospective employees may be asked whether they are bondable. An employer can purchase a **surety bond** for a specific amount from an insurance carrier. If a bonded employee should embezzle or otherwise abscond with funds, the employer can collect from the insurance carrier, up to the amount of the bond. However, the employer must have filed a complaint against the alleged dishonest employee in order to collect on the bond. If the insurance company pays the bond, it will then seek to recover the amount from the offending employee.

♦ ♦ ♦ ♦ Employment Paperwork

Once employed, the new worker will be asked to provide certain information so that the employer may comply with federal and state regulations. Complete records for every employee must include:

- Social Security number.

- Number of exemptions claimed.

- Gross salary.

- Deductions for Social Security, Medicare, and federal, state, and city taxes.

- Withholding for state disability insurance, state unemployment tax, and health care plans, if applicable.

The law requires employers to withhold specified amounts from employees' pay and to keep records of and send these sums to the proper income tax center. The amount to be withheld is based on the employee's total salary, the number of exemptions he or she claims, marital status, and the length of the pay period involved.

Health care practitioners who are self-employed do not have to deduct withholding, but they must make quarterly city, state, and federal income tax payments. Self-employed individuals must also pay Social Security taxes (FICA), via a self-employment tax percentage that is higher than the rate paid by individuals who are not self-employed. The difference lies in the fact that a self-employed individual is making both the employer and the employee contribution.

Employers must provide each employee with a Form W-2, Wage and Tax Statement, by January 31 of each year. The W-2 shows the following information:

- Employer's tax identification number.

- Employee's Social Security number.

- Total earnings (wages and other compensation) paid by the employer.

- Amounts deducted for income tax and Social Security.

- Amount of advance earned income credit payment, if any.

Most employers want the workplace to be as pleasant and safe for employees as it can possibly be. However, it is still the employee's responsibility to know the employment legalities most likely to affect him or her and to work within this legal framework to help ensure a satisfying and productive employer-employee relationship.

Applying Knowledge

Answer the following questions or complete the following statements in the spaces provided.

1. Under the concept of employment-at-will, who has the right to terminate employment?

   _____

2. What evidence may be produced to substantiate a wrongful discharge claim?

   _____

3. List three federal laws that protect employees from potential discrimination.

   _____

   _____

   _____

4. Title VII of the _____ Act makes sexual discrimination illegal.

   _____ is considered a form of sexual discrimination.

5. What federal office can be contacted to report any charges or complaints of employment discrimination?

   _____

6. _____,"something for something," is a form of sexual harassment. Another form of sexual harassment is behavior toward an employee that creates a(n) _____ that interferes with an employee's work performance.

7. _____ laws allow an injured employee to file a claim with the state or federal government instead of _____ . However, employees are required to accept this compensation as a(n) _____ for on-the-job illness or injury.

8. For what three reasons may an ex-employee be denied unemployment compensation?

   _____

   _____

   _____

9. What information is given on the employee's Form W-2?

   _____

   _____

   _____

   _____

   _____

10. What government publication is the primary source for locating OSHA standards?

   _____

Write "T" or "F" in the space provided to indicate whether you think each of the following statements is true or false.

_____11. OSHA standards require an employer to provide a safe workplace, to inform employees about hazards, to keep certain records, and to post an annual summary of accidents.

_____12. Employers have no responsibility for providing safety training or appropriate safety equipment for employees.

_____13. OSHA requires an employee to comply with all applicable OSHA standards, to follow safety rules, and to use protective equipment when necessary.

_____14. CDC guidelines divide tasks for health care workers into two groups. Examples of Category I tasks include phlebotomy and urinalysis.

_____15. An improper question asked by an employer in a preemployment interview will, in itself, give the applicant grounds for legal challenge if he or she is not hired.

_____16. Manufacturers of potentially hazardous chemicals must supply, on request, a Material Safety Data Sheet (MSDS) for a specific product.

_____17. The Centers for Disease Control and Prevention enforce regulations concerning universal precautions in the medical office.

Match each description that follows with the correct term by writing the appropriate letter in the space provided.

_____18. Established the EEOC.

_____19. Makes it illegal to discriminate because of pregnancy, childbirth, or related medical conditions.

_____20. Protects employees aged 40 or older.

_____21. Protects employees who engage in union or other organizational activities.

_____22. Regulates private pension funds and employer benefit programs.

_____23. Requires equal pay for equal work.

_____24. Ensures a safe work environment.

_____25. Regulates child labor and provides for minimum wages and overtime pay.

_____26. Provides for Medicare, unemployment insurance, disability, and OASI, through FICA funding.

_____27. Protects the disabled and mentally ill.

_____28. Provides minimum federal standards for quality laboratory testing.

a. Wagner Act
b. Social Security Act
c. Fair Labor Standards Act
d. Equal Pay Act
e. Civil Rights Act of 1964
f. Age Discrimination in Employment Act
g. Occupational Safety and Health Act
h. Rehabilitation Act
i. Employee Retirement Income Security Act
j. Pregnancy Discrimination Act
k. Clinical Laboratory Improvement Amendments

Use your critical-thinking skills to answer the questions that follow the case study.

You are a surgical assistant in a large hospital. Whenever you work with a certain surgeon she tells off-color jokes to you and your coworkers and makes blatantly suggestive comments to workers of the opposite sex. One coworker tells you that he might quit his job because he is married and the surgeon's behavior makes him so uncomfortable that he dreads coming to work.

29. **Is the surgeon's behavior illegal or simply in bad taste? Explain your answer.**

   _____

   _____

   _____

   _____

   _____

30. **Do you or your coworkers have grounds for a sexual harassment complaint? Explain your answer.**

   _____

   _____

   _____

   _____

   _____

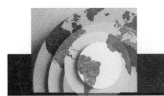

Internet Activities

Complete the activities and answer the questions that follow.

31. Find the government Web site for sexual harassment. Click on "FAQs" and list two common questions about sexual harassment.

   _____

   _____

32. Visit the fedeal government's OSHA Web site. Click on "Enforcement." What are the rules the government must follow regarding negotiation and filing lawsuits?

   _____

   _____

33. Access the Web site for OSHA. Find the location of the OSHA office for your area. What is the office's address? Under what circumstances, as a health care worker, might you want to contact OSHA?

   _____

   _____

   _____

THE BEGINNING OF LIFE AND CHILDHOOD

Objectives

After studying this chapter, you should be able to:

1. Define genetics and heredity.
2. Distinguish between DNA, chromosomes, and genes.
3. List several situations in which genetic testing might be appropriate.
4. Discuss genetic discrimination.
5. Define cloning and explain why it is a controversial issue.
6. Discuss some of the pros and cons of genetic engineering.
7. Explain why stem cells are useful for scientific research.
8. Distinguish between mature and emancipated minors and discuss situations in which such minors might legally make their own health care decisions.

Key Terms

- amniocentesis
- chromosome
- cloning
- DNA
- emancipated minors
- gene
- gene therapy
- genetic counseling
- genetic discrimination
- genetic engineering
- genetics
- genome
- heredity
- heterologous artificial insemination
- homologous artificial insemination
- Human Genome Project
- in vitro fertilization
- mature minors
- *parens patriae*
- stem cells
- surrogate
- xenotransplantation

The Influence of Technology on the Beginning of Life

Health care practitioners have always had to make informed decisions based on legal and ethical principles and on personal values. But in today's technological world the task becomes even more difficult, perhaps especially when those decisions apply to the beginning of life and to childhood.

Genetics

genetics *The study of heredity.*

heredity *The process by which organisms pass genetic traits on to their offspring.*

DNA *Deoxyribonucleic acid. The combination of proteins called nucleotides that comprises an organism's chromosomes.*

chromosome *Microscopic structures found within the nucleus of plant and animal cells that carry genes responsible for the organism's characteristics.*

gene *A tiny segment of DNA found on a cell's chromosomes. Each gene holds the formula for making a specific molecule.*

genome *All the genetic information necessary to create a human being or any other organism.*

Genetics was often in the news from the mid-1990s into the twenty-first century, as scientists published the results of experiments in genetics research. **Genetics,** as you probably remember from earlier science courses, is the study of **heredity,** or how traits are passed from one generation to the next.

As a result of genetic research, improved science education, and extensive media coverage of genetics procedures and issues, health care practitioners and members of the general public have become familiar with the term **DNA** (deoxyribonucleic acid). DNA is the combination of proteins called nucleotides that comprises each human **chromosome.** Forty-six chromosomes (23 pair) are found inside the nucleus of every human cell except egg and sperm cells, which have 23 chromosomes each. We inherit half of our chromosome complement from our mother and half from our father. These 46 chromosomes carry the genes responsible for all our human characteristics, from eye, skin, and hair color to height, body type, and intelligence. Each **gene** is a tiny segment of DNA that holds the formula for making a specific molecule.

The genes that make up the human **genome**—all the genetic information necessary to create a human being—are responsible for all the cells, organs, tissues, and traits that make up each individual. Some of these genes are also responsible for the more than four thousand genetic diseases that can afflict human beings, including cystic fibrosis, sickle cell anemia, hemophilia, Huntington's disease, Down's syndrome, Tay-Sachs Disease, multiple sclerosis, some forms of cancer, and other diseases.

Check Your Progress

1. The science that studies inherited traits (heredity) is _____ .

2. The threadlike structures inside cell nuclei that are comprised of DNA and carry an organism's genes are _____ .

3. All the genes necessary to replicate a human being make up the _____ .

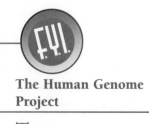

Genetic Testing ◆ ◆ ◆ ◆

Like fingerprints, each individual's DNA is unique to that person, so DNA testing has become a reliable method of identifying the source of body fluids and tissues left at crime scenes, determining parentage, and testing for other genetic information. Specially trained technicians perform DNA tests. The tests are conducted from samples of solid tissues, such as hair roots or skin, and from bodily fluids such as blood, semen, or saliva.

In addition to forensic use and tracing lineage, genetic testing has made it possible for individuals to determine whether they carry a gene for an inherited disease and for expectant parents to determine, through **amniocentesis,** whether a developing fetus shows signs of abnormalities. During amniocentesis the physician withdraws a sample of amniotic fluid (the fluid surrounding the developing fetus inside the mother's womb) from a woman's pregnant uterus. The fluid is then tested for genetic or other conditions that may lead to abnormal development of the fetus. Down's syndrome is one inherited condition that is often detected through amniocentesis.

Individuals who come from families in which certain inherited diseases have appeared may opt for genetic testing to confirm or rule out the presence of a disease-causing gene. For example, Huntington's chorea runs in families, but symptoms typically do not develop until individuals reach middle age. Since the disease is incurable, debilitating, and fatal, affecting the brain and the nervous system, adults who have relatives who have developed the disease may opt to be tested in order to plan for any eventuality.

On the other hand, individuals with a family history of incurable inherited diseases may opt not to be tested, simply to preserve peace of mind. Health care practitioners should refer any patient who undergoes genetic testing to a **genetic counselor.** Genetic counselors can explain test results and help patients deal with difficult questions concerning those results.

Some inherited diseases for which genetic tests are available include:

- Cystic fibrosis, a disease that affects the production of mucus and is eventually fatal.

- Down's syndrome, a disease that causes mental retardation and other physical problems.

- Fragile X disease, a common source of mental retardation.

- Gaucher's disease, a condition affecting fat metabolism.

- Hemochromatosis, an iron storage disorder and the most commonly occurring inherited disease.

- Huntington's chorea, an untreatable, ultimately fatal disease of the brain and nervous system.

- Mucopolysaccaridosis (MPS), a metabolic disorder that causes skeletal deformities and usually mental retardation.

- Phenylketonuria (PKU), a metabolic disorder for which all newborns are tested; it results in mental retardation if left untreated.

- Sickle-cell anemia, a malformation of the red blood cells most often diagnosed in African Americans.

- Some forms of breast, ovarian, and colon cancer.

- Spinocerebellar ataxia, a rare disorder that eventually destroys the brain's cerebellum.

- Tay-Sachs, a lipid metabolism disorder that affects some people of Jewish descent.

As genetic testing has become more widely available and more reliable, use of test results has become an important issue. For example, if a couple learns through amniocentesis that the fetus the mother is carrying will be born with Down's syndrome, should they consider aborting the fetus? Should the young man who learns he has the gene for Huntington's chorea opt not to marry, to avoid taking the chance of passing the gene on to offspring? And will the woman who learns she has one of two genes known to predispose her to breast cancer live her life any differently than she would had she not been tested?

VOICE OF EXPERIENCE

Genetic Research: Checks and Balances

Carma is an oncology certified RN with a masters degree in health administration. She is also the research administrator for the Human Gene Therapy Department of a Midwestern health system. The Human Gene Therapy Department where Carma works is a private facility funded by grants and the sponsoring health system. According to Carma, the mission of her department is "to advance and apply the science of gene therapy for cancer." The department does laboratory research and performs clinical trials for the use of gene therapy.

In one clinical trial, scientists at Carma's department genetically altered a virus to be used in targeting ovarian cancer cells. Two additional projects deal with breast cancer. One involves developing a breast cancer vaccine and the other uses radioactive iodine to target breast cancer cells, much like radioactive iodine is used to treat thyroid cancer.

Carma says that data provided by the Human Genome Project has helped further the work of her department. "We still don't know, though, how genes are linked," she emphasizes. "For example, two of the genes that cause breast cancer have been identified, but since we are not sure how genes interact, if we alter those genes to not cause cancer, there could be a cascade of other effects."

Carma's facility does not do genetic testing, but she stresses that such testing should not be done without genetic counseling. Carma also emphasizes that many checks and balances exist for gene therapy research and clinical trials. "Gene therapy protocols within our department must be approved by the Institutional Review Board (IRB), a local group composed of scientific and medical personnel as well as chaplains and other lay people. Any research project involving humans in any way (physically as well as psychologically) needs approval from the IRB." Any gene therapy protocol is also subject to FDA approval.

An ethical concern in genetic research, Carma adds, is to question whether a project should be done just because it is possible. "Just because we can do it doesn't always mean we should do it," she emphasizes.

Genetic testing has also raised the issue of privacy. For instance, should employers and health and life insurance companies have access to genetic test results? How can individuals be certain that information about their genetic makeup is not shared with unknown sources?

Clearly, advances in genetics and genetic testing have led to difficult ethical, social, and medical questions for patients and their families and for health care practitioners.

◆ ◆ ◆ ◆ Genetic Testing and Discrimination

genetic discrimination *Differential treatment of individuals based on their actual or presumed genetic differences.*

With the increased ability to identify genetic differences comes increasing concern for the proper use of such information. The term **genetic discrimination** describes the differential treatment of individuals based on their actual or presumed genetic differences.

Harvard Medical School's Lisa N. Geller and her colleagues conducted a comprehensive and often-quoted study of genetic discrimination throughout the 1990s. The study found that a number of institutions were reported to have engaged in genetic discrimination, including health and life insurance companies, health care providers, blood banks, adoption agencies, the military, and schools. Geller's study included individuals at risk for or related to people with hemochromatosis, phenylketonuria (PKU), mucopolysaccaridosis (MPS), and Huntington's chorea.

Out of 917 respondents who returned questionnaires for Geller's study, 455 said they had experienced genetic discrimination. In one case a health maintenance organization had covered the medical expenses of a child since birth but refused to pay for occupational therapy after she was diagnosed with mucopolysaccaridosis, claiming that the condition was pre-existing.

In another case a 24-year-old woman was denied life insurance due to her family history of Huntington's chorea and the fact that she had not been tested for the presence of the gene. If she agreed to be tested and was found not to carry the gene, the insurance company would issue her a policy.

Geller also reported that in several cases medical professionals reportedly pressured patients at risk for having children with serious genetic conditions to undergo prenatal diagnostic testing or to decide against having children.

There are now laws in place to prevent genetic discrimination. By the end of the year 2000, 39 states had laws prohibiting discrimination in health insurance based on genetic tests, and 15 states had passed laws forbidding genetic discrimination in employment. In addition, the Health Insurance Portability and Accountability Act (HIPAA) passed in 1996 prevents health insurers from denying coverage based on genetic information. HIPAA, however, applies only to individuals moving between group health insurance plans. (Chapter 2 discusses HIPAA in detail.)

The Americans with Disabilities Act (ADA) of 1990, discussed in Chapter 8, also offers some protection against genetic discrimination in the workplace. It protects against discrimination those who have a genetic condition or disease or who are regarded as having a disability. Under a 1995 ruling by the Equal Employment Opportunities Commission, the ADA applies to anyone who is discriminated against on the basis of genetic information relating to illness, disease, condition, or other disorders. Provisions of the ADA do not cover insurance companies.

In February 2000, then President Bill Clinton signed an executive order banning the federal government from using genetic data in employment decisions. Under the order the government cannot request or require job applicants or employees to take genetic tests. The government is also prohibited from using information from genetic tests in hiring or promotion decisions.

◆ ◆ ◆ ◆

Genetic Engineering

genetic engineering *Manipulating DNA within the cells of plants and animals, to ensure that certain harmful traits will be eliminated in offspring and that desirable traits will appear and be passed on.*

Our increased body of knowledge about DNA, chromosome structure, and the basis of heredity has allowed scientists to manipulate DNA within the cells of plants and animals to ensure that certain traits will appear and be passed on. This is called **genetic engineering.** Because the chemical composition of DNA is nearly identical throughout the plant and animal kingdoms, genes can often be interchanged among plants and animals to transfer desirable characteristics to different species. Through this process, for example, genes from a species of Arctic flounder have been added to strawberry plants to make them better able to withstand cold temperatures. Genetic engineering has also created corn and soybean crops that are resistant to insect-borne diseases, "golden" rice with increased beta carotene content, and bacteria that can devour oil spilled into oceans.

However beneficial a genetic engineering project may sound, controversy is almost guaranteed as a new project is announced. Objections may be raised on the religious or moral grounds that humans simply should not tamper with the time-honored progression of life as dictated by nature. Or opponents may fear that the process will harm the environment by releasing genetically engineered superspecies that may crowd out naturally occurring species and lead to the eventual disappearance of many original organisms. Critics may also fear that the undisclosed addition of genes to plants or animals ingested by humans can have unforeseen effects. For instance, some fear that genes from peanut plants added to a product might cause harmful reactions in unsuspecting consumers who are allergic to peanuts.

Clearly, if genetic engineering is to truly benefit society, scientists and governments must consider the objections and fears of consumers and the general public and proceed with research in a manner that takes these concerns into account.

Cloning

cloning *The process by which organisms are created asexually, usually from a single cell of the parent organism.*

One type of genetic engineering that has become extremely controversial is **cloning.** The word *clone* comes from the Latin root meaning "to cut from." A clone is an organism grown from a single cell of the parent, and it is genetically identical to the parent. In other words, the genes and chromosomes found in each cell's nucleus are the same in clone and parent. Identical twins are clones. So are all the cells in our bodies, except for eggs and sperm.

The term *cloning* became familiar to the general public with the birth of Dolly, a Finn Dorset sheep, in July 1996. Dolly was the product of scientists at the Roslin Institute near Edinburgh, Scotland. Her birth was controversial because she was the world's first mammal cloned from an adult parent cell. That is, Dolly was not the product of union of egg and sperm but was created from a single cell scraped from the inside of her six-year-old mother's udder. Scientists used a process called nuclear transfer to clone Dolly from the udder cell.

Since Dolly's birth scientists have cloned cattle, goats, mice, monkeys, and pigs. One objective of the cloning of farm and laboratory animals is to breed genetically identical animals that can produce substances useful in medicine, such as insulin and growth hormone. Another objective in cloning farm animals is the consistent production of prime, low-fat meat.

A third objective of animal cloning is to clone animal tissues and organs for human medical use. Because pigs are similar to humans in organ size and other biological aspects, an objective in cloning them is to grow a potential source of organs and tissue for transplanting into human patients. Transplanting animal tissues and organs into humans is called **xenotransplantation.** Research in this area is continuing, but at least two major problems make the process difficult. Animal cells produce a sugar that human cells do not, causing a severe immune rejection reaction in humans when animal tissues are transplanted. In addition, scientists have found that human cells can be infected with some viruses found in animals.

Many animal-rights proponents object on ethical grounds to using animals in this way. They argue that animals should be allowed to exist in nature without being subjected to experiments for the benefit of humankind.

Recent successes in animal cloning have led to the important question, Should we extend our cloning knowledge to clone human embryos, even if solely for research purposes?

xenotransplantation *Transplanting animal tissues and organs into humans.*

◆ ◆ ◆ ◆ ## Human Stem Cell Research

stem cells *Early embryonic cells that have the potential to become any type of body cell.*

Early stage human embryos, called blastocysts, consist of about 20 cells and are considered valuable for research because they are composed of **stem cells.** These early embryonic cells are called stem cells because they have the potential to become any type of body cell, including bone, blood, muscle, brain, thyroid, liver, and other cell types. Interest in this type of research remains intense because stem cells have shown promise for treating patients with a wide variety of medical problems. For example, stem cells that develop into neuronal tissue could be used to treat patients with Parkinson's and Alzheimer's diseases, as well as patients with strokes, spinal cord injuries, and other neurological diseases. Stem cells that become pancreatic islet cells might help those with diabetes. Skin tissue grown from stem cells could replace burned tissue, and cultivated cardiac tissue might help damaged arteries and hearts.

Most embryos used in stem cell research in the United States are the frozen products of in vitro fertilization that were not used to produce a pregnancy and are destined to be destroyed. However, a private research facility in the United States—Advanced Cell Technology in Worcester, Massachusetts—announced in November 2001 that scientists there had cloned a human embryo for use in stem cell research.

Opponents to human embryonic stem cell research argue that regardless of how the embryos were created, they are potential human beings with inherent rights to ethical and legal protection. Others argue that because the embryos are not growing within a uterus, they are not subject to the same protection as fetuses, and as most would be destroyed anyway, the good that could come from such research far outweighs any downside.

Because of the controversy over using human embryonic cells in research, scientists are searching for other sources of stem cells that do not require the destruction of human embryos. For example, stem cells have been recovered from umbilical cord and placenta, and some adult human body tissues, such as bone marrow and fat, have been found to function as stem cells.

◆ ◆ ◆ ◆ Legislation Banning Cloning

In August 2000 the U.S. government announced that it would allow publicly funded scientists to conduct research using human embryo cells, but only under guidelines proposed by the National Institutes of Health. The guidelines did not permit government-funded scientists to create embryos for research. In a statement issued in August 2001, President George W. Bush announced that scientists could be eligible for government funding to conduct research on 60 existing stem cell lines obtained from embryos that had already been destroyed. They could not, Bush reiterated, use federal funds to clone human embryos for research.

By the end of 2000, several states had passed legislation banning human cloning. As of November 2001 the U.S. Congress was considering similar legislation.

◆ ◆ ◆ ◆ Gene Therapy

gene therapy *Treating harmful genetic diseases or traits by eliminating or modifying the harmful gene.*

Researchers are optimistic that **gene therapy** will prove effective against some hereditary diseases. The treatment involves rewriting or rearranging bits of genetic code inside a patient's cells to suppress the expression of harmful effects. Retroviruses have been used to deliver altered DNA to a patient's cells, because these kinds of viruses normally infect cells by copying part of their DNA into the genetic code of a host cell. The harmful DNA in virus cells is replaced with genes intended to help treat a disease, such as cystic fibrosis or certain types of brain cancer. The research is promising, but there are difficulties with the technique. First, the viral DNA can trigger the formation of antibodies in the patient's blood that cause harmful side effects. Second, the virus may deliver its payload to a section of DNA in the recipient cell that is inert. And finally, the viral DNA may disrupt the patient's DNA in a harmful, rather than helpful, manner.

Other gene therapy methods are in the works that avoid the disadvantages of viruses. For instance, researchers have injected normal DNA directly into diseased tissue. In other clinical trials DNA and its mirror image, RNA, were injected into cells containing the gene that causes sickle cell anemia. The technique showed promise but has not yet been used inside the human body.

Gene therapy may emerge as an effective defense against hereditary diseases, but the research is still in its infancy.

YOU BE THE JUDGE

In 1984 John Moore, an Alaskan businessman, was treated at the University of California at Los Angeles (UCLA) for a rare cancer. During his treatment a doctor and researcher discovered that tissue from Moore's spleen produced a blood protein that encourages the growth of cancer-fighting white blood cells.

Without Moore's knowledge or consent, university scientists created a cell line from his tissue. They obtained a patent on their invention, which was estimated to be worth about $3 billion in potential profits. Moore later learned that his tissue had been used in this way and he sued UCLA, claiming that only he could own his tissue. The California Supreme Court ruled against Moore in 1990, saying that he had no property right over his own body tissues. This court's decision set precedent for allowing scientists to patent genes and tissues used in or created through research.

Since Moore's suit, some states have passed laws defining DNA ownership. For example, a 1995 Oregon law declared that a person owned his or her DNA and that of any children. In 2001, however, Oregon legislators were considering changing the law so that genetic information would no longer be considered private property once it is separated from a person's identity through encryption or anonymous research. The new law would also stridently protect genetic privacy.

In your opinion, should genes be considered private property? Why or why not?

_____

Should individuals receive payment if they turn over ownership of genes to researchers? Why or why not?

_____

Should scientists or drug companies be allowed to patent genes as they do other discoveries and inventions? Why or why not?

_____

Check Your Progress

4. The process of manipulating the DNA of organisms to produce desired results is called

_____ .

5. Define *genetic discrimination*. _____

_____

6. Circle the letter for the phrase that best defines *cloning:*
   a. an illegal medical procedure
   b. a form of genetic testing
   c. a scientific process that produces new organisms, identical to the parent, without the union of sperm and egg

Conception and the Beginning of Life

There is no legislated right to have children in the United States, but American couples may bear as many children as they wish. In fact, American couples who have difficulty conceiving may opt to use the services of infertility clinics.

◆ ◆ ◆ ◆ ## Infertility

When couples have difficulty conceiving and consult physicians who specialize in infertility problems, diagnoses are made and appropriate treatment recommended. Several options for infertile couples exist, depending on the type of fertility problem:

in vitro fertilization (IVF) *Fertilization that takes place outside a woman's body, literally, "in glass," as in a test tube.*

- **In vitro fertilization.** In the process of **in vitro fertilization (IVF),** eggs and sperm are brought together outside of the body, in a test tube or petri dish. When fertilization takes place, the resulting embryo can then be frozen in liquid nitrogen for future use or implanted in the female uterus for pregnancy to occur.

homologous artificial insemination *The husband's sperm is mechanically injected into his wife's vagina to fertilize her eggs.*

heterologous artificial insemination *Donor sperm is mechanically injected into a woman's vagina to fertilize her eggs.*

- **Artificial insemination.** This process involves the mechanical injection of viable semen into the vagina. If the husband's sperm cells are used to fertilize the wife's eggs, the process is called **homologous artificial insemination.** If the husband's sperm cells are not viable, a donor's sperm may be used to fertilize the wife's eggs; this is called **heterologous artificial insemination.**

surrogate *A woman who becomes pregnant, usually by artificial insemination or surgical implantation of a fertilized egg, and bears a child for another woman.*

- **Surrogacy.** If a woman cannot carry an embryo to term, the couple may elect to contract with a **surrogate.** A surrogate is a woman who agrees to carry a child to term for a couple, most often in exchange for a fee. If the surrogate is not genetically related to the embryo, the type of surrogacy is called *gestational* surrogacy. If the surrogate contributes eggs to produce the embryo or is related to either husband or wife, the type of surrogacy is called *traditional* surrogacy. (In one much-publicized case in the United States, a woman carried her own grandchild to term for her married daughter, who was born without a uterus.) Traditional surrogacy differs from gestational surrogacy in that a traditional surrogate is genetically related to the fetus she carries.

Infertility treatments can cost several thousand dollars, with no guarantee of success. Most insurance plans do not cover expenses for infertility treatments or for contracting with a surrogate mother to bear a child. The law has been slow to catch up with technology, but many states have passed legislation regulating infertility clinics and surrogacy. Health care practitioners dealing with infertility should check state laws for current regulations.

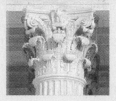

Baby M—A Traditional Surrogacy Case

In 1985 a woman signed a contract agreeing to serve as a surrogate for a couple who could not conceive. She was then medically inseminated with the husband's sperm and a pregnancy resulted. When the child was born in March 1986, the surrogate mother refused to give up the infant. The genetic father sued for violation of the surrogacy contract. The contract specified that the genetic father and his wife held custody and that the surrogate would terminate her parental rights. The trial court, considering the best interests of the child, affirmed the validity of the contract. In March 1987 an appellate court terminated the surrogate mother's parental rights and gave full custody of the then one-year-old Baby M to her genetic father and his wife. The genetic father's wife legally adopted the baby.

In re Baby M, 537 A.2d 1227 (N.J. 1988).

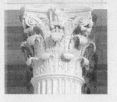

Gestational Surrogacy Contract Held Valid

A married couple was unable to have a child because the wife had undergone a hysterectomy. The wife's ovaries had not been removed, however, and could still produce eggs, so the couple opted for gestational surrogacy. They entered into a surrogacy contract with a woman who agreed to relinquish her parental rights after the child was born in exchange for a $10,000 fee and a paid life insurance policy. The wife's eggs were fertilized in vitro with the husband's sperm, and the resulting embryo was implanted into the surrogate's uterus. While she was still pregnant, the surrogate demanded immediate payment and threatened not to relinquish the child when it was born. The couple who had contracted with the surrogate filed a lawsuit seeking a legal determination that the surrogate had no parental rights to the baby. The surrogate countersued and the court consolidated the two cases.

A trial court found for the married couple. It determined that the couple were the child's "natural parents" and held that the surrogate had no parental rights to the child. An appellate court and the state Supreme Court upheld this decision.

Johnson v. Calvert, 851 P.2d 776 (Cal. 1993).

◆ ◆ ◆ ◆ Adoption

Adoption is also an option for couples who want to raise children. All 50 states have laws regulating adoption. Certain areas of federal law may also affect some aspects of the parent-child relationship established by adoption. For example, the Adoption Assistance and Child Welfare Act of 1980, the Child Abuse Prevention and Treatment and Adoption Reform Act, and the Indian Child Welfare Act all contain provisions that pertain to adoptive parents and their children.

Generally, any adult who shows the desire to be a fit parent may adopt a child. Depending on state law, married and unmarried couples may adopt jointly, and single people may adopt through a process called single-parent adoption. Some states list special requirements for adoptive parents, such as requiring an adoptive parent to be a specified number of years older than the child. There may also be state requirements concerning residency. Any adult who wishes to adopt will need to check state law before proceeding, and if potential adoptive parents use an adoption agency, they will also have to meet any agency requirements.

Some single individuals or couples may have a more difficult time qualifying as adoptive parents than others. For example, single men, gay singles, and homosexual couples may not specifically be prevented from adopting by state law but they may have a more difficult time meeting state and agency requirements than a married couple. All states strive to find placements that meet the best interest of the child, so in some cases potential adoptive parents may be asked additional questions about lifestyle and why they want to adopt. (See p. 212 for a more thorough explanation of "best interest of the child.")

Generally couples can adopt a child of a different race. Adoptions of Native American children, however, are governed by the Indian Child Welfare Act, and the act's provisions outline specific rules and procedures that must be followed if the adoption of a Native American child is to be approved.

There are several different types of adoptions, depending on services used and whether or not a blood or marital relationship exists between adoptive parents and children.

- Agency adoptions occur when state-licensed or regulated public or private adoption agencies place children with adoptive parents. Charities or religious or social service organizations often operate private agencies. Adoption agencies usually place children who have been orphaned or whose parents have lost or relinquished parental rights through abuse, abandonment, or inability to support.

- Independent or private adoptions are arranged without the involvement of adoption agencies. Potential adoptive parents may hear of a mother who wants to give up her child, or they may advertise in newspapers or on the Internet to find such a mother. At some point in the process an attorney must be involved to ensure the legality of the adoption. A few states prohibit independent adoptions. In states in which independent adoptions are allowed, they are usually strictly regulated.

- Identified adoptions are those in which adopting parents locate a birth mother, or vice versa, then ask an agency to take over the adoption process. Prospective parents who find a birth mother willing to give up her child can bypass the long waiting lists that most agencies maintain for adoptions and can perhaps be better assured that the adoption will proceed orderly and legally.

- International adoptions occur when couples adopt children who are citizens of foreign countries. In these procedures, adoptive parents must not only meet requirements of the foreign country where the child resides, they must also meet all U.S. state requirements and U.S. Immigration and Naturalization Service rules for international adoptions.

- Relative adoptions are those in which the child is related to the adoptive parent by blood or marriage. Stepparent/stepchild and grandparent/grandchildren adoptions fall within this category.

Rights of Children

parens patriae *A legal doctrine that gives the state the authority to act in a child's best interest.*

Common law has established the rights of parents to make health care decisions for minor children. However, in some circumstances, under the doctrine of **parens patriae,** the state may act as the parental authority. This doctrine is the legal principle that grants the state the broad authority to act in the child's "best interest." *Parens patriae*—literally, "the state as parent"—allows the state to override parental decisions alleged to go against the best interests of children. It also allows the state to remove abused or neglected children from the custody of offending parents.

◆ ◆ ◆ ◆ **Best Interest of the Child Concept**

When alternatives are available for child placement or for determining medical treatment for minor children, the common standard is the "best interest of the child." In other words, which alternative will best safeguard the child's growth, development, and health? This standard is used in child placement situations. It is also used when legal authorities must work with health care practitioners to determine the least harmful and most appropriate treatment for an ailing child.

◆ ◆ ◆ ◆ **Rights of the Newborn**

Rights of newborns became a public issue as the result of two highly publicized court cases in the 1980s. The first case involved a baby boy, born in Bloomington, Indiana, in April 1982. The baby was born with Down's syndrome and tracheoesophageal fistula. Down's syndrome is a congenital condition resulting in mild to severe mental retardation. Tracheoesophageal fistula is a birth defect that leaves a hole between the trachea and esophagus. Babies born with this condition cannot eat or drink properly. This condition can be repaired surgically, but the Indiana baby's parents decided against it. Since many Down's syndrome children grow up to live relatively normal lives, physicians attending the baby sought a court order to perform the surgery. However, the local court upheld the parents' right to privacy and to make decisions for their child. Food, water, and surgical treatment were withheld from the child, and after six days he died. To protect the family's privacy, the baby was referred to in court papers and newspaper articles as "Baby Doe."

In reaction to the Baby Doe case, the U.S. Department of Health and Human Services issued a notice to physicians and hospitals that, under authority of the Rehabilitation Act of 1973, they could lose federal funds if they withheld food or lifesaving medical treatment from disabled newborns. The HHS notice evolved into federal regulations posted in hospitals encouraging anyone who knew of a case where a disabled newborn had been denied lifesaving medical care to call a federal hot line. When calls were received, government agents were sent to investigate. The regulations were challenged in court and overturned in 1983 by a federal judge on grounds that HHS did not wait the required 30 days before implementing the regulations.

After the 1983 court decision, the Department of Health and Human Services issued a second set of regulations, this time under the authority of the 1974 Child Abuse Prevention and Treatment Act. Physicians who withheld treatment from disabled newborns could now be accused of child abuse and neglect. Under state law child protective services could investigate such complaints.

A second case involving a handicapped infant, called the "Baby Jane Doe" case, was litigated under the new federal regulations. A baby girl with spina bifida was born in October 1983 in Port Jefferson, New York. Spina bifida is a birth defect in which the developing fetus's spinal cord fails to fuse properly. A sac or cyst filled with cerebrospinal fluid, called a meningomyelocele, forms over the defective area of the spinal cord. The part of the spinal cord inside the cyst does not develop properly, often resulting in paralysis of the infant's lower body. The condition also causes a buildup of spinal fluid inside the brain (hydrocephalus). The resulting pressure on the infant's brain can cause mental retardation. Physicians told the New York baby's parents that without surgery she could probably survive no longer than two years. With surgery to repair the spinal cord and drain fluid from the brain, she could possibly survive for 20 years. If she survived, however, she would most certainly be paralyzed from the waist down and would suffer from epilepsy and recurring infections of her bladder and urinary tract. She would also probably be severely mentally retarded.

The parents had two choices. They could opt for conservative treatment, which meant surgery would not be performed but the baby would receive antibiotics and would be kept comfortable. Or surgery could be performed. The parents decided against surgery and the baby eventually died.

A right-to-life attorney in Vermont challenged in court the parents' decision, but New York courts upheld the parents' right to make medical decisions in the "best interest" of their child. An appeals court ruled that the attorney had no legal standing to contest the parents' decision.

In their final form, federal regulations concerning severely disabled newborns allowed parents and physicians several treatment options. Under the existing Child Abuse Amendments (U.S. Code, Title 42, Section 5106g), physicians may decide against giving food and water if they believe such treatment is not appropriate and if the infant's parents agree. Physicians may legally withhold treatment from infants who:

• Are chronically and irreversibly comatose.

• Will most certainly die and for whom treatment is considered futile.

• Would suffer inhumanely if treatment were provided.

The above court cases raised many ethical questions that have yet to be answered: Should the federal government have intruded into physicians' treatment decisions? Is it ever in an infant's "best interest" to die, or should medical treatment be administered regardless of the probable outcome? Is quality of life an issue that can ethically be considered? Who should decide among treatment options for disabled newborns if the parents are unwilling or unable to make such decisions?

7. Adoptions are regulated primarily by _____ .

8. Name four types of adoptions.

_____   _____

_____   _____

9. Under existing Child Abuse Amendments, physicians may, with the consent of parents, withhold treatment for infants who:

_____

_____

_____

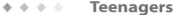

Teenagers

The above court cases and resulting federal regulations apply to infants, who cannot make decisions for themselves. Common law has dictated that parents have a right to decide what medical care their young children receive, but states also recognize that some older minors have the capacity to consent to their own medical care. For instance, teenagers considered mature or emancipated minors may give consent for medical treatment.

mature minors *Individuals in their mid- to late teens who, for health care purposes, are considered mature enough to comprehend a physician's recommendations and give informed consent.*

emancipated minors *Individuals in their mid- to late teens who legally live outside of parents' or guardians' control.*

Mature minors are individuals in their mid- to late teens who are considered mature enough to comprehend a physician's recommendations and give informed consent. Most states allow mature minors to seek medical treatment without the consent of a parent or guardian in certain critical areas, such as mental health, drug or alcohol addiction, treatment for sexually transmitted diseases, pregnancy, and contraceptive services.

Emancipated minors legally live outside of their parents' or guardians' control. A judge may issue an emancipation order at the request of parents or a minor child after certain important factors have been considered:

• Does the minor live at home with parents or other supervising adults, or is he or she living independently? If living at home, does he or she pay for room and board?

• Does the minor have a job, and does he or she spend his or her earnings without parental supervision?

• Does the minor pay his or her own debts?

• Is the minor claimed as a dependent on the parents' tax return?

The court may declare minors emancipated if one or more of the following criteria are met:

• They are self-supporting.

• They are married, provided the marriage is legal. In most states persons under the age of 18 must have parental consent and be at least 16 to marry. Emancipation is not forfeited if the minor divorces or is separated or widowed.

- They are serving in the armed forces.

Emancipated minors do not usually gain all the rights of adults. Some limits still apply, such as the legal age for purchasing alcohol or tobacco products, voting age, mandatory school attendance age (unless married), and other legal age restrictions.

Minors have the same constitutional rights as adults, including the right to privacy. This is especially relevant for the increasing number of adolescents in the United States who are sexually active. Many hesitate to seek birth control or family planning counseling if they must inform or seek consent from their parents.

No state explicitly requires parental involvement for a minor to obtain any of the services listed above. In some states, however, laws leave the decision about whether to inform parents that minor sons and daughters have received or are seeking contraceptives, prenatal care, or STD services to the discretion of the treating physician, based on the best interest of the minor.

In addition to the ability to consent to these specific services, laws in some states give minors the right to consent to general medical and surgical care under some circumstances, such as being a parent themselves, being pregnant, or reaching a certain age.

Several states also allow minors who are parents to consent to medical care for their children. In many states mothers who are minors may also legally place their children for adoption without the consent or knowledge of the minor mothers' parents.

In many states minors seeking an abortion must involve at least one parent in the decision. This means that teenagers who do not tell their parents about a pregnancy must either travel out of state or obtain approval from a judge—a process known as "judicial bypass"—in order to obtain an abortion. Currently the trend is toward state and federal legislation making it increasingly difficult for minors to obtain an abortion without parental involvement.

For exact legal restrictions regarding minors, health care practitioners should check statutes in the state in which they practice.

Check Your Progress

10. Define the term *mature minor.*

_____

11. Name three criteria that must be met if a minor is to be declared emancipated:

_____

_____

_____

12. What effect do the above designations have on a minor's health care decisions?

_____

13. In what treatment areas are minors most likely to make their own health care decisions?

_____

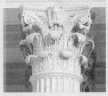

Judge Rules That Minor May Consent to Her Own Medical Treatment

Nancy, a 17-year-old Kansas girl, gave permission for a doctor to transplant some skin from her wrist to her finger. Her mother later sued on Nancy's behalf, on the grounds that Nancy was a minor.

Nancy's mother had been hospitalized for major surgery. After the operation Nancy accompanied her mother to her hospital room. A nurse asked Nancy to wait in the hallway. She didn't notice that Nancy's hand was resting on the wall near the door jamb, with her right ring finger in the space between the door and the jamb. As the nurse closed the door, Nancy cried out in pain. The door had closed on her finger, severing the tip.

Nancy was taken to the emergency room, where a doctor decided to graft a small piece of skin from Nancy's wrist over the raw tip of her finger. Nancy's mother was still recovering from her surgery, and it would be hours before she could give consent for her daughter's treatment. Nancy's parents were divorced, and her father lived in another city. To spare Nancy a long, uncomfortable wait, the emergency room physician called the girl's family physician and received his agreement that he should treat Nancy.

When Nancy's mother recovered, she sued the hospital, claiming that the nurse had been negligent in causing her daughter's injury and that the doctor had not obtained proper consent to treat her minor daughter.

The nurse was not found negligent. Regarding the question of consent, the Kansas Supreme Court ruled that Nancy "was of sufficient age and maturity to know and understand the nature and consequences of the 'pinch graft' utilized in the repair of her finger."

Younts v. St. Francis Hosp. and School of Nursing, 205 Kan. 292, 469 P.2d 330, 338 (1970).

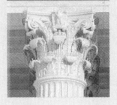

Osteopath Sued for Treating Minor

A 17-year-old girl was diagnosed with a herniated disc. The girl's parents rejected the orthopedic physician's recommendation that surgery be performed. On a day when the teenager's back pain was especially severe, she remembered that her father had once seen a local osteopath for back pain.

The girl drove herself to the osteopath's office, told him her father had been his patient, gave him her name, and told him of her diagnosis of a herniated disc. The osteopath said the girl did not have a herniated disc and treated her with manipulations of the neck, spine, and legs. (Because the osteopath was legally blind, he limited his practice to manipulative treatments of the skeletal system.)

Immediately after leaving the osteopath's office, the girl experienced pain when she walked. She later developed urinary retention problems and was catheterized in a local hospital's emergency room. The original diagnosing orthopedic physician performed surgery on the girl's herniated disc, but she still had trouble walking and with bladder and bowel control. Her parents filed suit against the osteopath for malpractice, battery (failure to obtain parental consent), and failure to obtain informed consent.

The Tennessee Supreme Court ultimately found:

1. Medical treatment may be provided without parental consent to mature minors.

(continued)

2. The minor in question, at 17 years, 7 months of age, had the capacity to consent and did consent.
3. The osteopath complied with the appropriate standard of care in providing the minor with sufficient information for her informed consent.
4. No battery occurred in the osteopath's treatment of the minor.
5. A directed verdict by a lower court on the medical malpractice claim was appropriate, because the plaintiff failed to present expert testimony on local standard of care.

Caldwell v. Bechtol, 724 SW 2d, 739 (Tenn. 1987).

In certain cases the legal right of a minor to decline medical treatment has been upheld.

Court Case

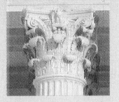

Minor Says No to Surgery

Believing they were acting in the best interests of a minor, a county health department in New York State tried to obtain the court's permission to seek surgery for a 14-year-old boy who had a cleft palate and upper lip.

The boy's father would not consent to surgery for his son because he believed that forces in the universe would heal all ailments. Influenced by his father, the boy refused the offer of surgery for his condition.

The court ruled that the boy could not be forced to have surgery. He could turn down the procedure, because his cooperation would be needed for the speech therapy that would follow. A majority of the judges saw less harm in letting him wait until he was an adult and could make the choice for himself than in pursuing surgery.

In the Matter of S., 309 N.Y. 80, 127 N.E. 2d 820 (1955).

Court Case

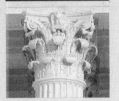

Minor's Informed Consent Not Necessary

A Texas physician was sued for failing to secure informed consent from a minor patient before performing an abortion.

In 1974 a 16-year-old girl's mother told her physician that her daughter was retarded and had been raped. The mother gave her written permission for her minor child to have an abortion, which the physician performed. The physician did not know that in reality the girl was not retarded and had not been raped. She had conceived the child with her boyfriend.

Sixteen years later the patient examined her medical records and realized that she had undergone an abortion. She sued the physician, claiming that she had not given informed consent for the procedure. In 1974 Texas law did not require that a minor give informed consent before an abortion. Since the physician had obtained informed consent from a parent, as required by law at that time, a trial court held and an appeals court affirmed that he was entitled to summary judgment.

Powers v. W.F. Floyd, 904 S.W.2d 713 (Texas Ct. of App., May 10, 1995; rehearing overruled May 24, 1995).

Applying Knowledge

Answer the following questions in the spaces provided.

1. Define *genetics*.
   _____

2. Define *DNA*.
   _____

3. List three situations in which DNA testing might be indicated.
   _____

   _____

   _____

4. Name two federal laws that help prevent genetic discrimination in employment and among health insurers.
   _____

   _____

5. Name two goals of the Human Genome Project.
   _____

   _____

6. Match the following definitions with the terms they define:

   _____A person is treated differently from others because of his or her genetic makeup.

   _____An experimental treatment for hereditary diseases.

   _____The manipulation of DNA to produce desired results in organisms.

   _____A procedure used to reveal the presence of a disease-causing gene or genes.

   a. genetic testing

   b. gene therapy

   c. genetic discrimination

   d. genetic engineering

7. Define *cloning.*

_____

8. Define *xenotransplantation.*

_____

9. Cloning is a form of _____ .

10. Why do many people fear the prospect of cloning?

_____

11. Explain why stem cells are valued for certain types of scientific research.

_____

Match the following terms with their correct definitions:

_____**12.** The use of a husband's sperm to fertilize his wife's eggs.

_____**13.** An arrangement between an infertile couple and a woman who agrees to carry their child to term.

_____**14.** Eggs and sperm are brought together outside of the body, in a test tube or petri dish.

_____**15.** Involves the mechanical injection of viable semen into a woman's vagina.

_____**16.** A woman who agrees to be a surrogate is genetically related to the child she will carry.

_____**17.** The use of a sperm donor to fertilize a woman's eggs.

_____**18.** A surrogate is not genetically related to the child she will carry.

a. homologous artificial insemination

b. traditional surrogacy

c. artificial insemination

d. heterologous artificial insemination

e. gestational surrogacy

f. in vitro fertilization

g. surrogacy

19. Define the doctrine of *parens patriae.*

_____

20. *Parens patriae* is the basis for the _____ consideration.

21. The most current federal regulations concerning severely disabled newborns take their authority from which federal law?

_____

22. Teenagers classified as _____ or _____ can generally make their own health care decisions.

23. A physician who treats a minor without parental consent risks being charged with _____ .

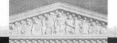

Case Studies

Use your critical-thinking skills to answer the questions that follow the case study.

As reproductive technology advanced, headlines announcing "Couple Battles Over Frozen Embryos" became more and more commonplace. For example, in the 1980s a man went to court and succeeded in preventing his ex-wife from using their frozen embryos to become pregnant. He maintained that after he and his wife divorced he no longer wanted to become a parent and should not be forced to do so against his will.

In 1998 a divorced woman in New Jersey won a legal battle with her ex-husband over custody of seven frozen embryos the couple created in vitro while still married. The wife wanted to have the embryos destroyed, whereas the ex-husband argued his right to adopt his own embryos to be implanted in a future partner or donated to an infertile couple.

24. **In your opinion, should frozen embryos be considered property to be awarded during a divorce? Why or why not?**

_____

_____

25. **Should a man who loses custody of frozen embryos in a lawsuit be responsible for child support if his ex-wife is implanted with the embryos and becomes pregnant at a later date? Explain your answer.**

_____

_____

26. **Should the husband or wife who wins custody of frozen embryos be allowed to destroy them, against the wishes of the ex-husband or ex-wife? Why or why not?**

_____

_____

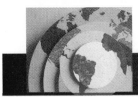

Internet Activities

Complete the activities and answer the questions that follow.

27. Find the Web site for the Human Genome Project. What is the current status of the project?

_____

_____

28. The American Society for Reproductive Medicine publishes guidelines for health care practitioners, for patients, and for egg and sperm donors that, if followed, can help ensure that infertility procedures are ethically performed. Find the organization's Web site and list five of their guidelines.

_____

_____

_____

_____

_____

29. Locate the Web site on the Internet for Planned Parenthood of America. What special section of the site addresses teenagers? How might this site be useful to teenagers or their parents?

_____

_____

_____

10

BIOETHICS: SOCIAL ISSUES

Objectives

After studying this chapter, you should be able to:

1. Explain why bioethical issues need to be addressed in a code of ethics.

2. Compare ethical standards recommended for physicians with those for the health care profession you plan to practice.

3. Relate the American Medical Association's *Fundamental Elements of the Patient-Physician Relationship* to your own professional standards.

4. Discuss any differences you see between ethical standards or guidelines and laws relevant to medical practice.

5. Relate each bioethical issue discussed to a relevant chapter in this text.

Key Terms

- **advance directive**

- **anencephaly**

- **biotechnology**

- **do-not-resuscitate (DNR) order**

- **euthanasia**

- **germ line therapy**

- **somatic cell therapy**

Bioethical Issues

biotechnology *Applied biological science.*

This chapter discusses bioethics—moral issues that have arisen as a result of advances in **biotechnology** and biological/medical research. To health care practitioners, bioethical issues are as important as laws governing medical practice and health care. In fact, ethical principles are often more compelling than the law.

AMA Ethical Guidelines

Physicians and other health care practitioners are bound not just by state and federal laws but also by the same ethical standards. As discussed in Chapter 1, the Judicial Council of the American Medical Association publishes an ethics guide for physicians, titled *Code of Medical Ethics: Current Opinions with Annotations,* to provide guidance in a wide variety of situations associated with medical practice. Although the ethical conduct of physicians is the focus of this guide, the standards are applicable to any health care practitioner.

Chapters 10 and 11 present an overview of the ethical issues discussed in the AMA's *Code of Medical Ethics.* The guidelines are applicable to every topic discussed in this text. They are presented here to serve as a basis for discussion and as a foundation for forming personal codes of ethics that will guide you, as a health care practitioner, in making ethically sound professional decisions. Keep in mind as you read Chapters 10 and 11 that the AMA ethical guidelines summarized are not law but deal solely with what the AMA considers ethical conduct for physicians. In fact, state and federal law may differ somewhat from an ethical principle. For example, state law in most cases does not require physicians to routinely inquire about physical, sexual, and psychological abuse as part of a patient's medical history, but the physician may feel an ethical duty to his or her patient to do so. Figure 10-1 presents what patients have a right to expect in their relationships with their physicians.

The following paragraphs summarize the AMA's position on ethical standards to be applied in a variety of situations physicians and other health care providers may face.

◆ ◆ ◆ ◆ Abortion

The AMA's *Code of Medical Ethics* does not prohibit physicians from performing abortions as long as such procedures are "in accordance with good medical practice and under circumstances that do not violate the law."

◆ ◆ ◆ ◆ Mandatory Parental Consent to Abortion

Physicians should know the law in their state on parental involvement to be sure that their procedures are consistent with their legal obligations. They should encourage minors to discuss their pregnancy with their parents or with other trusted adults, but if patients are reluctant to do so, physicians should not feel compelled to require them to involve their parents before making the decision to undergo an abortion.

Figure 10-1
**Fundamental Elements of the
Patient-Physician Relationship**

Physicians recognize that the health and well-being of patients depends on a cooperative effort between physician and patient. They also recognize that patients share with physicians the responsibility for their own health care. "Physicians can best contribute to [the patient-physician] alliance by serving as their patients' advocate and by fostering these rights:

1. "The patient has the right to receive information from physicians and to discuss the benefits, risks, and costs of appropriate treatment alternatives. Patients should receive guidance from their physicians as to the optimal course of action. Patients are also entitled to obtain copies or summaries of their medical records, to have their questions answered, to be advised of potential conflicts of interest that their physicians might have, and to receive independent professional opinions.
2. "The patient has the right to make decisions regarding the health care that is recommended by his or her physician. Accordingly, patients may accept or refuse any recommended medical treatment.
3. "The patient has the right to courtesy, respect, dignity, responsiveness, and timely attention to his or her needs.
4. "The patient has the right to confidentiality. The physician should not reveal confidential communications or information without the consent of the patient, unless provided for by law or by the need to protect the welfare of the individual or the public interest.
5. "The patient has the right to continuity of health care. The physician has an obligation to cooperate in the coordination of medically indicated care with other health care providers treating the patient. The physician may not discontinue treatment of a patient as long as further treatment is medically indicated, without giving the patient reasonable assistance and sufficient opportunity to make alternative arrangements for care.
6. "The patient has a basic right to have available adequate health care. Physicians, along with the rest of society, should continue to work toward this goal. Fulfillment of this right is dependent on society providing resources so that no patient is deprived of necessary care because of an inability to pay for the care. Physicians should continue their traditional assumption of a part of the responsibility for the medical care of those who cannot afford essential health care. Physicians should advocate for patients in dealing with third parties when appropriate."

"Fundamental Elements of the Patient-Physician Relationship", pp. xv and xvi of the American Medical Association's *Code of Medical Ethics: Current Opinions with Annotations,* Chicago, 2000.

Court Case

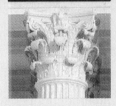

Landmark Case Legalizes Abortion

In 1970 a single woman in Texas became pregnant. She had difficulty finding work because of her pregnancy and feared the stigma of an illegitimate birth. Under the fictitious name "Jane Roe," the woman sued Henry Wade, the district attorney in Dallas County, Texas, claiming that she had limited rights to an abortion and seeking an injunction against the Texas statute prohibiting abortion except to save woman's life.

(continued)

It took three years for the case to reach the United States Supreme Court, which struck down the Texas statute. The ruling came too late for Jane Roe to have the abortion she originally sought, of course, but it affected the rights of all women who would seek abortions from that time on. The Court held that the constitutional right to privacy includes a woman's decision to terminate a pregnancy during the first trimester (three months), but states could impose restrictions and regulate abortions after that.

In reaching its decision, the court reviewed the medical and legal history of abortion, including the AMA's *Code of Medical Ethics,* which stated then, as it does now, that a physician is not prohibited from performing an abortion in accordance with good medical practice and consistent with local law.

Roe v. Wade, 410 U.S. 113, 144 n.39 (1973).

◆ ◆ ◆ ◆ ## Abuse of Spouses, Children, Elderly Persons, and Others at Risk

Because family violence occurs too frequently in today's society, physicians should routinely inquire about physical, sexual, and psychological abuse as part of a patient's medical history. Physicians should be familiar with protocols for treating abuse, laws regarding the reporting of abuse, and community resources available for victims of abuse.

Physicians must comply with laws regarding the reporting of abuse and are ethically obligated to report such incidents even when not specifically required by law to do so. When the patient is a mentally competent adult, however, the physician should not disclose an abuse diagnosis to spouses or any other third party without the consent of the patient.

Physicians are, however, ethically obligated to intervene. Actions can include suggesting the possibility of abuse to an adult patient; discussing safety methods available, such as reporting to police or other authorities; discussing community resources for victims of abuse; providing support; and documenting incidents for future reference.

Court Case

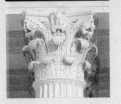

Psychologist's Testimony Admitted in Child Abuse Case

After a licensed clinical psychologist reported a patient's admission of sexual misconduct with a child, the patient was convicted of a lewd act with a child and child molestation or annoyance. The court held that the psychologist's testimony was properly admitted, since a state law requiring the reporting of actual or suspected child abuse expressly made the psychotherapist-patient privilege inapplicable.

People v. Stritzinger, 1137 Cal. App. 3d 126, 186 Cal. Rptr. 750, 752 rev'd 34 Cal. 3d 505, 668 p.2d 738, 194 Cal. Rptr. 421 (1983).

Allocation, Cost, and Service Issues

Allocation of Limited Medical Resources

Physicians must place the benefit of patients above policies for allocating limited medical resources. Therefore, treating physicians should not make allocation decisions. Decisions regarding the allocation of limited medical resources should consider only the likelihood of benefit, the urgency of need, the change in quality of life, the duration of benefit, and in some cases, the amount of resources required for successful treatment. Nonmedical criteria, such as the ability to pay, age, social worth, perceived obstacles to treatment, the patient's contribution to illness, or past use of resources, should not be considered.

Futile Care

Physicians are not ethically obligated to deliver care that, in their professional judgment, will not benefit their patients. Patients should not be given treatments simply because they demand them. Denial of treatment should be based on ethical principles and acceptable standards of care, not the concept of "futility," which cannot be adequately defined.

Medical Futility in End-of-Life Care

When further medical intervention to prolong a patient's life becomes futile, physicians are obligated to shift the intent of care toward comfort and closure. To help with decisions regarding futility, all health care institutions should adopt a policy on medical futility. In addition, policies on medical futility should follow a due process approach that includes:

- Advance deliberation and negotiation between patient, proxy, and physician on what constitutes futile care for the patient and what limits are acceptable for the physician, patient, family, and possibly the institution.

- Joint decision making among the physician, patient, and proxy, whenever possible.

- Negotiation when disagreements arise.

- Involvement of institutional ethics committees when possible and appropriate.

- Transfer to another physician or institution, if possible, when disagreements cannot be resolved.

The Provision of Adequate Health Care

Society is obligated to provide access to adequate health care for everyone, regardless of ability to pay. Physicians should help with policy-making decisions to achieve this goal. In determining what constitutes "adequate levels of health care," the following considerations should be weighed:

- Degree of benefit (difference between treatment and no treatment).

- Likelihood of benefit.

- Duration of benefit.

- Cost.

- Number of people who will benefit.

Unnecessary Services

Physicians should not provide, prescribe, or seek payment for medical services they know are unnecessary.

Capital Punishment and Treatment of Prisoners

Capital Punishment

An individual's opinion on capital punishment is his or her personal moral decision. As health professionals committed to preserving life, physicians should not participate in legally authorized executions. Such participation includes actions that (1) would directly cause the death of the condemned; (2) would assist, supervise, or contribute to the ability of another individual to directly cause the death of the condemned; or (3) could automatically cause an execution to be carried out on a condemned prisoner.

Physician participation in an execution also includes prescribing or administering tranquilizers and other psychotropic agents and medications that are part of the execution procedure, monitoring vital signs on site or from a remote location, attending or observing an execution in the capacity of a physician, and giving technical advice regarding the execution.

Court-Initiated Medical Treatments in Criminal Cases

Physicians can ethically participate in court-initiated medical treatments if such treatments are therapeutically beneficial and therefore not a form of punishment or a means of social control. The court has the authority to identify criminal behavior but cannot make a medical diagnosis or determine the type of medical treatment to be administered.

The physician who will administer treatment must be able to conclude, in good conscience and to the best of his or her professional judgment, that informed consent was given voluntarily to the extent possible.

Court Case

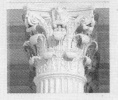

Execution of Insane Prisoner

Louisiana attempted to bypass a prohibition against executing insane prisoners by forcibly medicating a condemned prisoner. The court held that this violated the prisoner's right to privacy and constituted cruel and unusual punishment. The court also held that involuntary administration of medication is not medical treatment but constitutes a part of capital punishment and is contrary to the AMA's *Code of Medical Ethics.*

State v. Perry, 610 So.2d 746, 753 (1992).

Write "T" or "F" in the blank to indicate whether you think the statement is true or false.

_____ 1. The AMA's *Code of Medical Ethics* prohibits physicians from performing abortions.

_____ 2. According to the AMA's code of ethics, physicians are *not* ethically obligated to routinely inquire about physical, sexual, and psychological abuse as part of a patient's medical history.

_____ 3. Ethical standards must always follow the law exactly.

_____ 4. Allocation of limited medical resources should not depend on a patient's ability to pay.

_____ 5. State laws may vary, but ethical standards for various situations can apply, regardless of the law.

◆ ◆ ◆ ◆ **Research-Related Issues**

Clinical Investigation

When physicians engage in the clinical investigation of new drugs and procedures, they should use the following guidelines:

- Participation in clinical investigation should be limited to activities that are part of a systematic program competently designed, under accepted standards of scientific research, to produce data that are scientifically valid and significant.

- The subjects involved in a clinical investigation deserve the same concern and caution for their welfare, safety, and comfort as patients under the care of a physician and not participating in a clinical investigation.

- Minors or mentally incompetent persons may be used as subjects in clinical investigations only if mentally competent adults would not be suitable subjects for the investigation, and only if legally authorized representatives of the subjects give written and informed consent.

- In clinical investigations intended primarily as treatment, a physician-patient relationship exists and the best interest of the patient must be primary. Voluntary written consent must be obtained from the patient or from a legally authorized representative. Informed consent includes a disclosure that the physician intends to use an investigational or experimental drug or procedure, an explanation of the drug or procedure to be used, risks and benefits, an offer to answer questions, and a disclosure of alternative drugs or procedures that may be available.

- If the investigation is primarily for scientific knowledge, subjects' welfare, safety, and comfort must be safeguarded. Subjects must give written consent. Subjects should be informed that an investigative drug or procedure is to be used, told the risks or benefits of the drug or procedure, and assured that all questions will be answered.

- Subjects must voluntarily consent to be used in a clinical investigation. The overuse of institutionalized persons in research is unethical. The institution conducting the research is responsible for maintaining ethical standards and for the proper training and conduct of scientists involved.

- With the consent of subjects/patients, physicians engaged in research are encouraged to share results through the media, but unwarranted fanfare or sensationalism is unethical.

Court Case

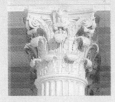

Experimental Treatment

A 26-year-old man afflicted with a primitive neuroectodermal tumor, a rare form of brain cancer, volunteered to participate in an oncologist's study. The physician wanted to treat the patient with high-dose chemotherapy and a supportive autologous bone marrow transplant. The estimated cost was $130,000.

The patient's insurance company said the bone marrow transplant was experimental and refused payment. The patient sought a restraining order and preliminary injunction to force the insurance company to pay for the treatment.

The court ruled in favor of the insurance company, stating that there was not enough scientific data to establish the proposed therapy as a safe and effective course of treatment for the patient's condition. Therefore, the treatment was considered "experimental and investigative" and was expressly excluded under the terms of the patient's insurance policy.

Watts v. Massachusetts Mutual Life Insurance Co., 892 F.Supp. 737 (D.C., N.C., July 11, 1995).

Court Case

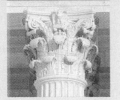

Physician Sues for Wrongful Discharge

A physician was employed by a pharmaceutical company to do research and was discharged when she refused to continue research she viewed as medically unethical. She sued the pharmaceutical company for wrongful discharge, claiming that as an employee-at-will she had a cause of action. A trial court granted summary judgment to the pharmaceutical company.

An appeals court held that an employee has a cause of action when discharged contrary to a clearly mandated public policy. However, the court affirmed summary judgment because human testing was not imminent and because plaintiff failed to demonstrate the existence of a clear public policy based on any statements of medical ethics to support her refusal to continue work on a controversial drug. The dissent argued that the Opinions and Reports of the AMA's Judicial Council did provide a clear expression of public policy and that the plaintiff's failure to specifically cite them was merely a technical defect.

Pierce v. Ortho Pharmaceutical Corp., 84 N.J. 58, 417 A.2d 505, 516, 518 (N.J., 1980).

Fetal Research Guidelines

The following guidelines are provided for physicians engaged in fetal research:

- Activities should be part of a competently designed program, conducted in accordance with accepted standards of scientific research, to produce scientifically valid and significant data.

- When appropriate, properly performed clinical studies on animals and nongravid (not pregnant) humans should precede any fetal research project.

- Investigators should show the same care and concern for the fetus as a physician would in providing fetal care or treatment in a nonresearch setting.

- All applicable federal and state laws should be followed.

- Fetal material should not be purchased.

- Competent peer review committees, review boards, or advisory boards should be available to protect against possible abuses.

- Written, informed consent should be obtained if research is for the treatment of the fetus or the gravid (pregnant) female. Informed consent includes information about alternative treatments or methods of care. Simpler, safer treatments should be pursued if possible.

Patenting the Human Genome

A patent grants the holder the right, for a limited amount of time, to prevent others from commercializing his or her inventions. The patent system also fosters information sharing. Patenting of human genetic material is a controversial matter. Opponents argue that the patenting of such material sets a troubling precedent for ownership of human life. Others argue, however, that DNA sequences do not constitute human life, and it is unclear whether such material is uniquely human.

Since genetic research holds great promise for achieving new medical therapies, the AMA Council on Ethical and Judicial Affairs concludes that granting patent protection should not hinder the goal of developing new beneficial technology. The council offers the following guidelines:

- Patents on processes, such as isolating and purifying gene sequences, do not raise the same ethical concerns as patents on the substances themselves and are therefore preferable.

- Substance patents on purified proteins present fewer ethical problems than patents on genes or DNA sequences and are thus preferable.

- Patent descriptions should be carefully constructed to ensure that the patent holder does not limit the use of a naturally occurring form of the substance in question. This includes patents on proteins, genes, and genetic sequences.

Gene Therapy

As discussed in Chapter 9, gene therapy involves rewriting or rearranging bits of genetic code to suppress the expression of harmful effects. The AMA's *Code of Medical Ethics* further defines gene therapy as "the replacement or modification of a genetic variant to restore or enhance cellular function or to improve the reaction of non-genetic therapies."

somatic cell therapy *A procedure in which human cells other than germ cells (eggs and sperm) are genetically altered.*

germ line therapy *A procedure in which a replacement gene is put into human gametes, resulting in expression of the new gene in the patient's offspring.*

Two types of gene therapy have been identified: (1) **somatic cell therapy,** in which human cells other than germ cells (eggs and sperm) are genetically altered, and (2) **germ line therapy,** in which a replacement gene is inserted in human germ cells, resulting in expression of the new gene in the patient's offspring.

The goal of gene therapy is to alleviate suffering and disease by remedying disorders for which other therapies are unsatisfactory. The welfare of the patient should be primary. Genetic manipulation simply to enhance "desirable" characteristics not related to disease is unacceptable.

Genetic Counseling

Genetic counseling and testing are most appropriate for prospective parents whose genetic histories indicate an elevated risk for genetic disorders.

Primary areas of prenatal genetic testing include (1) screening prospective parents for genetic disease before conception; (2) analyzing preembryos before implanting when artificial reproduction techniques are used; and (3) in utero testing after conception, including ultrasonography, amniocentesis, fetoscopy, and chorionic villus sampling. Written informed consent must be obtained from the patient before any of these genetic tests are performed.

Physicians should be aware that when a genetic defect is found in the fetus, parents may request or refuse an abortion.

VOICE OF EXPERIENCE

Nurses Can Play an Important Role in Genetic Counseling

Sharon, RN, Ph.D., FAAN (Fellowship in the American Academy of Nursing), is a nurse practitioner, psychologist, and university assistant professor. She practices and teaches on the West Coast. She has researched and written about numerous topics, including the nurse's role in genetic counseling.

"I think the nurse has a powerful role in a variety of ways," Sharon says. "Not only in case findings, suggesting to families when genetic testing might be useful, but also in preparing individuals for genetic testing and afterwards helping them sort through things they might not have understood."

"Nurses can help the tests make sense to people," she continues, and they can listen carefully as they take patient histories. For example, if a patient remarks, "My cousin has a child with Down's syndrome. I wonder if I could have a baby like that?" the nurse can impart information about genetic testing that can help patients make decisions.

Genetic counseling helps patients process the information obtained from genetic testing, Sharon explains. Such counseling before genetic testing can also help patients examine family histories and traits, to determine whether or not testing might be helpful. She suggests that families take family histories, old Bibles, photographs, and other items for the genetic counselor to examine. "The more information the family can take with them, the better evaluation and information they get," she concludes.

Genetic Testing by Employers

As a result of the Human Genome Project, more inherited diseases will be identified. One potential use of genetic testing to detect these diseases will be screening of potential workers by employers. The AMA's position on such screening is that it would generally be inappropriate to exclude workers with genetic risks of disease from the workplace. Tests may reveal the likelihood for an individual to develop a genetic disease, but this does not mean that the disease always develops. Consequently, use of genetic testing to screen employees would result in unfair discrimination against individuals with positive test results.

There may be a role for genetic testing, however, to exclude from the workplace workers who have a genetic susceptibility to injury. The following conditions would need to be met:

- The disease develops so rapidly that serious and irreversible injury would occur before harm could be prevented.

- The genetic testing is highly accurate, with the risk of false negative or positive test results substantially reduced.

- Data has demonstrated that the genetic abnormality results in an unusually high susceptibility to occupational injury.

- It would require undue cost to protect susceptible employees.

- Testing must be performed only with the informed consent of the employee or applicant for employment.

Insurance Companies and Genetic Information

Physicians should not participate in genetic testing by health insurance companies to predict a person's predisposition for disease. It may be necessary for physicians to keep separate files for genetic testing results so that such results are not sent to insurance companies when fulfilling requests for patient medical records. Physicians should tell insurance companies when medical results are sent that they do not include genetic testing results, whether or not the patient has undergone genetic testing.

Genetic Testing of Children

Before children are tested for genetic diseases, the benefit should outweigh the disadvantages. If a child is at risk for a genetic condition and preventive or therapeutic measures are available, genetic testing is appropriate and should be offered. (In some cases it is required.) If a child is at risk for a genetic condition with pediatric onset for which preventive or therapeutic measures are not available, parents should have discretion to decide about genetic testing. Genetic testing for carrier status should be deferred until the child reaches maturity, the child needs to make reproductive decisions, or reproductive decisions need to be made for the child. Genetic testing of children for the benefit of a family member should be performed only if the testing can prevent substantial harm to a family member. This information should not be disclosed to third parties, and the test results should be kept in a file separate from the medical record to prevent mistaken disclosure.

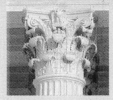
Physician Not Liable for Failure to Test

A woman gave birth to a baby with Tay-Sachs disease. She and her husband then sued a university and a physician for failure to test the couple for Tay-Sachs, an inherited disease most common among individuals of Jewish descent.

The couple did not reveal to a genetic counselor, in counseling sessions, that either of them was of Jewish descent. Therefore, the physician did not recommend genetic testing for Tay-Sachs disease. After other testing the wife was informed that she was carrying a healthy baby boy. However, ten months after the baby's birth, he was diagnosed with Tay-Sachs disease.

Affirming summary judgment in favor of the physician and the hospital, a California appellate court said the parents presented no expert testimony on the circumstances under which genetic testing for Tay-Sachs disease was indicated. The physician and hospital presented evidence by an expert who stated that the parents did not meet the profile that warranted a Tay-Sachs screening test and that it was within the standard of care not to perform the test.

Munro v. Regents of the University of California, 263 Cal. Rptr. 878 (Cal. Ct. of App., Nov. 16, 1989).

◆ ◆ ◆ ◆ **Genetic Engineering**

The federal Recombinant DNA Advisory Committee and the Food and Drug Administration supervise and regulate gene splicing, recombinant DNA research, chemical synthesis of DNA, and other genetic engineering research. As genetic engineering technology becomes commonplace in treating human disorders, the following ethical guidelines should be followed:

- Procedures performed in a research setting should conform to the guidelines on clinical investigation as set forth by the Judicial Council of the AMA.

- Usual and customary standards of medical practice and professional responsibility are required when nonresearch procedures are performed.

- Full discussion with the patient of proposed procedures and written, voluntary, informed consent are required.

- Viral DNA containing a replacement or corrective gene must not contain hazardous or unwanted viruses.

- Inserted DNA must function normally within the recipient cell to prevent metabolic damage.

- Effectiveness of gene therapy should be thoroughly evaluated.

- Such procedures should be used only when simpler, safer treatments are unavailable.

- Guidelines and considerations should be periodically reviewed as scientific information advances.

6. "Medical futility" implies that further medical treatment will not be beneficial to the patient. The AMA recommends that policies on medical futility should follow a due process approach that includes which five factors?

_____

_____

_____

_____

_____

7. In cases in which patients have been abused, the AMA states that physicians are "ethically obligated to intervene." List three ways this might be accomplished.

_____

_____

_____

8. Distinguish between somatic cell gene therapy and germ line gene therapy.

_____

_____

_____

9. What remedy is proposed for preventing confidential patient information about genetic testing from being used by insurance companies and possibly employers to discriminate against a person based on genetic test results?

_____

_____

_____

◆ ◆ ◆ ◆ Assisted Reproduction

Artificial Insemination by Known Donor

Women considering artificial insemination by husband, partner, or other known donor should be counseled about screening tests available for infectious and genetic diseases, including HIV infection. Disclosure of a full medical history and appropriate diagnostic screening should be recommended to donors and recipients but is not required.

Informed consent should include a discussion of alternative methods and disclosure of risks, benefits, and the likely success rate of the method proposed. Additional information should include screening, costs, and procedures for maintaining confidentiality. Prospective parents should be informed of the laws regarding the rights of children conceived by artificial insemination as well as laws about parental rights and obligations.

If the donor and the recipient are married, resultant children will have all the rights of a child conceived naturally. If the parents are not married, the recipient will be considered the sole parent of the child except in cases in which both the donor and the recipient agree to recognize a paternity right.

Choosing sperm to manipulate the gender of a resulting child is appropriate only for purposes of avoiding a sex-linked inheritable disease and not for gender preference. If semen is frozen and the donor dies before it is used, the frozen semen should not be used or donated for purposes other than those intended by the donor. If the donor died without leaving any instructions, the remaining partner may reasonably use the semen for artificial insemination, but not for donation to someone else.

Artificial Insemination by Anonymous Donor

Complete medical histories must be taken for all anonymous sperm donors, and they must be screened for infectious or inheritable diseases. Frozen semen should be used for artificial insemination because it enables the donor to be tested for HIV infection at the time of donation and again before the semen is used. Physicians should rely on the guidelines provided by professional organizations such as the American Society of Reproductive Medicine, the Centers for Disease Control and Prevention, and the Food and Drug Administration in determining intervals between initial and final HIV tests.

Physicians should keep permanent records of donors in order to:

- Exclude individuals who test positive for infectious or inheritable diseases.

- Limit the number of pregnancies resulting from a single donor source, thus avoiding future consanguineous marriages or reproduction.

- Notify donors of screening results that indicate the presence of an infectious or inheritable disease.

- Notify donors if a child born through artificial insemination has a disorder that may have been transmitted by the donor.

Informed consent should include the disclosure of alternative methods, risks, benefits, the likely success rate of the method proposed, and costs. Recipients and donors should be informed of the reasons for screening and confidentiality. They should also know whether nonidentifying and identifying information about the donor is accessible, and they should be informed of any legal ramifications regarding artificial insemination by an anonymous donor.

The consent of the recipient's husband is ethically appropriate if he is to become the legal father of the resultant child. Anonymous donors cannot assume the rights or responsibilities of parenthood for children born through artificial insemination, nor should they be required to do so.

It is not unethical to offer artificial insemination as a reproductive option for single women or women who are part of a homosexual couple.

Selecting sperm to manipulate the gender of a resulting child is ethical only for purposes of avoiding a sex-linked inheritable disease.

It is inappropriate to offer compensation to donors over and above reimbursement for time and actual expenses.

Surrogate Mothers

As discussed in Chapter 9, surrogate motherhood involves the artificial insemination of a woman who agrees, usually in exchange for a fee, to bear a child and to give the child to the child's father by surrendering her parental rights. The father's wife, who is usually infertile, adopts the child.

Surrogacy arrangements have generated many ethical, social, and legal problems. The AMA's Judicial Council recommends that surrogacy contracts, though permissible, should grant the birth mother the right to void the agreement within a reasonable period of time after the child's birth. Custody would then be determined according to the child's best interests. Gestational contracts, on the other hand, should not be voidable.

In Vitro Fertilization

The technique of in vitro fertilization and embryo transplantation offers certain couples previously incapable of conception the opportunity to bear a child. Because of serious ethical and moral concerns, however, any fertilized egg that has the potential for human life and that will be implanted in the uterus of a woman should not be subjected to laboratory research.

All fertilized ova that are not used for implantation and that are kept for research purposes should be subject to the guidelines for research and medical practice expressed earlier in the section "Fetal Research Guidelines." The highest standards of medical practice should also apply.

Frozen Preembryos

The process of freezing preembryos produced during in vitro fertilization offers infertile couples the ability to preserve embryos for future implantation, thus increasing the odds that they will be able to bear a child or children. The practice, however, has also posed serious ethical and legal questions regarding decision-making authority over the preembryos and the appropriate uses of preembryos.

The donors of eggs and sperm are the logical persons to exercise control over frozen preembryos. They should be able to use the preembryos themselves or to donate them to others, but not to sell them. Preembryos not intended for implantation should be available for research, in accordance with the Judicial Council's guidelines on fetal research. The preembryos may also be allowed to thaw and deteriorate. Donors should have an equal say in the use of their preembryos and, therefore, the preembryos should not be available for use by either provider individually or changed from their frozen state without the consent of both providers.

Written informed consent of both gamete providers should be obtained before any disposition of preembryos is made. Advance agreements are recommended for deciding disposition of frozen preembryos in the event of divorce or other changes in circumstances but should not be mandatory.

Preembryo Splitting

Splitting in vitro fertilized preembryos may result in multiple genetically identical siblings.

The procedure of preembryo splitting should be available, with the agreement of both egg and sperm donors. The procedure may greatly increase the chances of conception for an infertile couple and can reduce the number of invasive procedures necessary for egg retrieval and hormonal stimulation. But possibilities exist for ethically questionable practices, such as using identical frozen preembryos many years after one child was born and raised or selling embryos for a child with desirable characteristics. However, the Judicial Council has determined that benefits of the procedure to infertile couples or couples whose future reproductive function will be reduced far outweigh the risks of abuse.

Human Cloning

Cloning, as discussed in Chapter 9, creates cells and organisms with identical genetic composition. Physicians should help educate the public about the limits of human cloning as well as the current ethical and legal protections that would prevent abuse of human cloning. These include the following:

- Using human cloning as an approach to terminal illness or mortality is based on the mistaken notion that one's genotype largely determines one's individuality. Cloned offspring are not identical in every way to clone-parents.

- Current ethical and legal standards prohibit human cloning without an individual's permission.

- Current ethical and legal standards hold that a human clone would be entitled to the same rights, freedoms, and protections as other individuals in society.

Physicians should not participate in human cloning at this time because harms and benefits of the process are not yet known and further investigation and discussion are necessary.

◆ ◆ ◆ ◆ **Organ and Tissue Donation and Transplantation**

Commercial Use of Human Tissue

The rapid growth of biotechnology has led to the commercial availability of products derived from human tissue. Physicians considering the use of such products should:

- Obtain written informed consent from patients for the use of their organs or tissues in clinical research.

- Disclose all potential commercial applications to the patient before taking a profit on products developed from biological materials.

- Avoid using human tissue and its products for commercial purposes without the informed consent of the patient who provided the original cellular material.

- Remember that profits from the commercial use of human tissue and its products may be shared with patients, via lawful contractual agreements.

- Conform to ethical standards when offering patient diagnostic and therapeutic options and not be influenced in any way by the commercial potential of the patient's tissue.

Financial Incentives for Organ Donation

Physicians should encourage the voluntary donation of organs for transplantation, but it is unethical to participate in a plan that pays a donor. Organ donors may, however, be reimbursed for expenses incurred in connection with removal of an organ.

The Judicial Council suggests that in the future, contracts to prospective donors may be issued to allow the donor's family or estate to receive some financial remuneration after the donor's organs have been retrieved and judged medically suitable for transplantation. These conditions should apply:

- Only the potential donor and no other third party may opt to accept financial incentives for cadaveric organ donation (organs harvested for transplantation after the donor has died). The potential donor must be a competent adult when the decision to donate is made and must not have committed suicide.

- The financial incentive should not be a large amount but should be the lowest amount possible to encourage organ donation. A state agency should administer the incentive.

- Payment should be made only after the organs have been retrieved and judged medically suitable for transplantation. Suitability should be determined by procedures outlined by the Organ Procurement and Transplantation Network.

- Incentives should not be considered when allocating donated organs. The distribution should continue to be based on medical need.

Mandated Choice and Presumed Consent for Cadaveric Organ Donation

Ethically appropriate strategies for requiring individuals to express their preferences regarding organ donation include indicating the desire to be an organ donor on drivers' licenses or performing some other state-mandated task. A system of presumed consent, in which individuals are assumed to consent to organ donation after death unless otherwise specified, raises serious ethical concerns.

Organ Procurement Following Cardiac Death

A number of safeguards must be followed in procuring cadaveric organs for transplant:

- Consent for withdrawal of life support and organ retrieval must be voluntary. If for any reason undue influence on surrogates is suspected, a full ethics consultation should be required.

- There must be no conflict of interest among the health care team. Professionals providing end-of-life care should be separate from the transplant team.

- Assessment programs should evaluate the success and acceptability of organ removal following withdrawal of life support.

- In situ (inside the body) preservation of cadaveric organs is ethically permissible only with the prior consent of the decedent or his or her surrogate decision maker.

- Recipients of procured organs should be informed of the source of the organs, as well as any potential defects in the organs, so that they may decide, with their physicians, whether to accept the organs.

- Clinical criteria should be developed to ensure that only medically acceptable organs are used in transplantation.

Organ Transplantation Guidelines

The following guidelines should be used in considering transplantation of organs:

- The physician's primary concern must be the health of the patient. Care must be taken to protect the rights of both organ donors and recipients.

- When cadaveric organs are to be transplanted, the donor's death shall have been determined by at least one physician other than the recipient's physician. Death shall be determined based on currently accepted and available scientific tests.

- The proposed procedure should be fully discussed with the donor and the recipient or with responsible relatives or representatives. Consent must be fully informed and voluntary, with concern for the patient overriding any interest in advancing scientific knowledge.

- Only physicians with appropriate knowledge and competence should perform transplant procedures, and the procedures should be performed only in medical institutions with adequate facilities.

- Recipients should be determined according to the Judicial Council's guidelines on allocation of limited medical resources.

- Organs should be considered a national resource, and geographic priorities should be prohibited except when transportation of organs would threaten their suitability for transplantation.

- Patients should be placed on a single waiting list for each organ.

Medical Applications of Fetal Tissue Transplantation

The following safeguards should apply, so that the decision to have an abortion is not influenced by the decision to donate fetal tissue.

- The Judicial Council's guidelines on clinical investigation and organ transplantation should be followed.

- The decision to undergo an abortion should be made before any discussion of transplanting fetal tissue.

- The safety of the pregnant woman should be foremost in decisions regarding the technique used to induce abortion as well as the timing of the abortion regarding gestational age of the fetus.

- Payment is not made for fetal tissue, beyond reimbursement for reasonable expenses.

- The donor cannot designate the recipient of fetal tissue.

- Health care personnel involved in the termination of pregnancy cannot participate in the transplantation or receive benefit from the fetal tissue obtained.

- Written informed consent should be obtained from both the donor and the recipient, in accordance with applicable law.

anencephaly *A congenital deformity in newborns characterized by absence of the brain and spinal cord.*

Anencephalic Neonates as Organ Donors

Anencephaly is a congenital absence of most of the brain, skull, and scalp. Infants born with this condition differ from other brain-damaged persons in that they lack past consciousness and have no potential for future consciousness. Physicians may provide anencephalic neonates with life-support therapies necessary to sustain organ viability until determination of death is made, in accordance with accepted medical standards, relevant law, and regional organ procurement organization policy.

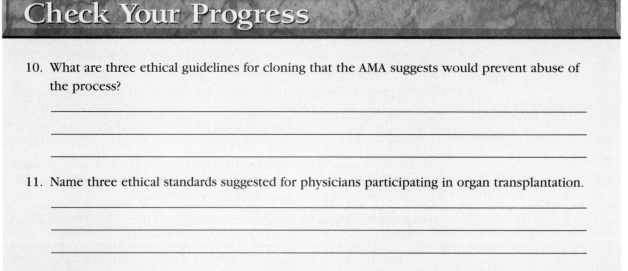

Check Your Progress

10. What are three ethical guidelines for cloning that the AMA suggests would prevent abuse of the process?

_____

_____

_____

11. Name three ethical standards suggested for physicians participating in organ transplantation.

_____

_____

_____

12. Define *anencephaly.*

_____

_____

_____

Hospital Conditions of Participation in Organ Donor Programs

A law passed in 1998, called Hospital Conditions of Participation (COP), established requirements for all U.S. hospitals participating in organ donor programs. These hospitals must:

• Have an agreement with an organ procurement organization (OPO) and must contact the OPO about all deaths.

(continued)

Fetal Umbilical Cord Blood

Hematopoietic stem cells from human umbilical cord blood have been used as an alternative to bone marrow transplantation. Such cells are obtained by clamping the umbilical cord immediately after delivery. Ethical concerns raised by the use of such tissue include the following:

1. Normal clamping procedures should be followed so that the neonate is not deprived of blood too soon.

2. Parents must be fully informed of the risks involved and must give written consent.

3. If the child-donor is at risk for an illness that is treated by bone marrow donation, the child should not be used as a donor, and his or her blood should be stored for possible future use.

- Have an agreement with a designated eye and tissue bank.
- Provide the option to donate organs and tissues or to decline donation. The person requesting donation must be either an OPO representative or an OPO-trained "designated requestor."
- Work with the OPO and tissue or eye banks to educate staff, and take part in death reviews to identify potential donors and provide donor management.
- Provide information to the Organ Procurement and Transplantation Network (OPTN), the Scientific Registry, and OPOs.

The Use of Minors as Organ and Tissue Donors

Use of minors as organ and tissue donors should be limited. They should be used as sources only when medical risks are low or moderate, as in blood, skin, or bone marrow donation. Parental consent and sometimes court authorization is necessary. Transplantation must present a "clear benefit" to the minor source, which means meeting the following requirements:

- Ideally the minor should be the only possible source.

- A transplant should be determined with some degree of medical certainty to represent a substantial benefit, beyond merely increasing the comfort of the recipient.

- The transplant must have a reasonable chance of success.

- Minors should be allowed to serve as sources only for close family members.

- Psychological or emotional benefits to both donor and recipient should be considered.

- It must be determined that the potential source does not have underlying conditions that create undue risk.

◆ ◆ ◆ ◆   **Choices for Life or Death**

Quality of Life

In making treatment decisions for seriously disabled newborns or for other persons seriously disabled by injury or illness, the primary concern must be for the welfare of the patient. It is permissible to consider quality of life, as defined by the patient's interests and values, when deciding about life-sustaining treatment.

Court Case

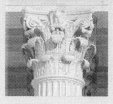

Disabled Woman Seeks Relief

In California, Elizabeth Bouvia, severely disabled from cerebral palsy, was hospitalized and fed by means of a nasogastric tube. She was not comatose or terminally ill, but she said she wanted to die and asked to have her feeding tube removed. When the hospital refused on the grounds that removal of the tube would cause Bouvia's death, she sued.

The court held that Bouvia was a competent adult, and therefore the decision to remove the feeding tube that kept her alive was hers to make.

Although Elizabeth Bouvia won her lawsuit and the nasogastric feeding tube was removed, she did not die. After the feeding tube was removed she was cared for in her home and no longer needed a feeding tube to receive nourishment.

Bouvia v. Superior Court of Los Angeles County, 179 Cal. App.3d 1172, 225 Cal. Rptr. 297 (Ct. App. 1986).

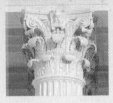
Withholding or Withdrawing Life-Sustaining Medical Treatment

Physicians are committed to sustaining life and relieving suffering. Where the performance of one duty conflicts with the other, the patient's wishes should prevail. Physicians are required by the principle of patient autonomy to respect a competent patient's decision to forgo life-sustaining treatment, which prolongs life without reversing the underlying medical condition. Life-sustaining treatment includes, but is not limited to, mechanical ventilation, renal dialysis, chemotherapy, use of antibiotics and other drugs, and artificial nutrition and hydration.

Surrogate decision makers should be designated for incompetent patients who may be eligible for life-sustaining treatment. Surrogates may make substituted decisions, based on what the patient would most likely have decided. Patients' advance medical directives can help proxies make decisions regarding life-sustaining treatment. In the following situations, institutional or judicial review or intervention may be required for incompetent patients:

- There are no available family members willing to make decisions for the patient.

- There is a dispute among family members, and no decision maker was designated in the **advance directive.**

- A health care provider believes the family's decision is not what the patient, if competent, would want.

- A health care provider believes the decision is clearly not in the patient's best interest.

advance directive *A document that makes one's wishes known concerning medical life-support measures in the event that one is unable to speak for oneself.*

euthanasia *The practice of willfully ending life in an individual with an incurable disease or condition.*

Euthanasia

The Judicial Council defines **euthanasia** as "the administration of a lethal agent by another person to a patient for the purpose of relieving the patient's intolerable and incurable suffering." The council states that

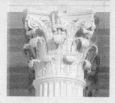
Landmark Case: Right-to-Die

In 1976 the parents of Karen Ann Quinlan obtained permission from a New Jersey court to remove their daughter from a respirator. Karen Ann had been in an irreversible coma for eight years, after allegedly ingesting an unknown combination of alcohol and drugs. Karen Ann's father, as her guardian, had asked her physicians to remove the respirator believed to be sustaining her life. The physicians refused, and the Quinlans sued for their daughter's right to die. A lower court held for the physicians, but on appeal judges allowed Karen Ann's respirator to be disconnected. She continued to live via a feeding tube and died in June 1985.

In re Quinlan, 70 N.J. 10, 49, 355 A.2d 647, 668 (1976).

euthanasia is incompatible with the physician's role as healer, would be difficult to control if made public policy, and would pose serious societal risks. Instead of practicing euthanasia, physicians should be sensitive to the needs of dying patients. Patients should not be abandoned when cure is impossible and should continue to receive emotional support, comfort care, adequate pain control, respect for their autonomy, and effective communication.

Physician-Assisted Suicide

Physician-assisted suicide occurs when a physician, aware that a patient may commit suicide, provides the necessary means (for example, a prescription for drugs) or information (for example, a lethal dosage) for the suicide to occur.

Physician-assisted suicide is incompatible with the physician's role as healer and may ultimately do society more harm than good. Alternatives for physicians are the same as those stated in the previous section, "Euthanasia."

Treatment Decisions for Seriously Ill Newborns

A physician's primary concern should be for the best interest of the newborn. Factors that should be weighed regarding life-sustaining treatment for newborns include:

1. The chance that therapy will succeed.

2. Risks involved with treatment and nontreatment.

3. The degree to which therapy, if successful, will extend life.

4. Pain and discomfort associated with the therapy.

5. Anticipated quality of life for the newborn with and without treatment.

Physicians must fully inform parents of seriously ill newborns concerning the nature of treatments, therapeutic options, and the expected prognosis with and without therapy. Counseling services and the opportunity to speak with other parents in similar situations should be available to parents. When conflicts arise, ethics committees or infant review committees should be consulted. These committees should also be consulted when referring cases to appropriate public agencies if parents' decisions are judged not to be in the best interests of the infant.

Do-Not-Resuscitate Orders

When patients suffer cardiac or respiratory arrest, efforts should be made to resuscitate them except when circumstances indicate that cardiopulmonary resuscitation (CPR) would be inappropriate or not in accord with the best interests or desires of patients.

Patients at risk of cardiac or respiratory failure should be encouraged to express in advance their wishes regarding CPR. Their written directives should be part of their medical records. Physicians are ethically obligated to honor patients' wishes.

If patients are incompetent, decisions regarding CPR should be made by designated surrogate decision makers, based on the previous expressed wishes of the patient or, if the patient's preferences are unknown, in accordance with the patient's best interests.

do-not-resuscitate (DNR) order *Orders written at the request of patients or their authorized representatives that cardiopulmonary resuscitation not be used to sustain life in a medical crisis.*

If the attending physician believes it is inappropriate to administer CPR, he or she may enter a **do-not-resuscitate (DNR) order** into the patient's medical record. CPR should be considered inappropriate if it cannot be expected either to restore cardiac or respiratory function or to meet established ethical criteria. If possible, the physician should inform the patient or the patient's designated decision maker of the basis for and content of the DNR order. Physicians should also discuss alternatives, such as obtaining a second opinion, consulting a bioethics committee, or transferring care to another physician.

DNR orders apply only to resuscitative efforts in case of cardiopulmonary arrest and should not preclude other procedures that may be medically appropriate.

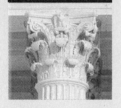

Court Case

Physician's Duty to Provide CPR Tested in Court

A physician was convicted of attempted murder of a terminally ill patient, and intentional and malicious second-degree murder of another terminally ill patient, for failure to provide CPR. A higher court reversed the physician's convictions, stating that the jury that convicted the physician could not disregard the testimony of several physicians who concurred with the defendant-physician's treatment of the deceased patients.

State v. Naramore, 25 Kan. App. 2d 302, 965 P.2d 211, 214, 216.

Optimal Use of Orders-Not-to-Intervene and Advance Directives

Advance care planning should be encouraged so physicians can tailor end-of-life care to a patient's express wishes. Improvement strategies for end-of-life planning include the following:

- Patients and physicians should make use of advisory as well as statutory documents.

- Advisory documents should be based on validated worksheets, ensuring that preferences for end-of-life treatment are elicited and recorded and are appropriate to medical decisions.

- Physicians should discuss, in advance if possible, the patient's preferences with the patient and the patient's proxy.

- Central repositories should be established for completed advisory documents, state statutory documents, and proxy and primary physician identification so the patient's wishes are readily available in emergencies.

- Health care facilities should honor, and physicians should use, orders on the Doctor's Order Sheet to indicate patient wishes regarding end-of-life medical treatments.

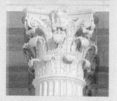

Court Case

Dental AIDS Patient Sues for Discrimination

A patient cracked a tooth in a car accident and went to a dental clinic to have the tooth extracted. Before the extraction procedure began, the dentist became concerned over whether or not to use general anesthesia since the patient had a functional heart murmur. The dentist and patient disagreed, so the dentist tried to reach the patient's physician for a consultation. The physician was not available, but the medical director of the hospital where he was on staff substituted. The director asked the patient for permission to inform the dentist that he was HIV-positive.

The patient reluctantly agreed, after which the dentist refused to treat him. The only alternative the dentist offered was referral to a "special clinic for HIV." The patient accepted the referral. The facility to which he was referred did not treat HIV-positive patients but served the medically indigent and mentally ill.

The patient sued the dentist under the Americans with Disabilities Act and the New Jersey Law Against Discrimination. He charged that the dentist's action had caused him shame, anger, helplessness, rejection, and depression.

The dentist did not defend against the charges, and the patient won by default. The trial court said the patient had established a *prima facie* case for discrimination under both the Americans with Disabilities Act and the New Jersey law. The court held that clearly the patient was HIV-positive and had been refused dental treatment on that basis.

The court awarded attorney fees to the patient and $82,000 in damages.

D. B. v. Bloom, 896 F. Supp. 166 (D.C., N.J., Aug. 15, 1995).

HIV Testing

Testing for human immunodeficiency virus (HIV) is appropriate and should be encouraged for diagnosis and treatment of HIV infection or medical conditions affected by HIV. In order to limit the public spread of HIV infection, physicians should encourage voluntary testing of patients at risk for infection.

Physicians should see that patient autonomy and confidentiality are respected as much as possible when conducting HIV testing.

Patients must give informed consent specifically for HIV testing. Patient autonomy and confidentiality must be respected whenever possible. Limits to confidentiality should be explained to the patient before consent for testing is given. Exceptions to confidentiality are appropriate to protect others from infection. If a physician knows that an HIV-positive person is putting others at risk, he or she is ethically obligated to (1) attempt to persuade the infected patient to stop endangering the third party; (2) if persuasion fails, notify authorities; and (3) if authorities take no action, notify the third party.

When a health care worker is at risk for HIV infection because of exposure to body fluids, it is acceptable to test the patient for HIV infection even if the patient refuses to give consent. When being tested without consent, the patient should receive the customary pretest counseling, in accordance with the law.

It is unethical to refuse to treat a person who is HIV-positive or who refuses to be tested for HIV. If the patient refuses to be tested and knowledge of HIV status is vital to medical treatment, the physician may elect to transfer care of the patient to another physician who is willing to treat under the patient's expressed conditions.

Information from Unethical Experiments

A human studies review board should evaluate the ethics of any proposed experiments using human subjects before the experiments are performed.

Authors, peer reviewers, and editors of medical texts that publish results of experimental studies are responsible for revealing that the data are from unethical experiments. Publications should adopt a standard regarding publication of data from unethical experiments.

Based on scientific and moral grounds, data obtained from cruel and inhumane experiments, such as the Nazi experiments and the Tuskegee Study, should never be published or cited. In those rare cases where no other data exist and human lives could be lost without the use of such data, publication or citation is permissible.

YOU BE THE JUDGE

A California surgeon used an innovative surgical procedure to treat a patient with duodenal ulcer disease. The surgery bypassed the ulcer by removing the lower portion of the patient's stomach and the ulcerated duodenum. The physician then attached the remaining part of the stomach to a healthy part of the small intestine. A "T" incision was used to close the duodenal stump, but the suture line on the stump leaked, and more surgery was needed to repair it.

The patient sued the surgeon for malpractice, claiming that the "T" incision used to close the duodenal stump breached the standard of care. Experts testified that the "T" incision satisfied the standard of care but was an "innovative" technique and not the usual way of handling the condition.

A lower court found the surgeon not liable, but an appellate court ordered a new trial. The court said that the new jury should not be instructed that the procedure was an approved method of treatment, since the treatment had been used in the small bowel but not in a duodenal operation.

State medical association spokespersons, physicians, and other health care practitioners feared that when the decision became known it would have "a chilling effect" on using experimental procedures on patients when other techniques have proven ineffective.

In your opinion, should the decision that the surgeon was not liable have been upheld by the appellate court? Why or why not? _____

_____

_____

Should physicians and other health care practitioners ever be allowed to use experimental procedures and techniques? Explain your answer.

_____

_____

_____

What ethical guidelines should apply when physicians and other health care practitioners consider using experimental treatment?

_____

_____

_____

Applying Knowledge

Write "T" or "F" in the blank to indicate whether you think the statement is true or false.

_____ 1. A physician may ethically participate in a legal execution.

_____ 2. A treating physician should not make medical treatment allocation decisions.

_____ 3. A physician has both a legal and an ethical responsibility to report suspected child abuse.

_____ 4. Ethically, informed consent for artificial insemination is not required from both husband and wife.

_____ 5. It is ethical for physicians to prescribe treatment or services deemed financially beneficial to themselves, regardless of the general opinion of the medical community.

_____ 6. In organ transplantation, a recipient's rights are to be considered paramount to the donor's.

_____ 7. It is never ethical for fetal tissue to be used in transplant procedures.

Match each of the following definitions with the correct term by writing the appropriate letter in the spaces provided.

_____ 8. A rapidly advancing science that includes recombinant DNA technology and the development of medical products from human tissue.

_____ 9. The landmark case that legalized abortion in the United States.

_____10. Care that in a physician's best professional judgment cannot benefit the patient.

_____11. A landmark right-to-die case.

_____12. Moral issues that have arisen as a result of advances in biotechnology and biological/medical research.

_____13. Written documents that have evolved to serve as moral guidelines for those entrusted with providing care to the sick.

_____14. Involves rewriting or rearranging bits of genetic code to suppress the expression of harmful effects.

_____15. A voluntary act that causes the death of a patient who has a terminal disease or condition.

_____16. A physician's order, entered into a patient's medical record, prohibiting the use of cardiopulmonary resuscitation (CPR) in the event of cardiac arrest.

a. advance directive

b. euthanasia

c. bioethics

d. genetic counseling and testing·

e. _Roe v. Wade_

f. gene therapy

g. futile care

h. do-not-resuscitate (DNR) order

i. codes of ethics

j. somatic cell therapy

k. patent

l. life-sustaining treatment

m. _In re Quinlan_

n. germ line therapy

o. biotechnology

_____17. A document expressing a hospital patient's wishes concerning CPR and other life-sustaining treatment, should cardiac arrest occur.

_____18. Grants the holder the right, for a limited amount of time, to prevent others from commercializing his or her inventions.

_____19. The procedure by which human cells other than germ cells (eggs and sperm) are genetically altered.

_____20. The procedure by which a replacement gene is inserted in human germ cells, resulting in expression of the new gene in the patient's offspring.

_____21. Two procedures that are most appropriate for prospective parents whose genetic histories indicate an elevated risk for genetic disorders.

Answer the following questions in the spaces provided.

22. What legal and ethical issues does HIV testing pose for physicians and other health care professionals?

_____

_____

_____

_____

23. What ethical issues are raised by the practice of using medical treatments that involve fetal tissue and stem cells from human umbilical cord blood?

_____

_____

_____

_____

24. List five ethical guidelines concerning clinical investigation.

_____

_____

_____

_____

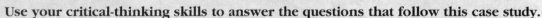

Case Studies

Use your critical-thinking skills to answer the questions that follow this case study.

An organ procurement organization (OPO) staff member recently asked the American Medical Association's Ethics Forum how to deal with physicians who fail to maintain patient's functions to allow for organ donation. The staff member told of a case where a patient's family had indicated its willingness to allow donation, but the surgeon failed to notify the OPO of the patient's imminent death and no action was taken to optimize organ donation. Therefore, the patient's organs could not be used.

25. **What ethical considerations should guide physicians regarding donation of a patient's organs?**

   _____

   _____

   _____

26. **In your opinion, should legal action be taken against those who would unethically and illegally override a patient's wishes concerning willingness to donate organs? Explain your answer.**

   _____

   _____

   _____

27. **What should constitute adequate proof that a patient wants to donate his or her organs?**

   _____

   _____

   _____

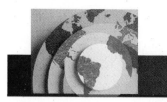

Internet Activities

Complete the activities and answer the questions that follow.

28. Visit the Web site for the Midwest Bioethics Center. Find the page, "What is Bioethics?"
Who invented the term and when? _____
According to the Center, what is the current standard of bioethics? _____
_____

29. Do an Internet search for "Tuskegee Study." Explain why the study is mentioned in the *Code of Medical Ethics* as an "unethical study." In your opinion, are unethical studies still being conducted? Give an example from the news.

_____

_____

_____

_____

_____

_____

INTERPERSONAL RELATIONSHIPS AND PRACTICE MATTERS

11

Objectives

After studying this chapter, you should be able to:

1. Discuss ethical concerns involving a physician's relationship with other professionals.
2. Explain ethical responsibilities dealing with advertising, telecommunications, media, and confidentiality.
3. Identify ethically acceptable fees and charges.
4. Discuss ethical guidelines concerning medical records.
5. Discuss ethical guidelines concerning a physician's practice.
6. Identify ethical issues dealing with professional rights and responsibilities.

Key Terms

- conflict of interest
- contingent
- Federal Trade Commission Act
- fee splitting
- lien
- limited practitioner

- professional courtesy
- referral
- sexual misconduct
- staff privileges
- waiver

Ethics and the Business of Health Care

Health care practitioners must be guided by ethics in dealing with patients, colleagues, and others. They must also be aware of the ethical issues inherent in operating a business in the health care field. For example, is it proper for physicians and other health care practitioners to advertise their services? What information about a patient may a medical assistant or other health care practitioner release to the media without breaching confidentiality? Is it ethical for health care practitioners to own a financial interest in laboratories, nursing homes, or other health care facilities? May a nurse, medical assistant, or other health care practitioner question a physician's order?

Summarized in this chapter are ethical guidelines for interprofessional relationships and other practice matters taken from the AMA's *Code of Medical Ethics: Current Opinions and Annotations.* Again, the guidelines refer to the ethics for various situations and are not laws, which will vary with states. As you read the guidelines, refer back to relevant sections of each chapter in the text.

Interprofessional Relationships

As the number of specialists in health care has increased, so has the number of questions concerning the relationship of physicians to other trained practitioners. The following pointers can help workers function smoothly as members of a medical team.

◆ ◆ ◆ ◆ Nonscientific Practitioners

Nonscientific practitioners are those who have no training or licensure in medical science but profess to heal through other, nonscientific means. It is unethical for a physician to practice any treatment that has no scientific basis and is dangerous, is calculated to deceive the patient by giving false hope, or may cause the patient to delay in seeking proper care.

State laws may also prohibit a physician from aiding and abetting an unlicensed person in the practice of medicine, aiding and abetting persons providing services beyond the scope of their licenses, or entering into joint patient treatment with such persons.

◆ ◆ ◆ ◆ Nurses

Physicians and nurses share a mutual ethical concern for patients. When nurses carry out the orders of attending physicians, they are fulfilling their duty to provide reasonable care. The physician has an ethical obligation to respond to a nurse's concern when orders appear to the nurse to be in error or contrary to customary medical and nursing practice. The ethical physician should neither expect nor insist that nurses follow orders contrary to standards of good medical and nursing practice. In emergencies, when prompt action is necessary and the physician is not immediately available, a nurse may be justified in acting contrary to the physician's standing orders to ensure patient safety. Such occurrences should not be considered a breakdown in professional relations.

Allied Health Professionals

Physicians often work with other members of the health care team, including nurses, physician's assistants, optometrists, medical assistants, and other health care practitioners. These guidelines can further professional relationships:

- Physicians may ethically employ or work in consultation with allied health professionals as long as they are appropriately trained and duly licensed to perform services requested.

- Physicians have an ethical obligation to ensure that their patients' medical and surgical conditions are appropriately evaluated and treated.

- Physicians may teach in recognized schools for allied health professionals for the purposes of improving educational quality and preparing allied health professionals to engage in their professions within the limits prescribed by law.

- It is unethical and inappropriate to substitute the services of an allied health professional for those of a physician when the allied health professional is not appropriately trained and duly licensed to provide the requested medical services.

Referral of Patients

referral *The act of recommending to a patient the diagnostic or therapeutic services of another physician.*

limited practitioner *A provider licensed to provide specific treatment or treatments specific to certain body parts.*

Physicians may ethically make **referrals** for diagnostic or therapeutic services to other physicians, limited practitioners, or other providers of health care services lawfully providing such services. **Limited practitioners** are those licensed to provide specific treatments or treatments specific to certain body parts. Examples of such practitioners include chiropractors, podiatrists, and optometrists. Other providers of health care services include physical therapists, speech and occupational therapists, and so forth. When referrals are made, physicians should be confident that the services will benefit the patient and will be performed competently and in accordance with accepted scientific standards and legal requirements.

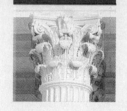

Court Case

Physician Accused of Soliciting Bribes

A physician accused of soliciting bribes in return for referring patients to a Medicaid provider moved to dismiss the indictment alleging mail fraud and violations of the Medicaid antikickback statute. The court denied the physician's motion to dismiss the indictment, noting that the physician's fiduciary duty under the "Referral of Patients" section of the AMA's *Code of Medical Ethics* supported an intangible rights mail fraud charge.

United States v. Neufeld, 908 F. Supp. 491, 500.

◆ ◆ ◆ ◆ Chiropractic

A physician may ethically associate professionally with chiropractors provided that the physician believes that such association is in the patient's best interest. A physician may refer patients to a chiropractor legally permitted to furnish such diagnostic or therapeutic services. Physicians may also teach in recognized schools of chiropractic.

◆ ◆ ◆ ◆ Sports Medicine

The professional responsibility of the physician who serves in a medical capacity at athletic contests or sporting events is to protect the health and safety of the athletes. Physicians should be guided solely by medical considerations and should not be controlled or influenced by spectators, event promoters, or even injured athletes.

Check Your Progress

1. Define *chiropractor.*

   _____
   _____

2. Define *sports medicine specialist.*

   _____
   _____

3. Regarding nonscientific practitioners, state laws generally prohibit physicians from which type of activities?

   _____
   _____

4. If the customary dosage of a medication is 0.5 cc to 1 cc and a physician's written order reads "3 cc," is the nurse responsible for carrying out the order ethically bound to question it? Explain your answer.

   _____
   _____

◆ ◆ ◆ ◆ Sexual Harassment and Exploitation Between Medical Supervisors and Trainees

Sexual harassment as a legal issue is discussed in Chapter 8. Health care practitioners should be aware that, even though sexually suggestive behavior may not have crossed the line legally, any form of sexual harassment or exploitation between medical supervisors and trainees, employers and employees, coworkers, or medical practitioners and patients is unethical.

As explained in Chapter 8, sexual harassment has occurred when:

- Such conduct interferes with an individual's work or academic performance or creates an intimidating, hostile, or offensive work environment.

- Accepting or rejecting such conduct affects employment decisions or academic evaluations concerning an individual.

Sexual relationships between medical supervisors and trainees are not acceptable, even when consensual, because of the unequal power and status between the individuals involved and because such relationships can adversely affect patient care. The supervisory role should be terminated if the parties involved wish to pursue their relationship.

◆ ◆ ◆ ◆ Hospital Relations

The AMA's *Code of Medical Ethics* addresses the following issues regarding hospital relations:

Admission Fee

It is unethical for physicians to charge a separate fee for securing the admission of patients to a hospital. Physicians should derive their incomes from medical services rendered.

Compulsory Assessments

It is improper for medical staff membership or privileges to be conditioned on compulsory assessments for any purpose. Self-imposed assessments by vote of the medical staff are acceptable.

Billing for Housestaff and Student Services

Physicians may ethically charge patients for services performed by residents or students under the physician's direct supervision.

Economic Incentives and Levels of Care

The welfare of patients always takes priority over economic interests of the hospital. Hospital staff members are obligated to perform within licensing laws and accreditation requirements. It is unethical to provide unnecessary treatment, inadequate treatment, or treatment performed solely to increase income.

Organized Medical Staff

It is ethical for the organized medical staff to act as a group for the purpose of dealing with the hospital's governing board and others as long as applicable laws are not violated and patient care does not suffer.

Physician-Hospital Contractual Relations

There are many financial agreements and contracts between physicians and hospitals that are mutually beneficial and ethical. For example, the physician may be a hospital employee, a hospital-associated medical specialist, or an independent practitioner with staff privileges. Physicians may be employed by hospitals for fixed annual salaries, for hourly wages, or pursuant to other similar arrangements relative to the professional services, skill, education, expertise, or time involved.

Staff Privileges

staff privileges *The right to practice at a particular hospital.*

Decisions regarding hospital privileges should be based on the training, experience, and demonstrated competence of candidates. The granting of **staff privileges** should not be based on numbers of patients admitted to the facility or the economic or insurance status of the patient. Neither should personal friendships, antagonisms, jurisdictional disputes, or fear of competition affect these decisions. The welfare of the patient should be paramount when physicians are involved in the granting, denying, or termination of hospital privileges.

Communications and Confidentiality Issues

Following are guidelines from the AMA's *Code of Medical Ethics* related to communications and confidentiality issues relevant to medical practice.

◆ ◆ ◆ ◆ Advertising

Physicians may ethically advertise their services and provide services to members of managed care plans that advertise for subscribers as long as the claims are true and are not deceptive. It is deceptive for prepaid or managed care plans to advertise the services of a renowned physician if that physician's services are not available to all plan members or subscribers.

◆ ◆ ◆ ◆ Direct-to-Consumer Advertisements of Prescription Drugs

Physicians should encourage studies that examine whether direct-to-consumer advertising of drugs improves the communication of health information, enhances the patient-physician relationship, and imparts accurate information about risks, precautions, adverse reactions, and costs.

When patients request drugs they have seen advertised, physicians should deny requests for inappropriate prescriptions and educate patients about the drugs and other treatment options.

Physicians should be concerned that direct-to-consumer advertising does not raise false expectations. Ideally, such advertising should enhance consumer education, convey an accurate and responsible health education message, refer patients to their physicians for more information, identify the target population at risk, and discourage self-diagnosis and self-treatment.

◆ ◆ ◆ ◆ Advertising and Publicity

Federal Trade Commission Act *A federal statute that established the Federal Trade Commission (FTC), which prohibits unfair or deceptive acts in advertising and other trade areas.*

There are no restrictions on advertising by physicians if such advertising is not deceptive and is consistent with federal regulatory standards that apply to commercial advertising. Section 5 of the **Federal Trade Commission Act,** for example, specifies that claims made must be explicitly (expressed) and implicitly (implied) truthful and not misleading.

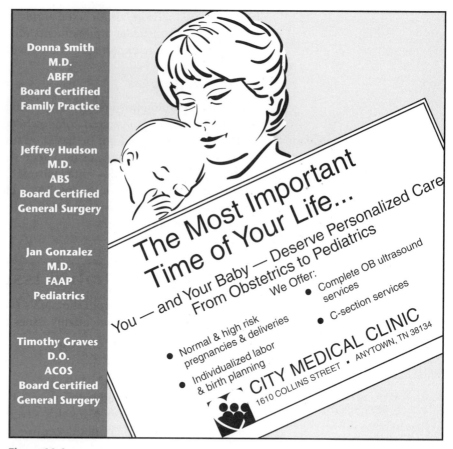

Figure 11-1
Sample Physicians' Advertisement

Physicians' advertisements may include mention of educational background, basis of fee determination (including charges for specific services), credit and payment plans, and any other relevant, nondeceptive information. Figure 11-1 illustrates a sample advertisement by a group of physicians.

Testimonials from patients concerning a physician's skill or the quality of his or her services are questionable, since they may not reflect the results that other patients with similar conditions generally experience. Statements that a physician has a truly exclusive or unique skill or remedy are also misleading, since physicians are ethically obligated to share medical advances. Similarly, statements that a physician has successfully treated a large number of certain types of cases may also be misleading, since they imply a certain result and may create unjustified expectations.

Physician Advisory or Referral Services by Telecommunication

Physicians in today's health care environment frequently provide advisory services through telephone, facsimile, or computer, all of which are outside the traditional physician-patient relationship. Telecommunication advisory services can be useful sources of medical information for the public, but certain guidelines should apply. In general, physicians and other health care professionals providing information via telecommunication should not diagnose or prescribe and should make limitations of the service clear to users.

Physician referral services can be most useful to the public if referrals are based on medical considerations and not on fees collected from physicians who enroll.

YOU BE THE JUDGE

As use of the Internet has exploded, patients are turning to Web sites to find health information. Some sites offer services that were once available only during a face-to-face encounter between patient and physician. For example, in mid-2001 three of Boston's top hospitals launched a service to sell second opinions online. Massachusetts General Hospital, Dana Farber Cancer Institute, and Brigham and Women's Hospitals offer links on their homepages to the "Partner's Online Specialty Consultation" site.

The service was launched to provide physician consultations for patients who may question a diagnosis or treatment approach. It also sought to ease the long waits that can occur when patients need to schedule appointments with specialists and to help prevent hospital overcrowding.

Patients could not access the consultation service directly. They contacted primary care physicians, who were to formally request the assessment. Fees for the service were set at $600 per case, which was not covered by insurance providers. Upon payment of the fee, a patient's registration form and all relevant medical records were forwarded to a designated specialist. Within three business days the primary care physician would hear from the specialist, and he or she could then discuss results with the patient.

In your opinion, is the service operating within ethical standards for medical care? Explain your answer.

_____

_____

_____

Do you believe the $600 fee is reasonable for such a service? Explain.

_____

_____

_____

At what point, in your estimation, does providing medical information over the Internet constitute a physician-patient relationship? Does the consultation service described above meet this criteria? Why or why not?

_____

_____

_____

_____

Kimberly is a physical therapist and an instructor in the physical therapy program at a small university in a rural area of a Northwestern state. Although there has long been a stigma attached to advertising by physicians and other health care providers, Kimberly sees public attitudes toward advertising in her area changing in today's health care environment.

"Now there is more competition in the health care marketplace," Kimberly states. "Physical therapists are starting to think, 'Why aren't we advertising?' " A physical therapist, for example, "can inform the public regarding where you are located, and any specialty practiced."

"I think advertising [by health care practitioners] is becoming more acceptable," Kimberly adds. "But health care marketing is different than for other businesses. People in health care businesses don't advertise the same way." For example, price is not usually mentioned in health care service ads (a half-price ad for medical services would repel rather than entice consumers), but, increasingly, other aspects of a provider's services are advertised to the public.

In addition, direct-to-consumer drug advertising on television and in print media "is affecting the way physicians practice to some degree," Kimberly says, "because patients will come in and say, 'I think this drug will help me,' without really knowing anything about the drug. They just saw a 30 to 60 second [television] commercial spot about it. This could change prescription patterns."

As medical service advertising becomes more prevalent, however, accuracy, honesty, and patient welfare should never be compromised.

[*Note:* Acceptance and prevalence of health care practitioners' advertising may vary with different areas of the country. For example, residents of more populated Eastern and Southeastern states may have long been familiar with and accepting of the practice, whereas residents of less populated states are more recently becoming familiar with health care practitioner ads.]

Communications Media:
Standards of Professional Responsibility

Physicians or others acting as their spokespersons may not release to the media information about a specific patient without that patient's consent or the consent of the patient's authorized representative. The physician may cooperate with the media but may release only authorized information or information that is public knowledge. When patients or their authorized representatives consent to the release of medical information, physicians may assist the representatives of the media in every way possible to ensure that the medical news is accurate and is released promptly.

Requests for statements regarding injuries sustained in assaults or other police matters should be referred to the proper authorities.

Certain news that is part of the public record, such as deaths, may be released without the consent of the patient or his or her representative.

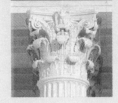

Court Case

Release of Medical Records to the Media Violates Confidentiality

A patient entered a nursing home in 1987 after falling into a chronic vegetative state. Her parents petitioned to remove life support. A trial court granted permission for artificial hydration and nutrition to be discontinued. The patient was then transferred from the nursing home to a hospital.

Two weeks later a Christian fellowship group, alleging abuse by the patient's parents and health care providers, filed a petition seeking guardianship of the patient. The group's attorney was granted temporary guardianship and a 21-day stay on the order allowing withdrawal of life support.

During the 21-day period of the stay, the group sent copies of sections of the patient's medical records to various local media outlets to publicize the case for maintaining her life support.

The group's attorney was then subject to action by the state disciplinary commission for transmitting the patient's medical records to the media without proper authorization. In 1995 the Supreme Court of Indiana ordered that the attorney be publicly reprimanded for disclosing the patient's confidential medical records.

In the Matter of Patti Sue Mullins, 649 N.E.2d 1024 (Ind. Sup. Ct., May 9, 1995).

◆ ◆ ◆ ◆ Confidentiality

In order to ensure proper medical treatment, a patient must feel free to tell a physician everything pertinent to his or her case. Therefore, strict confidentiality is imperative. The physician may not release confidential information without the patient's consent unless legally required to report certain incidents, as in the following examples:

- A patient threatens to inflict bodily harm to another person or to himself or herself and may reasonably be expected to carry out the threat.

- A patient has a reportable, communicable disease, such as tuberculosis, hepatitis, or AIDS.

- A patient has a gunshot or knife wound.

- The physician is subpoenaed to give testimony in a court of law about a patient's medical record.

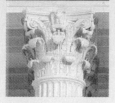
Confidential Care for Minors

Physicians who treat minors have an ethical duty to involve these patients in the medical decision-making process whenever feasible, thus promoting their autonomy. Physicians should encourage minors who request confidential services to involve their parents. However, when minors request contraceptive services, pregnancy-related care, or treatment for sexually transmitted disease, drug and alcohol abuse, or mental illness, physicians should recognize that requiring parental involvement may not be in the best interest of the health and well-being of the patient.

Where the law allows, physicians should permit competent minors to consent to their own medical care and should not notify parents without the patient's consent. Physicians may evaluate competence in most cases, but they may sometimes need to consult experts in adolescent medicine or child psychology.

Other Issues Regarding Confidentiality

Special circumstances often arise in which confidentiality becomes an issue of concern. Guidelines for the release of patient medical information in certain special circumstances are as follows:

- Confidentiality of HIV status on autopsy reports should be maintained whenever possible.

- A patient's history, diagnosis, treatment, and prognosis may be discussed with the patient's lawyer with the consent of the patient or the patient's lawful representative.

- Physicians may testify in court or before a worker's compensation board in any personal injury or related case.

- The confidentiality of computerized medical records must be as diligently protected as other medical records. Only authorized personnel should enter confidential medical information into computers. The release of medical data should be limited to only those individuals or agencies with a bona fide use for the data, and only the data necessary for that specific use should be released. Stringent security procedures should be in place to prevent unauthorized access to computer-based patient medical records.

- Physicians may not ethically divulge patient medical data to data collection firms for marketing purposes. Often, physicians are offered incentives such as computer hardware or software in return for agreeing to such an arrangement, but they must not release such information without the consent of the patient or his or her lawful representative. If permission is not obtained, physicians violate patient confidentiality. Where physicians are somehow compensated for such information, they may also violate AMA principles regarding gifts to physicians from industry. Finally, such arrangements harm the integrity of the physician-patient relationship.

- Physicians may disclose patient information concerning medical history, diagnosis, and prognosis to insurance companies only with the consent of the patient or his or her lawful representative.

- When physicians are employed by industry or as independent medical examiners to perform certain assessments of an individual's health or disability, the information obtained is confidential. Such information should not be released to a third party without the patient's written consent, unless required by law. Information released to employers or prospective employers should include only data relevant to the patient's ability to perform the work required by the job. When physicians treat patients for work-related illnesses or injuries, worker's compensation laws may dictate provisions for releasing medical information to the employer.

    Employee identities should be deleted whenever statistical information about employees' health is released.

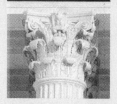

Court Case

Did the Consultant on an HIV Report Have a Duty to Warn?

In 1987 a patient tested positive for HIV. In a later, confirmatory test, the result was HIV-negative. The physician told the patient that the results meant the virus was not present in the blood sample used in the second test. The patient misinterpreted the physician's explanation and thought he was virus-free.

In 1988 the patient was again tested for HIV. A consultant hired by the physician reviewed the test results. In 1993 the patient and his wife sued the consultant for failing to notify the wife that the patient had tested positive for HIV. They claimed that the consultant's review of test results constituted a physician-patient relationship. The trial court disagreed and granted summary judgment to the consultant.

An appellate court affirmed the trial court's decision. The consultant had properly reviewed the patient's report for laboratory or typographical errors. Because there was no indication in the six-page report that the patient was HIV-positive, the consultant could not be held liable for failing to diagnose HIV or for failing to notify the patient's wife of such a diagnosis.

In re Sealed Case, 67 F.3d 965 (D.C., Oct. 27, 1995).

5. What federal regulatory standard must physicians who advertise their services follow?

_____

6. In what way should physicians confine their remarks when making statements to the media about a patient's condition?

_____

_____

7. List four situations in which physicians may release confidential information without a patient's consent.

_____

_____

_____

_____

Fees and Charges

contingent *Dependent on or conditioned by something else.*

A physician's fee should be based on the value of the service provided and not **contingent** on the outcome of a claim that does not relate to the value of the medical service.

A physician should not charge or collect an illegal or excessive fee. For example, a physician has illegally charged a patient if he or she accepts an assignment from Medicare, receives payment from the provider, and then charges the patient an additional amount. Fees should be based on the following factors:

- The difficulty or uniqueness of services performed and the time, skill, and experience required.

- Fees customary in the physician's locality for similar services.

- The total amount of charges involved.

- The quality of performance. This refers to level of skill and competence of the physician and does not mean that fees should be contingent on a particular treatment outcome.

   Additional guidelines concerning ethical fees include the following:

- When more than one physician is engaged in the care of a patient, each physician should charge separately for services, commensurate with the services performed. No physician should bill for services not rendered.

- A physician may charge a patient for a missed appointment or for one not canceled 24 hours in advance, but the patient should be informed in advance that such charges will be made.

- A physician should complete a standard insurance claim form for a patient at no extra charge. However, a charge for more complex or multiple forms may be made, in conformity with local custom.

- Physicians must comply with state and federal laws, such as the Truth-in-Lending Act, regarding interest and finance charges. Harsh or commercial collection practices are discouraged. Physicians who have problems with delinquent accounts may request that payment be made at the time of treatment or may add interest or other charges to these accounts, as long as the patient is notified in advance of the interest or finance charge. In hardship cases the Judicial Council of the AMA encourages physicians to drop these charges or to make other exceptions.

- When the charge for laboratory services cannot be sent directly to the patient, the referring physician's statement to the patient should indicate the actual charges for laboratory services, including the name of the laboratory as well as any separate charges for the physician's services.

fee splitting *Payment by one physician to another solely for the referral of a patient, or payment from a source for using its services or supplies.*

- **Fee splitting,** which involves payment by or to physicians solely for referring patients to other physicians, clinics, laboratories, hospitals, or other health care facilities, is unethical.

- Physicians may not ethically accept payment or other compensation from drug companies or device manufacturers in exchange for prescribing or recommending their products. It is also unethical for physicians to accept finder's fees for referring patients to research studies.

waiver *The act of intentionally relinquishing a known right, claim, or privilege.*

- Most health insurance programs impose patient co-payments. In cases of financial hardship, physicians may forgive or waive patient co-payments, but they should be sure that such a **waiver** is in accordance with applicable law and with agreements with insurers. In some cases routine forgiveness or waiver of co-payments may constitute fraud under state or federal law. For example, this would be the case for a clinic that advertises waiver of all patient co-payments and then performs unnecessary medical tests and sends statements to insurance companies for the tests.

lien *A charge against real or personal property for the satisfaction of a debt or duty owed by law.*

- In states with lien laws, physicians may file a **lien**—a hold or claim by one person on the property of another—as security for an unpaid fee, providing the fee is fixed in amount and not contingent on the patient's settling a claim against a third party.

◆ ◆ ◆ ◆ ## Professional Courtesy

professional courtesy *The practice of treating other physicians and their families free of charge or at a reduced fee.*

Professional courtesy refers to the provision of medical care to physician colleagues or their families for free or at a reduced rate. Professional courtesy is a long-standing tradition in the medical profession, but it is not ethically required. Physicians may use their own judgment in this matter.

Medical Records

Upon the request and proper written authorization of the patient, no physician should refuse to make records available to another physician treating the patient. These records cannot be withheld because of an unpaid bill.

The notes made by a physician in treating a patient are intended for his or her own use and belong to the physician. Statutes in most states, however, give patients access to their own medical records. Access to mental health records may be limited by law.

Physicians are obligated to retain patients' records that may reasonably be of future value to patients, based on the following guidelines:

- Medical considerations should determine how long and which records to keep. Operative notes and chemotherapy records should always be retained. A useful criterion regarding whether to keep parts of a record is whether a physician would need the information if seeing the patient for the first time.

- If a record is no longer medically useful, the physician should check state laws to see whether there is a requirement that records be kept for a specified period of time.

- Records should be kept for at least as long a time as the applicable statute of limitations for medical malpractice claims, and time should be measured from the last professional contact with the patient.

- For minor patients, the statute of limitations may not apply until they have reached the age of majority.

- Immunization records must always be kept.

- Records for patients covered by Medicare or Medicaid must be kept for at least five years.

- When discarding old records, all documents should be destroyed.

- If feasible, before a physician destroys old records, patients should be given the opportunity to claim the records or have them sent to another physician.

Court Case

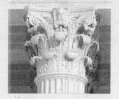

Psychologist Allowed to Testify

A New York appellate court ruled that a trial court acted properly in permitting a psychologist to testify on behalf of a patient. The pregnant patient experienced sharp abdominal pains that eventually necessitated surgery for removal of the fetus. The physician showed the patient a photo of the fetus he had removed. The patient filed suit against the physician for malpractice and emotional harm.

The trial court permitted testimony by the psychologist as an expert on the emotional injuries allegedly suffered by the patient. The appellate court held that the trial court did not abuse its discretion in allowing the psychologist to testify.

Shawe v. Addo-Yodo, 555 N.Y.S.2d 317 (N.Y. Sup. Ct., May 10, 1990).

◆ ◆ ◆ ◆   **Disposition of Medical Records**

When a physician leaves a group practice, retires, or dies, his or her patients should be notified. With patients' consent, records can then be forwarded to a new physician to ensure continued care.

The records of a deceased physician should not be destroyed but retained, subject to requests from patients that they be sent to another physician.

A practice may be sold either by the physician who owns it or by his or her estate. The "practice" includes office furniture, fixtures, equipment, office leasehold, and goodwill, which is the opportunity to take over the patients of the seller. When a practice is sold, active patients must be notified and given the opportunity to have their records forwarded to another physician of their choice.

A reasonable fee for duplicating records may be charged.

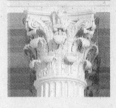

Court Case

Deceased Physician's Executor May Not Destroy Records

The executor of a deceased physician's estate refused to deliver the physician's medical records to his patients on the grounds that a provision in the decedent's will directed that all "office records" be destroyed. The deceased physician's former patients sued. The court ruled that, although a patient's records belong to the physician, it would be against public policy to permit their destruction.

The executor was ordered to make the records available to the patients' physicians at their request.

In re Culberton's Will, 57 Misc. 2d 391, 292 N.Y.S.2d 806, 808-10 (N.Y.Surr. 1968).

Practice Matters

Ethical guidelines for the treatment of and relationship with patients include the following:

- Physicians in management positions and other nonclinical roles, not directly involved in patient care, must place patient welfare before all other concerns.

- Physicians should recommend that patients obtain second opinions whenever they believe such opinions would be helpful to the patient.

- Physicians should provide information to enable patients to make intelligent choices and to give informed consent when necessary. Exceptions to informed consent are permitted only for cases in which the patient is incapable of consenting, and harm from failure to treat is imminent, or in which risk disclosure poses such a harmful psychological threat that it is medically contraindicated. In general, truthful disclosure to patients is fundamental to ethical treatment, without regard for any legal liability that might result.

- Both physicians and patients are free to accept or decline a physician-patient contractual relationship, except in those cases in which the need for emergency treatment precludes free choice. Once a physician accepts a case, he or she should not neglect the patient.

- Physicians are responsible for continuity of care for their patients. They cannot withdraw from a case without notifying the patient in advance, so that another physician may be obtained.

- A physician employed to perform surgery on a patient cannot substitute another surgeon without the patient's advance knowledge or consent.

- When patients need to be restrained to protect them from injuring themselves or others, restraints must be ordered by a physician, except in emergencies. Standing orders for restraints should be reviewed frequently. Physical and chemical restraints should be used only in a patient's best interest and not as punishment or for the convenience of the medical staff.

- Informing families of a patient's death is the attending physician's duty and should not be delegated to others.

- Physicians should not treat themselves or members of their immediate families, except in emergencies.

- It is unethical for any health care provider to be under the influence of a controlled substance, alcohol, or other substance that impairs ability while treating patients.

- Sexual contact between physicians and patients, while the physician-patient relationship exists, constitutes **sexual misconduct.**

- When deciding among treatments, physicians shall not use treatments that are scientifically invalid, illegal, or have no medical indication and offer no possible benefit to the patient.

- Physicians should consistently have authorized health professionals available as chaperones for patient examinations.

sexual misconduct *An unethical sexual relationship between medical supervisors and trainees or between health care providers and patients.*

Check Your Progress

8. Define *fee splitting*.

_____

_____

_____

9. Define *lien*.

_____

_____

_____

10. Define *professional courtesy*.

_____

_____

_____

◆ ◆ ◆ ◆ Conflicts of Interest

conflict of interest *A situation in which a person is faced with choosing between financial gain and his or her duty to provide the best possible medical care to patients.*

A physician must always try to avoid a **conflict of interest.** Following are examples:

- It is always unethical for physicians to place their own financial interests above the welfare of patients.

- Physicians engaged in biomedical research cannot ethically buy or sell the sponsoring company's stock until involvement ends and research results are published. In addition, financial remuneration received by researchers must be commensurate with efforts on behalf of sponsoring companies, and researchers should disclose any material ties to companies sponsoring research.

- Physicians are free to own interests in health care facilities, products, and equipment. However, if physicians do not directly provide patient care on-site, they generally should not refer patients to facilities in which they have an interest.

- Physicians who refer patients to home care providers should not accept payment for such referrals or for services in prescribing, monitoring, or revising treatment plans. Patients or their designated third-party payers should pay for these services.

- Physicians should not be influenced in prescribing drugs or medical products by a direct financial interest in a pharmaceutical firm or other medical products supplier. Physicians may own or operate pharmacies but generally may not refer patients to them.

- Gifts to physicians from companies within the medical industry are acceptable only if they are related to the physician's work (pens, notepads, and so forth). Drug samples for patient use are permissible. Cash payments should not be accepted, and no gifts should be accepted that have conditions attached.

- It is unethical for physicians to accept an offer of indemnity from lawsuits in exchange for prescribing certain drugs or products.

Court Case

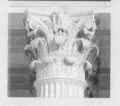

Medical Board's Decision on Referrals Is Upheld

Two physicians who shared a practice asked their state board of medicine to make a declaratory order concerning the referral of patients or patients' specimens to facilities in which the referring physician had a financial interest. The physicians wanted to know whether such a referral was a violation of state law. The board ruled that such a referral constituted "directing or requiring" the patient to use the facility in question and was in violation of state law prohibiting coercion in referral.

A trial court reversed the order, but an appellate court reinstated it. It found that the board had correctly interpreted a state statute preventing physicians from in any way arranging for or commanding a patient to use a facility in which said physicians had a financial interest.

Indenbaum v. Michigan Board of Medicine, 539 N.W.2d 574 (Mich. Ct. of App., Nov. 17, 1995).

Managed Care

Physicians practicing within managed care systems should:

- Continue to place the interests of patients first, regardless of allocation guidelines or gatekeeper directives for the plan.

- Maintain awareness of plan decisions about drug selection and work to ensure that formulary decisions reflect the needs of individual patients.

- Advocate for plan guidelines that are sensitive to patients' differences.

- Use appellate mechanisms within the plan for both patients and physicians to address disputes regarding medical care. In some cases, physicians may be obligated to initiate appeals on behalf of patients.

- Promote full disclosure of information to patients. Managed care plans should inform potential subscribers of limitations or restrictions before they enter the plan.

When managed care plans offer financial incentives to limit care, conflicts arise between physicians' financial interests and patients' needs.

Professional Rights and Responsibilities

A physician is free to choose his or her specialty, to limit practice to specialized services, and to choose whom he or she will serve, as long as there are no legal prohibitions and patients under the physician's care are not neglected.

Generally, both physicians and patients are free to enter into or decline the patient-physician contractual relationship. However, physicians who offer their services to the public may not decline to accept patients because of race, color, religion, national origin, sexual orientation, or any other basis that would constitute discrimination.

Physicians have an ethical duty to expose incompetent, corrupt, dishonest, or unethical conduct by members of the medical profession. Review should generally begin at the local level. If there is any question concerning the legality of an action, the situation may be referred to the proper authorities. An ethical health care professional abides by the laws regulating his or her profession and should not assist others in evading such laws.

A physician or medical student whose professional conduct is under review by a medical society tribunal, medical staff committee, or similar body composed of peers has the right to a fair and objective hearing. The fundamental aspects of a fair hearing include:

- A listing of specific charges.

- Adequate notice of the right to a hearing.

- The opportunity to be present and to rebut the evidence.

- The opportunity to present a defense.

Dilemmas of Health Care Professionals

In *Ethical Dimensions in the Health Professions* Third Edition © 1999 (W.B. Saunders Co.), author Ruth Purtilo outlines alternatives for health care professionals who see questionable behavior by coworkers:

- You may prevent possible serious offenses by talking to the coworker.
- You can elect to do nothing, but this decision could endanger coworkers or patients.
- To prevent further harm, you can act decisively to remove the person from his or her position. If this option is chosen, you must follow reporting procedures in order to protect the rights of all concerned.
- You should always document the behavior in question. In addition to confronting the alleged offender, resolving the situation may involve your dealing with supervisors, administrators, counselors, regulatory board members, risk managers, or representatives of professional associations. Once begun, you should see the process through.

Because the judgment handed down in a hearing can affect a physician's reputation, professional status, and livelihood, these principles of fair play apply in any situation in which one physician sits in judgment of the professional conduct of another.

If a patient who has a legal claim requests a physician's assistance, the physician should furnish medical evidence, with the patient's consent, in order to secure the patient's legal rights. Medical experts should confine their testimony to their field of medical expertise. Physicians cannot ethically accept fees that are contingent on the outcome of litigation.

Physicians who know that they have an infectious disease that poses a significant risk to others should not engage in any activity that risks transmission of the disease.

Physicians involved in accreditation (approval or certification) activities have an ethical responsibility to apply standards that are relevant, fair, reasonable, and nondiscriminatory. Standards should be based on quality patient care and should not be adopted or used as a means of economic regulation.

Any agreement between physicians that restricts the right of a physician to practice medicine for a given length of time or restricts practice in a given area is discouraged, since it is considered contrary to public interest. Competition should be encouraged, since ethical medical practice thrives best under free market conditions.

Physicians are obligated to share their knowledge and skills and to report research results. Sharing scientific information through presentation or publication is encouraged. The intentional withholding of such information is condemned. A physician may patent a surgical or diagnostic instrument he or she has discovered or developed. However, the patenting of medical procedures poses substantial risks to the effective practice of medicine by limiting the availability of new procedures to patients and should, therefore, be condemned.

Recent studies suggest that blacks are less likely than whites to receive certain surgical procedures or other therapies and that gender bias may be affecting medical decisions. Physicians have a responsibility to see that neither race nor gender is inappropriately used as a consideration in clinical decisions.

Applying Knowledge

Answer the following questions in the spaces provided.

1. What is the overriding, fundamental, ethical obligation of any health care provider?
   _____

2. A busy midtown clinic does not accept new patients who are enrolled in Medicaid programs. Is this practice legal and ethical? Explain your answer.
   _____
   _____

3. The same busy midtown clinic asks every patient to make an insurance co-payment at the time services are rendered. Is this practice legal and ethical?
   _____
   _____

4. Is it ethical for a physician to engage in, aid, or abet a nonscientific treatment? Why or why not?
   _____
   _____

5. Name two circumstances in which a physician may ethically charge for the completion of an insurance form.
   _____
   _____

6. A physician should not release confidential information without prior consent of the patient, unless required by law. Give three examples when this might occur.
   _____
   _____
   _____

7. List four safeguards to protect confidentiality of computerized medical records.
   _____   _____
   _____   _____

8. What is included in the selling price when a physician sells his or her practice?
   _____
   _____

9. List four guidelines for physicians to use when establishing fees for their services.
   _____
   _____
   _____
   _____

10. List five guidelines to be used in retaining a patient's medical records.

_____

_____

_____

_____

_____

Match each of the following statements with the correct term by writing the appropriate letter in the spaces provided.

_____**11.** Physicians may ethically employ or work in consultation with this group of professionals as long as they are appropriately trained and duly licensed to perform services requested.

_____**12.** Physicians may ethically make _____ for diagnostic or therapeutic services to other physicians, limited practitioners, or other providers of health care services lawfully providing such services.

_____**13.** Physicians may ethically charge patients for services performed by _____ under the physician's direct supervision.

_____**14.** Neither medical staff membership nor _____ should be dependent upon compulsory assessments.

_____**15.** Those health care providers licensed to provide specific treatments or treatments specific to certain body parts.

a. residents and students

b. referrals

c. allied health professionals

d. limited practitioners

e. staff privileges

Answer the following questions in the spaces provided.

16. Decisions regarding hospital privileges should be based on _____ of candidates.

17. Is it ethical for physicians to advertise their services? Explain your answer.

_____

_____

_____

18. Ideally, direct-to-consumer advertising of prescription drugs should accomplish what five goals?

_____

_____

_____

_____

_____

Review and Case Studies

19. List two guidelines that should apply when physicians and other health care professionals provide telecommunication advisory services.

_____

_____

20. Physicians should encourage minors who request confidential services to involve their parents. However, when minors request these services:

_____

_____

Physicians should recognize that requiring parental involvement may not be in the best interest of the health and well-being of the patient.

21. List five guidelines for the release of patient medical information in certain special circumstances.

_____

_____

_____

_____

_____

22. _____ refers to the provision of medical care to physician colleagues or their families for free or at a reduced rate.

23. List five ethical guidelines for physicians to follow in the treatment of and their relationship with patients.

_____

_____

_____

_____

_____

24. List two ethical guidelines concerning financial remuneration for physicians engaged in biomedical research.

_____

_____

25. Physicians who offer their services to the public may not decline to accept patients because of _____ or any other basis that would constitute discrimination.

Use your critical-thinking skills and your knowledge of legal and ethical principles to answer the questions that follow each of the case studies.

You are a CMA, and you have been asked by a patient not to report her diagnosis of chlamydia to the state authorities.

26. What legal and ethical issues are involved? How would you handle the situation?

_____

_____

_____

In the physician's office where you work as a CMA, drug samples are kept in a central location, and the cabinet is often packed full. These samples may not be dispensed without a prescription. On a busy day, a coworker asks you for samples of a specific sleep-inducing drug to take for her insomnia.

27. What legal and ethical issues are involved? How would you handle the situation?

_____

_____

_____

You are the supervising RN in a clinic. You report for work and find that an automated report has been generated for someone not recognized as a regular patient at the clinic. A laboratory technician finally admits his responsibility in the matter. The night before, after working hours, he brought a neighbor's child into the clinic. He swabbed the child's throat, performed a test for streptococcus bacteria, and noted that the test was positive. He then took samples of antibiotics from the storeroom for the child to take at home.

28. What legal and ethical principles are involved? How would you handle the situation?

_____

_____

_____

You are a medical assistant in a medical office. A laboratory technician with whom you work appears on a nationally televised talk show. After her appearance she brings to work a copy of the video for staff members to view together. During the interview the laboratory technician reveals that her lover fathered one of her children. The brother of that lover fathered another of her children. She says that she continues to maintain a sexual relationship with the brother, who is married. The man's wife is a known prostitute and IV drug user.

29. What legal and ethical questions are involved? How would you handle the situation?

_____

_____

_____

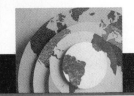

Internet Activities

Complete the activities and answer the questions that follow.

30. Visit the Web site for "The American Journal of Bioethics Online," published by the Center for Bioethics at the University of Pennsylvania. List two current articles posted that are relevant to this text's Chapters 10 and 11. Explain how the articles are relevant.

_____

_____

_____

_____

Under "Future Direction in Medical Ethics," list three issues destined to be of major importance in the future.

_____

_____

_____

Link to two additional Web sites under "Bioethics Related Journals." List two current articles from each journal that are relevant to the topics in this chapter.

_____

_____

_____

_____

DEATH AND DYING

Objectives

After studying this chapter, you should be able to:

1. Discuss accepted criteria for determining death.
2. Determine the health care professional's role in caring for the dying.
3. Explain differences between a living will, a health care proxy, and durable power of attorney.
4. Discuss the various stages of grief.
5. Begin to form a knowledge base for assisting dying patients and their family members through the grieving process.
6. Begin forming a personal philosophy concerning death and dying.

Key Terms

- active euthanasia
- brain death
- curative care
- durable power of attorney
- health care proxy
- hospice
- involuntary euthanasia
- living will
- palliative care

- passive euthanasia
- Patient Self-Determination Act
- terminally ill
- thanatology
- Uniform Determination of Death Act
- Uniform Rights of the Terminally Ill Act
- voluntary euthanasia

Attitudes Toward Death and Dying

Prior to the twentieth century, death was an intimate experience for most families. Antibiotics and chemotherapies had not yet been discovered; genetically engineered drugs, organ transplantation, and life-support machines were still science fiction; and infectious diseases periodically decimated populations. Nearly every husband and wife, mother and father, brother and sister had lost a loved one. Loved ones customarily died at home, surrounded by family members who bade them good-bye and then mourned their passing with funeral rituals and rites.

By the late twentieth century, individuals were more likely to die in the hospital, at least in the Western world. Once admitted to hospitals, the dying were isolated from family members and surrounded by machines designed to prolong life as long as possible. Consequently, modern technology has effectively hidden death from view, but in so doing it has also made the end of life a fearful prospect.

Attitudes toward death and dying vary with individuals, of course, but as each of us ages, we will likely begin to think of our own mortality and perhaps to wonder how the end will come. Will I die alone, in an impersonal, clinical hospital environment? Will my health care providers be so committed to preserving life that they prolong my dying to an irrational degree? Will I suffer in pain? Will I feel a sense of tasks left unfinished, goals left unrealized, or will I experience a peaceful letting go?

Because the fears associated with death and dying are universal, health care practitioners should evaluate their own attitudes in order to effectively and compassionately respond to dying patients and their families.

Determination of Death

Uniform Determination of Death Act *A proposal that established uniform guidelines for determining when death has occurred.*

brain death *Final cessation of bodily activity, used to determine when death actually occurs; circulatory and respiratory functions have irreversibly ceased, and the entire brain (including the brain stem) has irreversibly ceased to function.*

Modern medical technology and life-support equipment may keep a person's body "alive"—the heart may beat and blood may circulate—long after the brain ceases to function. This makes it difficult in some cases to determine the moment when death actually occurs. For this reason, in 1981 a **Uniform Determination of Death Act** was proposed by the President's Commission for the Study of Ethical Problems in Medicine and Biomedical Research, working in cooperation with the American Bar Association, the American Medical Association, and the National Conference of Commissioners on Uniform State Laws. Most states have adopted the act's definition of **brain death** as a means of determining when death actually occurs:

- Circulatory and respiratory functions have irreversibly ceased.

- The entire brain, including the brain stem, has irreversibly ceased to function.

Before pronouncing a comatose patient dead, physicians perform a series of tests to determine whether death has occurred. Death is indicated if the following signs are present. The patient:

- Cannot breathe without assistance.

- Has no coughing or gagging reflex.

- Has no pupil response to light.

- Has no blinking reflex when the cornea is touched.

- Has no grimace reflex when the head is rotated or ears are flushed with ice water.

- Has no response to pain.

Today the declaration of death occurs only when the last signs of brain activity are gone. Technically, death results from lack of oxygen. When deprived of oxygen, cells cannot maintain metabolic function and soon begin to deteriorate.

◆ ◆ ◆ ◆ ◆ **Autopsies**

After a patient is declared dead, family members (next of kin) may be asked to consent to an autopsy. An autopsy is a postmortem examination to determine cause of death or to obtain physiological evidence. Autopsies performed in hospitals may confirm or correct clinical diagnoses, thus providing a measure of quality assurance. Autopsy results can also highlight those cases in which diagnoses tend to be incorrect, or treatments tend to be ineffective, thereby adding to scientific knowledge and revealing areas that need further study. In cases of suspicious deaths, autopsy results can provide information to help law enforcement authorities, such as cause and time of death. (Legal requirements concerning autopsies are discussed in Chapter 7.)

Autopsies must be performed in cases in which the death is suspicious or due to homicide, but the number of autopsies performed in all other deaths each year has steadily declined. One reason that fewer autopsies are performed today is cost—insurance companies and government health care programs usually do not pay for autopsies. In addition, some clinicians argue that technological advances have made clinical diagnoses more accurate, so postmortem diagnoses are less essential. Another reason for the decline in autopsies is that in many smaller hospitals pathologists are not readily available.

Furthermore, even though autopsies can yield information that may clarify causes of death, save lives, or reassure survivors that their loved ones could not have been saved, family members are often reluctant to give consent. They may feel that their loved one has "suffered enough," that the physician already knows the cause of death, or that the procedure would interfere with viewing of the body during funeral rites. Health care practitioners may believe that these perceptions of autopsies are inaccurate, but they must remain sensitive to the beliefs and emotions of surviving family members.

YOU BE THE JUDGE

Recent reports indicating a continuing decline in the number of autopsies performed in the United States raise many ethical questions.

In your opinion, could the decline in the number of autopsies performed be partly due to the fact that their importance in advancing medical knowledge is not being properly conveyed to patients? How could a health care practitioner ethically and tactfully impart this information to a patient's next-of-kin?

_____

_____

_____

What might some of the reasons be for a physician's or other health care practitioner's reluctance to talk to patients' families about autopsies?

_____

_____

_____

In what ways might economic constraints have had an effect on the number of autopsies performed?

_____

_____

_____

Check Your Progress

1. Briefly explain how attitudes toward death and dying in the United States have changed over the years.

   _____

   _____

2. The _____ was proposed as a universal means of determining when death actually occurs.

3. Define *brain death*.

   _____

   _____

4. Name six signs for which physicians may test that indicate death has occurred.

   _____   _____

   _____   _____

   _____   _____

Teaching Health Care Practitioners to Care for Dying Patients

terminally ill *Referring to patients who are expected to die within six months.*

Although modern medicine has effectively prolonged the moment of death, in many cases it has dealt less conscientiously with compassionate, comfort care for **terminally ill** patients—those who are not expected to live beyond six months, usually because of an unrelenting chronic illness for which there is no cure.

- A 1995 study published in the *Journal of the American Medical Association* (JAMA) found that nearly four out of every ten terminally ill patients spend at least ten days in intensive care connected to life-sustaining machines. The same study found that half of patients who die in hospitals experience moderate to severe pain.

- In November 1996 the Robert Wood Johnson Foundation published results of the largest study ever conducted on patients near death. The six-year SUPPORT study of 9100 hospitalized patients showed that most physicians did not know their patients' end-of-life wishes or did not follow them, and that half of those patients who were conscious during the last three days of life died in pain.

- A survey by the Association of American Medical Colleges in 1998 found that 122 medical schools (96.1 percent) included information about death and dying as part of an existing course, but just 6 schools (4.7 percent) featured the subject as a separate required course. Fifty schools (39.4 percent) offered a course in death and dying as an elective.

- A survey of medical textbooks, published in the February 9, 2001, issue of the *Journal of American Medicine* (JAMA), showed that most "don't deal with the end of life," according to the article's lead author, Michael Rabow of the University of California at San Francisco medical school. Of the 50 top-selling textbooks that were reviewed, 56.9 percent did not discuss end-of-life care at all. The remaining books either covered the topic minimally (19 percent) or did include some helpful information on end-of-life care (24.1 percent).

- A report by the National Research Council and the Institute of Medicine issued in June 2001 states that U.S. physicians and hospitals are not prepared to handle the suffering of dying cancer patients. The report, "Improving Palliative Care for Cancer: Summary and Recommendations," says that federal research and training efforts have focused largely on treatment and finding cures while neglecting symptom control measures that could relieve a patient's suffering.

thanatology *The study of death and of the psychological methods of coping with it.*

Fortunately, the need to teach end-of-life care to physicians and other health care practitioners has been recognized. Increasingly, schools that train health care providers are offering courses in **thanatology**—the study of death and of the psychological methods of coping with death. In addition, many organizations exist that list their primary mission as advocacy for improved care for the dying and educating health professionals and the public about end-of-life issues. A sampling of such groups in mid-2001 included Finding Our Way, Partnership for Caring (formerly Choice in Dying), The Last Acts Campaign, Growth House, the Project on Death in

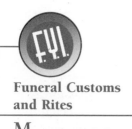

Funeral Customs and Rites

Many of today's funeral customs and rites originated in ancient times. Which of the following are still practiced in some form?

- Black has long been worn by undertakers, mourners, and pallbearers to show grief. In ancient times it was also used as a disguise to protect against malevolent spirits that might be lurking nearby.
- An early custom for mourners was to go barefoot and to wear sackcloth and ashes. This was said to discourage the dead from becoming envious, as they might be if mourners appeared at funerals wearing new clothes and shoes.
- Pagan tribes began the custom of covering the face of the deceased with a sheet because they believed that the spirit of the deceased escaped through the mouth. They often held the mouth and nose of a sick person shut, hoping to retain the spirit and thus delay death.

—continued

Uniform Rights of the Terminally Ill Act *A federal statute passed in 1989 to guide state legislatures in constructing laws to address advance directives.*

America, and Americans for Better Care of the Dying. Most provide living will and medical power of attorney forms and provide useful information to the public. Some routinely file *amicus curiae* (friend of the court) briefs in legal cases addressing end-of-life issues. Others are engaged in research, public advocacy, and education activities to improve the care of the dying and their families.

In 2001 the American Medical Association, perhaps the nation's most influential organization for physicians, implemented a program called Education for Physicians on End-of-Life Care (EPEC). The project was designed to educate all U.S. physicians on the essential clinical competencies required to provide quality end-of-life care.

Despite a conscious effort to improve training and attitudes regarding dying patients, end-of-life care remains one of the most emotionally trying for health care practitioners.

Landmark Events Concerning the Right to Die

The following events illustrate the increasing concern of federal and state legislatures and other groups over protection of the rights of the terminally ill.

- 1946—Committee of 1776 Physicians for Legalizing Voluntary Euthanasia is formed in New York State.

- 1967—Attorney Luis Kutner and members of the Euthanasia Society (later called Choice in Dying and then Partnership for Caring) devise the original living will.

- 1973—American Hospital Association creates the Patient's Bill of Rights.

- 1976—New Jersey Supreme Court's *Quinlan* decision establishes the primacy of patients' wishes over the state's duty to preserve life.

- 1976—California's Natural Death Act, the nation's first right-to-die statute, is signed into law.

- 1977—Laws dealing with the refusal of treatment are passed in Arkansas, Idaho, Nevada, New Mexico, North Carolina, Oregon, and Texas.

- 1984—The District of Columbia and 22 states have statutes that recognize advance directives.

- 1989—The **Uniform Rights of the Terminally Ill Act** serves as a guideline for state legislatures in constructing laws addressing advance directives.

- 1990—U.S. Supreme Court's *Cruzan* decision recognizes that the right to refuse medical treatment is guaranteed by the U.S. Constitution.

- 1990—Congress passes the Patient Self-Determination Act, the first federal act concerning advance directives.

- In earlier times traffic was halted for a funeral procession because any delay in transporting a soul might turn it into a restless ghost, reluctant to pass over into the next world.
- Wakes held today come from the ancient custom of keeping watch over the deceased, hoping that life would return.
- In England the dead were always carried out of the house feet first; otherwise, their spirits might look back into the house and beckon family members to come with them.
- Pagan beliefs concerning funeral wreaths held that the circle formed by the wreath would keep the dead person's spirit within bounds.
- The firing of a rifle volley over the deceased is similar to the tribal practice of throwing spears into the air to ward off spirits hovering over the deceased.
- In the past, holy water was sprinkled on the body to protect it from demons.

- 1992—Pennsylvania becomes the 50th state to enact advance-directive legislation.
- 1997—U.S. Supreme Court holds that state bans on physician-assisted suicide do not violate the U.S. Constitution. The Court leaves the decision up to each state on whether to ban physician-assisted suicide.
- 1997—Oregon's Death With Dignity Act is passed, making the state the first to permit physician-assisted suicide in certain circumstances.
- 1997—By this date 35 states have enacted statutes expressly criminalizing assisted suicide; 9 states criminalize assisted suicide through common law.
- 1998—The Death and Dying Task Force, a group made up of medical students, advocates for improved training for physicians regarding death and dying issues. Members of the group are concerned that medical school leaves them inadequately prepared to communicate with terminally ill patients and poorly equipped emotionally to deal with matters of death and dying.
- 2001—The California Supreme Court clarifies the right to die in a decision that states that the right to die does not extend to people who are conscious and in a twilight state, are unable to communicate or care for themselves, and have not left formal written directions for health care.

Court Case

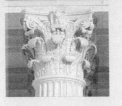

State Law Versus Patients' Right to Die

Several physicians in Washington State joined with a nonprofit corporation that provides information, assistance, and counseling to competent, terminally ill adult patients considering suicide to sue the state. The plaintiffs claimed that a state law making it a crime to aid anyone in attempting suicide was unconstitutional because it prevents terminally ill patients from exercising their protected liberty interests. An appeals court held that the choice of how and when to die is a liberty interest and that the statute violated the due process rights of competent, terminally ill adults who wished to hasten their deaths by obtaining medication prescribed by their physicians. The dissent stated that physician-assisted suicide is unethical, per the AMA's *Code of Medical Ethics.*

Compassion in Dying v. Washington, 1996 U.S. App. Lexis 3944, replacing 49 F.3d 596 (9th Cir. 1995).

5. Define *terminally ill.*

_____

_____

6. Define *thanatology.*

_____

_____

7. List five landmark events in the United States concerning the right to die and the year in which each occurred.

_____

_____

_____

_____

_____

_____

Caring for Dying Patients

When a patient suffers from a disease or condition that is clearly terminal and no longer treatable, help is still available and care should not stop.

◆ ◆ ◆ ◆ ## Palliative and Curative Care

curative care *Treatment directed toward curing a patient's disease.*

palliative care *Treatment of a terminally ill patient's symptoms in order to make dying more comfortable; also called comfort care.*

When it becomes evident that a patient's disease is incurable and death is imminent, palliative care may serve the dying patient better than curative care. **Curative care** consists of treatments and procedures directed toward curing a patient's disease. **Palliative care,** also called comfort care, is directed toward providing relief to terminally ill patients through symptom and pain management. The goal is not to cure but to provide comfort and maintain the highest possible quality of life. Going beyond relief of disease symptoms, palliative care includes relief of emotional distress and other problems so that a patient's last months and days may be as comfortable as possible.

Traditionally, in educational programs for health care practitioners, courses of study have placed more emphasis on curative care than on palliative care. Treatments included in curative care include surgery, chemotherapy, radiation therapy, and other treatments and procedures and may be used more aggressively as a patient's disease progresses. Since most physicians are taught to fight disease with every product and technique at their command, it is sometimes difficult for them to recognize or admit that curative care has failed or is no longer effective in treating a patient's disease. Through use of palliative care, health care providers can help relieve a dying patient's pain and emotional distress and ease the journey toward life's end.

Hospice Care

hospice *A facility or program (often carried out in a patient's home) in which teams of health care practitioners and volunteers provide a continuing environment that focuses on the emotional and psychological needs of the dying patient.*

Most physicians, hospitals, and social agencies can refer terminally ill patients to facilities or agencies that provide **hospice** care. A hospice in medieval times was a way station for travelers. In the twentieth century, as medical science prolonged death for increasing numbers of terminally ill patients, hospices, where the symptoms of terminal illness could be eased, were founded. The first hospice facilities were established in England in the 1960s as places where patients could go to die in comfort.

In the United States hospice care may be provided in facilities built especially for that purpose, in hospitals and nursing homes, or at home. Hospice care focuses on relieving pain, controlling symptoms, and meeting emotional needs and personal values of the terminally ill instead of targeting the underlying disease process. The hospice philosophy also recognizes that family members and other caregivers deserve care and support,

VOICE OF EXPERIENCE
Hospice Volunteer Cares for Dying Patients

Joyce is a hospice volunteer in a rural area in a Midwestern state. She received training through a hospital in a nearby city, then was interviewed by a hospice coordinator to determine her willingness to accept assigned patients.

"My first patient was a dear friend of my family," Joyce says. He was a nursing home resident and "was happy to have company."

As a volunteer, Joyce provides minimal physical care. (NHPCO states that "most hospice volunteers are trained to relieve the primary caregivers, do household chores and help bathe the patients.") Joyce says her services include doing "whatever the patients ask me to do. One day I might fix lunch, or feed the dog. Or a patient and I might just have coffee together. Often I do the dishes and straighten up the house." Sometimes she simply listens to her patient's concerns and provides comfort.

"One man I visited was quite fearful," Joyce recalls. "He knew that his end was coming soon, and he was afraid. I went to his house and simply took his hand and rested my head on his arm. It seemed meaningful to him. He settled down, as though the comfort was what he wanted and needed. . . . I still think of that man. He so appreciated what I did for him. I feel that I did as much as anyone could have done for him at that time, and that's often how I feel.

"When I am asked to go into a hospice situation I feel honored, because death and sickness is a private thing for families. When you are asked to take part in that, it's an honor to be there for those people. I know that we volunteers can bring hope and peace even in that difficult time, and that gives me satisfaction."

continuing even after the death of the patient. Hospice programs ease dying; they do not support active euthanasia or assisted suicide.

Bereavement services are also available through hospice care, to help patients discuss such issues as preparing a will and planning a funeral and to help surviving family members cope with grief and loss after the patient dies. Hospice programs generally provide bereavement services through discussion groups, follow-up visits from hospice personnel, and sometimes referral to appropriate mental health professionals.

Most in-home hospice programs are independently run, in a fashion similar to visiting nurse or home health care agencies. Patients receive coordinated care at home by multidisciplinary teams composed of physicians, nurses, social workers, home health aides, pharmacists, physical therapists, clergy, volunteers, and family members. Hospice teams meet regularly to work on patients' needs concerning pain and other serious symptoms, depression, family problems, inadequate housing, financial problems, or lack of transportation. The team then expands, amends, or otherwise revises each patient's care plan, as necessary.

For patients to be eligible for hospice care, physicians usually must certify that they are not expected to live beyond six months. Hospice care is now generally reimbursed by Medicare, Medicaid, and many private insurance companies and managed care programs.

According to the National Hospice and Palliative Care Organization (NHPCO), in 1999, 95 percent of the days of hospice service provided consisted of routine home care, 3 percent of the days were inpatient care, 1 percent was respite care, and 1 percent was continuous home care. NHPCO estimates that nearly 2.4 million individuals died in the United States in 1999, and one out of every four, or just over 600,000 people, died while receiving hospice care.

Planning Ahead

Patient Self-Determination Act *A federal law passed in 1990 that requires hospitals and other health care providers to provide written information to patients regarding their rights under state law to make medical decisions and execute advance directives.*

In today's health care environment, individuals are well-advised to be prepared for the time when they or their legal representatives may have to make decisions about medical treatment, including the use of life-sustaining measures. To address this concern, the federal **Patient Self-Determination Act** was passed in 1990 and took effect December 1, 1991. The act requires hospitals and other health care providers to provide written information to patients regarding their rights under state law to make medical decisions and execute advance directives. (Advance directives include the living will, durable power of attorney, and the health care proxy, which is simply a durable power of attorney for medical care.) The act also provides that:

- Health care providers will document in the patient's medical record whether he or she has executed an advance directive.

- Providers may not discriminate against an individual based on whether or not he or she has executed an advance directive.

- Providers must comply with state laws respecting advance directives.

- Providers must have a policy for educating staff and the community regarding advance directives.

Congress's action in passing this law was due, in large part, to the *Nancy Cruzan* case decided by the U.S. Supreme Court in June 1990.

As a result of the Patient Self-Determination Act, patients are encouraged to execute living wills or durable powers of attorney while still able to do so and before life-sustaining measures become necessary for life to continue.

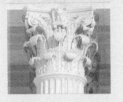
Check Your Progress

8. Distinguish between *palliative care* and *curative care*.

_____

_____

9. Define *hospice*.

_____

_____

Indicate with a "C" or a "P" whether each of the following actions constitutes a form of curative care or palliative care.

_____ 10. Allowing a patient who is terminally ill with lung and stomach cancer to self-administer morphine patches as needed for pain relief.

_____ 11. Radiation treatments after breast cancer surgery.

_____ 12. Surgical severing of certain nerves to relieve suffering for a patient terminally ill with cancer of the spine.

_____ 13. Counseling a terminally ill patient and his or her family concerning funeral arrangements and other end-of-life decisions.

_____ 14. Administering antibiotics to cure an infected tooth.

_____ 15. Cosmetic surgery for a teenaged patient whose face was burned in a fire.

Living Will

living will *An advance directive that specifies an individual's end-of-life wishes.*

A **living will** provides instructions directly to physicians, hospitals, and other health care providers involved in a patient's treatment. It may detail circumstances under which treatment should be discontinued, such as coma, brain death, or a terminal condition. It may also detail which treatments or medications to suspend (for example, invasive surgery, artificial nutrition or hydration, and measures that serve no purpose except to delay death) and which to maintain (for example, kidney dialysis and drugs for pain). In addition, it may list which "heroic measures" (for example, emergency surgery and CPR) should and should not be used. A living will may also indicate preferences regarding organ donation, autopsy, and alternative treatments. Living wills may designate an agent to carry out these wishes if the patient is incapable of making decisions.

Nearly all 50 states accept the validity of living wills, although they also specify various requirements that must be met. Standard state forms may be obtained from a number of sources for completion by individuals and their attorneys.

Generic living will forms may also be obtained from various sources, but users should be aware of any state-specific requirements. Copies of completed forms should be given to designated family members or agents and may be filed with medical records upon a patient's admission to the hospital. (See Figure 12-1.)

Durable Power of Attorney

durable power of attorney *An advance directive that confers upon a designee the authority to make a variety of legal decisions on behalf of the grantor, usually including health care decisions.*

The **durable power of attorney** is not specifically a medical document, but it may serve that purpose. It confers upon a designee the authority to

---

If the time comes when I am incapacitated to the point when I can no longer actively take part in decisions for my own life, and am unable to direct my physician as to my own medical care, I wish this statement to stand as a testament of my wishes. I _____ (name) request that I be allowed to die and not be kept alive through life-support systems if my condition is deemed terminal. I do not intend any direct taking of my life, but only that my dying not be unreasonably prolonged. This request is made, after careful reflection, while I am of sound mind.

_____
(Signature)

_____
(Date)

_____
(Witness)

_____
(Witness)

Figure 12-1
Sample Living Will

make a variety of legal decisions on behalf of the grantor. It takes effect when the grantor loses the capacity to make decisions, through either unconsciousness or mental incompetence. The document may place limits on the rights and responsibilities of the designee (usually an attorney or a spouse), and it may give specific instructions regarding the grantor's medical and other preferences. Standard forms are available and are governed by state law.

◆ ◆ ◆ ◆ Health Care Proxy

health care proxy *A durable power of attorney issued for purposes of health care decisions only.*

A **health care proxy,** or health care power of attorney, is a state-specific, end-of-life document. With it, individuals specify their wishes and designate an agent to make medical decisions for them, in the event that they lose the ability to reason or communicate. As with the living will, this document outlines specific types of care and treatment that should be permitted or excluded. It also carefully outlines the specific responsibilities and authority of the proxy. Some states prohibit attending physicians, hospital employees, or other health care providers from serving as proxies unless related to the patient by blood. Patients should name one or more alternates, in case the primary proxy cannot serve when called. (See Figure 12-2 on p. 290.)

◆ ◆ ◆ ◆ Do-Not-Resuscitate (DNR) Order

When admitted to a hospital, most patients are allowed by state law to specify that they are not to be revived if their heart stops. The request can be made via a standard do-not-resuscitate (DNR) order, which is then placed with the patient's chart. In some hospitals patients may also wear a bracelet alerting medical personnel to the existence of a DNR order.

◆ ◆ ◆ ◆ Organ Donor Directives

Patients may also want to make clear to hospital personnel that they wish to donate organs for transplantation or medical research in the event of their death. As discussed in Chapter 6, some states allow licensed drivers to fill out an organ donation form on the back of their licenses. Nondrivers, or residents of states where drivers' licenses do not include this information, may carry an organ donor card in their wallets specifying their desire to donate organs. Organizations such as the National Kidney Foundation, the United Network for Organ Sharing (UNOS), and the Living Bank provide donor registration materials in response to requests. In addition to having an organ donor card, patients should make clear to family members their wishes regarding organ donation in the event of their death.

I, _____ , designate and appoint:

Name: _____

Address: _____

Telephone Number: _____

to be my agent for health care decisions and pursuant to the language stated below, on my behalf to:

(1) Consent, refuse consent, or withdraw consent to any care, treatment, service or procedure to maintain, diagnose or treat a physical or mental condition, and to make decisions about organ donation, autopsy and disposition of the body;

(2) make all necessary arrangements at any hospital, psychiatric hospital or psychiatric treatment facility, hospice, nursing home or similar institution; to employ or discharge health care personnel to include physicians, psychiatrists, psychologists, dentists, nurses, therapists or any other person who is licensed, certified or otherwise authorized or permitted by the laws of this state to administer health care as the agent shall deem necessary for my physical, mental and emotional well-being; and

(3) request, receive and review any information, verbal or written, regarding my personal affairs or physical or mental health including medical and hospital records and to execute any releases of other documents that may be required in order to obtain such information.

In exercising the grant of authority set forth above my agent for health care decisions shall:

_____

The powers of the agent herein shall be limited to the extent set out in writing in this durable power of attorney for health care decisions, and shall not include the power to revoke or invalidate any previously existing declaration made in accordance with the natural death act.

The agent shall be prohibited from authorizing consent for the following items:

_____

The durable power of attorney for health care decisions shall be subject to these additional limitations:

_____

This power of attorney for health care decisions shall become effective immediately and shall not be affected by my subsequent disability or incapacity or upon the occurrence of my disability or incapacity.

Any durable power of attorney for health care decisions I have previously made is hereby revoked. This durable power of attorney for health care decisions shall be revoked in writing, executed and witnessed or acknowledged in the same manner as required herein.

Executed this _____ , at _____

                                          _____
                                          (Signature of principal)

State _____ County _____ S.S. No. _____

This instrument was acknowledged before me _____ (date) by _____ (name)

                                          _____
                                          (Signature of notary public)

Figure 12-2
Sample Health Care Proxy

Stages of Grief

Dr. Elisabeth Kubler-Ross, recognized for more than 20 years as an authority in the field of death and dying, was the first to list and describe the coping mechanisms of people who grieve. Such individuals experience five stages of grief, she maintained, not necessarily in any particular order, before coming to terms with the death of a loved one or the prospect of imminent death.

STAGE 1   This first stage is identified with feelings of denial and isolation. This is the it-can't-be-true stage, in which patients believe the physician's diagnosis must be a mistake, or relatives informed of a loved one's death deny that the person is gone. They may suggest that X rays or results of blood tests were somehow mixed up or that identities of accident victims were somehow mistaken. Denial is usually a temporary state, claims Kubler-Ross, and is soon replaced by partial acceptance. A terminally ill patient seldom continues to deny his or her disease until death comes, and grieving relatives realize all too soon that a loved one has, in fact, died.

STAGE 2   When denial can no longer be maintained, the patient or grieving relative progresses to anger, rage, and resentment. "Why me?" is the typical reaction. Patients are angry over the "betrayal" of once-healthy bodies and the loss of control over their lives. Grieving relatives may feel anger toward a God that took the loved one away. Even the terminally ill family member may feel the same anger at God for leaving others behind to bear the pain of loss. Anger is a normal reaction to death and may be expressed in different ways. For example, a bereaved person may yell at others or withdraw in sullen silence.

STAGE 3   Grieving individuals next respond with attempts at bargaining and guilt. Just as children continue to ask for a favor after parents have said no, patients may ask for "just enough time to see my daughter married" or "one more week at work before I have to quit." Something in the human psyche seems to believe, if only for a short time, that if we are "good," the "bad" will be taken away or postponed.

A corresponding experience for individuals grieving the loss of a loved one is guilt. The bereaved person may somehow feel responsible for the death, especially if the relationship with the deceased was not good. He or she might be tortured by thoughts of how things might have been different if only the loved one had lived.

STAGE 4   The fourth stage involves depression or sadness, which is the most expected reaction to loss. Patients coping with terminal illness may face not only physical pain and debilitation but also loss of financial security and inevitable changes in lifestyle—all of which can cause them to feel that their situation is hopeless. Individuals grieving the loss of a loved one may see no point in going on.

During this state bereaved persons may cry frequently or may be unable to cry at all, expressing their grief in body language—downcast eyes, shuffling steps, and stooped shoulders. Daily routines may be difficult or impossible to maintain. If depression continues for a prolonged period of time, health care providers, family members, or friends should help the bereaved person seek professional counseling.

STAGE 5   Finally, those experiencing the grieving process reach a stage of acceptance. At this point the bereaved person has finally accepted his or her loss. Terminally ill patients have come to terms with dying, and bereaved persons have accepted that the loved one is gone. For example, patients may write wills, complete advance directives, or plan funerals. A grieving spouse may finally decide to remove a deceased partner's clothing from a shared closet or to convert his or her office to a spare bedroom.

Grieving family members can now move on to the growth stage, in which they adjust daily routines or become involved in new activities and relationships.

Although the stages of grief have been universally observed, each person dealing with loss grieves differently. Bereaved persons may not show their grief. A stage may be skipped or returned to repeatedly during the grieving process. A combination of all of the emotions just described may be felt at the same time.

◆ ◆ ◆ ◆   **Finding Support**

People who are grieving can find support from a variety of sources. They can read books on the subject, attend a bereavement support group sponsored by a hospital or hospice, visit a counselor, talk with a member of the clergy, or talk with family members and friends.

Health care providers can be excellent sources of support for terminally ill patients and their families. Talking and listening are the most helpful activities others can perform, the experts advise. Do not force a conversation, but make yourself available to talk. Do not respond in kind if patients are angry and resentful. Talking about distress helps relieve it, and sensitive listening is effective in itself. Adapted from *"I Don't Know What To Say . . .": How to Help and Support Someone Who Is Dying* (Little, Brown and Company, 1989), oncologist Dr. Robert Buckman recommends the following when talking with a dying patient:

• Pay attention to setting. Sit down, relax, do not appear rushed, and act as though you are ready to listen.

• Determine whether or not the patient wants to talk. Ask, "Do you feel like talking?" before plunging into conversation.

• Listen well, and show that you are listening. Pay attention to the patient's words, without the distraction of planning your next remark.

• Encourage the patient to talk by saying, "What do you mean?" or "Tell me more."

• Remember that silence and nonverbal communication, such as grasping a hand or touching a shoulder, are also effective.

- Do not be afraid to describe your own feelings. It is permissible to say, "I find this difficult to talk about," or even, "I don't know what to say."

- Make sure you haven't misunderstood. You can ask, "What did it feel like?" or say, "You seem angry."

- Do not change the subject. If you are uncomfortable, admit it. Don't try to distract the patient by changing the subject to something less threatening, such as the weather.

- Do not give advice early. The time may come when the patient asks your advice, but it is usually not prudent to offer unsolicited advice, because it stops the dialogue.

- Encourage reminiscence. Sharing memories can be a wrenching experience, but it can also encourage patients to look positively at the past.

- Respond to humor. Humor allows patients to express fears in a non-threatening way. Do not try to cheer someone up with your own jokes, but if patients want to tell jokes or funny stories, humor them.

In short, the more you try to understand the feelings of others, the more support you will be able to give.

Applying Knowledge

Match each definition that follows with the correct term by writing the appropriate letter in the space provided.

_____ 1. One who has six months or less to live.

_____ 2. An irreversible condition that determines when death has occurred.

_____ 3. Care provided to relieve pain and make a patient's last days as comfortable as possible.

_____ 4. The range of emotions one feels in response to loss.

_____ 5. Care provided in an attempt to halt the disease process.

_____ 6. The study of death and its accompanying psychological aspects.

_____ 7. Greek for "good death."

a. grief

b. terminally ill

c. euthanasia

d. thanatology

e. palliative care

f. brain death

g. curative care

Answer the following questions in the spaces provided.

8. Distinguish between active euthanasia, passive euthanasia, and voluntary euthanasia.

_____

_____

_____

9. Technically, death results from what basic, biological cause?

_____

10. List the criteria for brain death.

_____

_____

11. List six tests that physicians can perform to determine whether death has occurred.

_____   _____

_____   _____

_____   _____

12. Distinguish between a living will, a health care proxy, and durable power of attorney.

_____

_____

_____

_____

_____

13. What is the philosophy behind the hospice movement?

_____

_____

14. What is the significance of the Uniform Rights of the Terminally Ill Act?

_____

_____

15. What is the significance of the Patient Self-Determination Act?

_____

_____

16. List Dr. Elisabeth Kubler-Ross's five stages of coping with a terminal illness.

_____

_____

_____

_____

_____

17. How do the stages apply to grief over the loss of a loved one?

_____

_____

18. What is the significance of the *Cruzan* case?

_____

_____

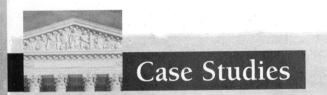

Use your critical-thinking skills to answer the questions that follow this case study.

You are a member of a hospital resource allocation committee that must decide which three out of seven critical patients will receive immediate live-saving surgery. The hospital has resources to save just three of the seven, but without surgery all seven patients will die. The situation is further complicated by the fact that a blizzard is raging outside and none of the patients can be transferred to another hospital. All seven are too critical to be moved by snowmobile.

19. Working alone or in a group, decide what criteria will be used to make the decisions. (Age, social standing, benefit to society, degree of physical deterioration?)

    _____

    _____

    _____

20. Obtain a list of the seven patients from your instructor, and choose three patients to receive immediate life-saving surgery. Write your decisions or discuss the rationale for your choices with the class.

    _____

    _____

    _____

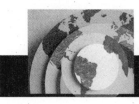

Internet Activities

Complete the activities and answer the questions that follow.

21. Visit the Web site for Partnership for Caring. Have there been changes in the advance directive laws in your state? If so, list the changes.

    _____

    _____

22. Visit the Web site for the National Hospice and Palliative Care Organization (NHPCO). List three of the most frequently asked questions about hospice care. Include the answers to those questions.

    _____

    _____

    _____

    _____

    _____

    _____

23. Visit the Web site for Healing Resources. List three links found at the site that might help the bereaved. Why might these resources prove helpful?

    _____

    _____

    _____

    _____

    _____

    _____

APPENDIX 1

STATE MEDICAL BOARDS

Alabama State Board of Medical Examiners

P.O. Box 946
Montgomery, AL 36101-0946
(street address 848 Washington Ave., 36104)
(334) 242-4116 / Fax: (334) 242-4155
(800) 227-2606
www.albme.org

Alaska State Medical Board

3601 C Street, Suite 722
Anchorage, AK 99503-5986
(907) 269-8163 / Fax: (907) 269-8196
www.dced.state.ak.us/occ/pmed.htm

Arizona Board of Medical Examiners

9545 East Doubletree Ranch Road
Scottsdale, AZ 85258
(480) 551-2700 / Fax: (480) 551-2704
www.bomex.org

Arizona Board of Osteopathic Examiners in Medicine and Surgery

9535 East Doubletree Ranch Rd.
Scottsdale, AZ 85258-5539
(480) 657-7703 / Fax: (480) 657-7715
www.azosteoboard.org

Arkansas State Medical Board

2100 Riverfront Dr., Suite 200
Little Rock, AR 72202-1793
(501) 296-1802 / Fax: (501) 296-1805
www.armedicalboard.org

Medical Board of California

1426 Howe Ave., Suite 54
Sacramento, CA 95825-3236
(916) 263-2389 / Fax: (916) 263-2387
(800) 633-2322
www.medbd.ca.gov

Osteopathic Medical Board of California

2720 Gateway Oaks Dr., Suite 350
Sacramento, CA 95833-3500
(916) 263-3100 / Fax: (916) 263-3117
www.docboard.org

Colorado Board of Medical Examiners

1560 Broadway, Suite 1300
Denver, CO 80202-5140
(303) 894-7690 / Fax: (303) 894-7692
www.dora.state.co.us/medical

Connecticut Medical Examining Board

P.O. Box 340308
Hartford, CT 06134-0308
(street address 410 Capitol Ave. MS13PHO)
(860) 509-7648 / Fax: (860) 509-7553
Licensing Information: (860) 509-7563

Delaware Board of Medical Practice

P.O. Box 1401
Dover, DE 19903
(street address 861 Silver Lake Blvd., Cannon Bldg., Suite 203, 19904)
(302) 739-4522 / Fax: (302) 739-2711
www.state.de.us/license/28/index.htm

District of Columbia Board of Medicine

825 North Capital St., NE, 2nd Floor
Washington, DC 20002
(202) 442-9200 / Fax: (202) 442-9431
www.dchealth.com

Florida Board of Medicine

4052 Bald Cypress Way, BIN #C03
Tallahassee, FL 32399-1753
(850) 245-4131 / Fax: (850) 922-3040
www.doh.state.fl.us

Florida Board of Osteopathic Medicine

2020 Capital Circle, SE, BIN # C06
Tallahassee, FL 32399-3253
(street address Northwood Centre,
1940 N. Monroe St., 32399-0757)
(850) 488-0595 / Fax: (850) 487-9874
www.doh.state.fl.us

Georgia Composite State Board of Medical Examiners

2 Peachtree St., NW, 6th Floor
Atlanta, GA 30303-3465
(404) 656-3913 / Fax: (404) 656-9723
www.medicalboard.state.ga.us

Guam Board of Medical Examiners

Health Professional Licensing Office
P.O. Box 2816
Hagatna, GU 96932
(011) 671-475-0251 / Fax: (011) 671-477-4733

Hawaii Board of Medical Examiners

Dept. of Commerce & Consumer Affairs
P.O. Box 3469
Honolulu, HI 96801
(street address 1010 Richards St., 96813)
(808) 586-3000 / Fax: (808) 586-2874
www.state.hi.us

Idaho State Board of Medicine

Statehouse Mail
P.O. Box 83720
Boise, ID 83720-0058
(street address 1755 Westgate Drive, Suite 140, 83704)
(208) 327-7000 / Fax: (208) 327-7005
www.bom.state.id.us

Illinois Department of Professional Regulation (licensure)

320 W. Washington St., 3rd Floor
Springfield, IL 62786
(217) 785-0800 / Fax: (217) 524-2169
www.dpr.state.il.us

Indiana Health Professions Bureau

402 W. Washington St., Room 041
Indianapolis, IN 46204
(317) 232-2960 / Fax: (317) 233-4236
www.ai.org/hpb

Iowa State Board of Medical Examiners

400 Southwest Eighth Street, Suite C
Des Moines, IA 50309-4686
(515) 281-5171 / Fax: (515) 242-5908
www.docboard.org

Kansas Board of Healing Arts

235 SW Topeka Blvd.
Topeka, KS 66603-3068
(785) 296-7413 / Fax: (785) 296-0852
www.ink.org/public/boha

Kentucky Board of Medical Licensure

Hurstbourne Office Park
310 Whittington Parkway, Suite 1B
Louisville, KY 40222-4916
(502) 429-8046 / Fax: (502) 429-9923
www.state.ky.us/agencies/kbml

Louisiana State Board of Medical Examiners

P.O. Box 30250
New Orleans, LA 70190-0250
(street address 630 Camp St., 70130)
(504) 524-6763 / Fax: (504) 568-8893
www.lsbme.org

Main Board of Licensure in Medicine

137 State House Station (U.S. mail)
2 Bangor St., 2nd Floor (delivery service)
Augusta, ME 04333
(207) 287-3601 / Fax: (207) 287-6590
www.docboard.org/me/me_home.htm

Maine Board of Osteopathic Licensure

142 State House Station
Augusta, ME 04333-0142
(207) 287-2480 / Fax: (207) 287-3015
www.docboard.org/me-osteo

Maryland Board of Physician Quality Assurance

P.O. Box 2571
Baltimore, MD 21215-0095
(street address 4201 Patterson Ave., 3rd Floor, 21215)
(410) 764-4777 / Fax: (410) 358-2252
www.docboard.org

Massachusetts Board of Registration in Medicine

10 West St., 3rd Floor
Boston, MA 02111
(617) 727-3086 / Fax: (617) 451-9568
(800) 377-0550
www.massmedboard.org

Michigan Board of Medicine

P.O. Box 30670
Lansing, MI 48909-7518
(street address 611 W. Ottawa St., 1st Floor, 48933)
(517) 373-6873 / Fax: (517) 373-2179
www.cis.state.mi.us/bhser

Michigan Board of Osteopathic Medicine and Surgery

P.O. Box 30670
Lansing, MI 48909-7518
(street address 611 W. Ottawa St., 1st Floor, 48933)
(517) 373-6873 / Fax: (517) 373-2179
www.cis.state.mi.us/bhser

Minnesota Board of Medical Practice

University Park Plaza
2829 University Ave., SE, Suite 400
Minneapolis, MN 55414-3246
(612) 617-2130 / Fax: (612) 617-2166
Hearing Impaired: 1-800-627-3529
www.bmp.state.mn.us

Mississippi State Board of Medical Licensure

1867 Crane Ridge Drive, Suite 200B
Jackson, MS 39216
(601) 987-3079 / Fax: (601) 987-4159
www.msbml.state.ms.us

Missouri State Board of Registration for the Healing Arts

P.O. Box 4
Jefferson City, MO 65102
(street address 3605 Missouri Blvd., 65109)
(573) 751-0098 / Fax: (573) 751-3166
www.ecodev.state.mo.us/pr/healarts/

Montana Board of Medical Examiners

P.O. Box 200513
Helena, MT 59620-0513
(street address 301 S. Park Ave., 4th Floor)
(406) 444-4284 / Fax: (406) 841-2362
www.discoveringmontana.com

Nebraska Health and Human Services Regulation and Licensure Credentialing Division

P.O. Box 94986
Lincoln, NE 68509-4986
(street address 301 Centennial Mall South, 68508)
(402) 471-2118 / Fax: (402) 471-3577
www.hhs.state.ne.us/

Nevada State Board of Medical Examiners

P.O. Box 7238
Reno, NV 89510
(street address 1105 Terminal Way, Suite 301, 89502)
(702) 688-2559 / Fax: (702) 688-2321
www.state.nv.us/medical

Nevada State Board of Osteopathic Medicine

2860 E. Flamingo Rd., Suite G
Las Vegas, NV 89121
(702) 732-2147 / Fax: (702) 732-2079

New Hampshire Board of Medicine

2 Industrial Park Drive, Suite 8
Concord, NH 03301-8520
(603) 271-1203 / Fax: (603) 271-6702
complaints (800) 780-4757
www.state.nh.us/medicine

New Jersey State Board of Medical Examiners

P.O. Box 183
Trenton, NJ 08625
(street address 140 E. Front St., 2nd Floor)
(609) 826-7100 / Fax: (609) 984-3930
www.state.nj.us

New Mexico State Board of Medical Examiners

Lamy Bldg., 2nd Floor
491 Old Santa Fe Trail
Santa Fe, NM 87501
(505) 827-5022 / Fax: (505) 827-7377
www.state.nm.us/nmbme

New Mexico Board of Osteopathic Medical Examiners

P.O. Box 25101
Santa Fe, NM 87504
(street address 2055 S. Pacheco, Suite 400)
(505) 476-7120 / Fax: (505) 827-7095
www.state.nm.us/rld

New York State Board for Medicine (Licensure)

Cultural Education Center, Room 3023
Empire State Plaza
Albany, NY 12230
(518) 474-3841 / Fax: (518) 486-4846
www.op.nysed.gov

New York State Board for Professional Medical Conduct (Discipline)

New York State Dept. of Health
Office of Professional Medical Conduct
433 River St., Suite 303
Troy, NY 12180
(518) 402-0855 / Fax: (518) 402-0966
www.health.state.ny.us/

North Carolina Medical Board

P.O. Box 20007
Raleigh, NC 27619-0007
(street address 1201 Front St., 27609)
(919) 326-1100 / Fax: (919) 326-1130
www.ncmedboard.org

North Dakota State Board of Medical Examiners

City Center Plaza
418 E. Broadway, Suite 12
Bismarck, ND 58501
(701) 328-6500 / Fax: (701) 328-6505
www.ndbomex.com

Northern Mariana Islands Medical Profession Licensing Board

P.O. Box 501458, CK
Saipan, MP 96950
(670) 664-4811 / Fax: (670) 664-4813
www.mariana-islands.gov.mp/

State Medical Board of Ohio

77 S. High St., 17th Floor
Columbus, OH 43266-0315 (for Fed Ex delivery use Zip 43215)
(614) 466-3934 / Fax: (614) 728-5946
(800) 554-7717
www.state.oh.us/med/

Oklahoma State Board of Medical Licensure and Supervision

P.O. Box 18256
Oklahoma City, OK 73154-0256
(street address 5104 N. Francis, Suite C., 73118)
(405) 848-6841 / Fax: (405) 848-8240
(800) 381-4519
www.osbmls.state.ok.us

Oklahoma State Board of Osteopathic Examiners

4848 N. Lincoln Blvd., Suite 100
Oklahoma City, OK 73105-3321
(405) 528-8625 / Fax: (405) 557-0653
www.docboard.org

Pennsylvania State Board of Medicine

P.O. Box 2649
Harrisburg, PA 17105-2649
(street address 124 Pine St., 17101)
(717) 787-2381 / Fax: (717) 787-7769
www.dos.state.pa.us

Pennsylvania State Board of Osteopathic Medicine

P.O. Box 2649
Harrisburg, PA 17105-2649
(street address 124 Pine St., 17101)
(717) 783-4858 / Fax: (717) 787-7769
www.dos.state.pa.us

Board of Medical Examiners of Puerto Rico

P.O. Box 13969
San Juan, PR 00908
(street address Kennedy Ave., ILA Bldg., Hogar del Obrero Portuario, Piso 8, Puerto Nuevo, 00920)
(787) 782-8989 / Fax: (787) 782-8733

Rhode Island Board of Medical Licensure and Discipline

Dept. of Health
Cannon Bldg., Room 205
Three Capitol Hill
Providence, RI 02908-5097
(401) 222-3855 / Fax: (401) 222-2158
www.docboard.org/ri/main.htm

South Carolina Department of Labor, Licensing and Regulation Board of Medical Examiners

P.O. Box 11289
Columbia, SC 29211-1289
(street address: 110 Centerview Drive, Suite 202, 29210)
(803) 896-4500 / Fax: (803) 896-4515
www.llr.state.sc.us/pol/medical

South Dakota State Board of Medical and Osteopathic Examiners

1323 S. Minnesota Ave.
Sioux Falls, SD 57105
(605) 334-8343 / Fax: (605) 336-0270
www.usd.edu/med/sdsma

Tennessee Board of Medical Examiners

1st Floor, Cordell Hull Bldg.
425 5th Ave. North
Nashville, TN 37247-1010
(615) 532-4384 / Fax: (615) 532-5369
www.state.tn.us/health

Tennessee Board of Osteopathic Examiners

425 5th Ave. North
1st Floor, Cordell Hull Bldg.
Nashville, TN 37247-1010 (37219 Fed Ex Zip Code)
(615) 532-4384 / Fax: (615) 532-5369
(888) 310-4650
www.state.tn.us/health

Texas State Board of Medical Examiners

P.O. Box 2018
Austin, TX 78768-2018
(street address 333 Guadalupe, Tower 3,
    Suite 630, 78701)
(512) 305-7010 / Fax: (512) 305-7008
Disciplinary Hotline (800) 248-4062
Consumer Complaint Hotline (800) 201-9353
www.tsbme.state.tx.us

Utah Department of Commerce Div. of Occupational & Professional Licensure

P.O. Box 146741
Salt Lake City, UT 84114-6741
(street address Heber M. Wells Bldg., 4th Floor,
    160 E. 300 South, 84102)
(801) 530-6628 / Fax: (801) 530-6511
www.commerce.state.ut.us

Vermont Board of Medical Practice

109 State St.
Montpelier, VT 05609-1106
(802) 828-2673 / Fax: (802) 828-5450
www.docboard.org/vt/vermont.htm

Virgin Islands Board of Medical Examiners

Virgin Islands Dept. of Health
48 Sugar Estate
St. Thomas, VI 00802
(340) 774-0117 / Fax: (340) 777-4001

Virginia Board of Medicine

6606 W. Broad St., 4th Floor
Richmond, VA 23230-1717
(804) 662-9908 / Fax: (804) 662-9517
www.dhp.state.va.us/

Washington Medical Quality Assurance Commission

P.O. Box 47866
Olympia, WA 98504-7866
(street address 1300 SE Quince St., 98501)
(360) 236-4800 / Fax: (360) 586-4573
www.doh.wa.gov

Washington State Board of Osteopathic Medicine and Surgery

P.O. Box 47870
Olympia, WA 98504-7866
(street address 1300 SE Quince St., 98501)
(360) 236-4943 / Fax: (360) 586-0745
www.doh.wa.gov

West Virginia Board of Medicine

101 Dee Drive
Charleston, WV 25311
(304) 558-2921 / Fax: (304) 558-2084
www.wvdhhr.org/wvbom

West Virginia Board of Osteopathy

334 Penco Rd.
Weirton, WV 26062
(304) 723-4638 / Fax: (304) 723-6273

Wisconsin Medical Examining Board

Dept. of Regulation & Licensing
P.O. Box 8935
Madison, WI 53708-8935
(street address 1400 E. Washington Ave., 53703)
(608) 266-2112 / Fax: (608) 267-0644
http://badger.state.wi.us

Wyoming Board of Medicine

211 W. 19th St., Colony Bldg., 2nd Floor
Cheyenne, WY 82002
(307) 778-7053 / Fax: (307) 778-2069

APPENDIX 2
EEOC FIELD OFFICES

To be automatically connected with the nearest EEOC field office, call:
Phone: 1-800-669-4000
TTY: 1-800-669-6820

Albuquerque District Office

505 Marquette St., NW
Albuquerque, NM 87102
Phone: (505) 248-5201
TTY: (505) 248-5240

Atlanta District Office

100 Alabama St., Suite 4R30
Atlanta, GA 30303
Phone: (404) 562-6800
TTY: (404) 562-6801

Baltimore District Office

City Crescent Bldg.
10 South Howard St.
3rd Floor
Baltimore, MD 21201
Phone: (410) 962-3932
TTY: (410) 962-6065

Birmingham District Office

Ridge Park Place
1130 22nd St., Suite 2000
Birmingham, AL 32205
Phone: (205) 731-0082/3
TTY: (205) 731-0095

Boston Area Office

John F. Kennedy Federal Bldg.
Government Center
4th Floor, Room 475
Boston, MA 02203
Phone: (617) 565-3200
TTY: (617) 565-3204

Buffalo Local Office

6 Fountain Plaza, Suite 350
Buffalo, NY 14202
Phone: (716) 551-4441
TTY: (716) 551-5923

Charlotte District Office

129 West Trade St.
Suite 400
Charlotte, NC 28202
Phone: (704) 344-6682
TTY: (704) 344-6684

Chicago District Office

500 West Madison St.
Suite 2800
Chicago, IL 60661
Phone: (312) 353-2713
TTY: (312) 353-2421

Cincinnati Area Office

550 Main St.
Suite 10019
Cincinnati, OH 45202
Phone: (513) 684-2851
TTY: (513) 684-2074

Cleveland District Office

1660 West Second Street
Suite 850
Cleveland, OH 44113-1454
Phone: (216) 522-2001
TTY: (216) 522-8441

Dallas District Office

207 S. Houston Street, 3rd Floor
Dallas, TX 75202-4726
Phone: (214) 655-3355
TTY: (214) 655-3363

Denver District Office

303 E. 17th Ave.
Suite 510
Denver, CO 80203
Phone: (303) 866-1300
TTY: (303) 866-1950

Detroit District Office

477 Michigan Ave., Room 865
Detroit, MI 48226-9704
Phone: (313) 226-7636
TTY: (313) 226-7599

El Paso Area Office

The Commons, Building C.
Suite 100
4171 N. Mesa St.
El Paso, TX 79902
Phone: (915) 832-6550
TTY: (915) 832-6545

Fresno Local Office

1265 West Shaw Ave.
Suite 103
Fresno, CA 93711
Phone: (559) 487-5793
TTY: (559) 487-5837

Greensboro Local Office

801 Summit Ave.
Greensboro, NC 27405-7813
Phone: (336) 333-5174
TTY: (336) 333-5542

Honolulu Local Office

300 Ala Moana Blvd.
Room 7123-A
P.O. Box 50082
Honolulu, HI 96850-0051
Phone: (808) 541-3120
TTY: (808) 541-3131

Houston District Office

1919 Smith Street, 7th Floor
Houston, TX 77002
Phone: (713) 209-3320
TTY: (713) 209-3367

Indianapolis District Office

101 W. Ohio St.
Suite 1900
Indianapolis, IN 46204-4203
Phone: (317) 226-7212
TTY: (317) 226-5162

Jackson Area Office

Dr. A.H. McCoy Federal Bldg.
100 West Capitol St., Suite 207
Jackson, MS 39269
Phone: (601) 965-4537
TTY: (601) 965-4915

Kansas City Area Office

400 State Ave., Suite 905
Kansas City, KS 66101
Phone: (913) 551-5655
TTY: (913) 551-5657

Little Rock Area Office

425 West Capitol Ave.
Suite 625
Little Rock, AR 72201
Phone: (501) 324-5060
TTY: (501) 324-5481

Los Angeles District Office

255 E. Temple, 4th Floor
Los Angeles, CA 90012
Phone: (213) 894-1000
TTY: (213) 894-1121

Louisville Area Office

600 Dr. Martin Luther King Jr.
   Place
Suite 268
Louisville, KY 40202
Phone: (502) 582-6082
TTY: (502) 582-6285

Memphis District Office

1407 Union Ave., Suite 521
Memphis, TN 38104
Phone: (901) 544-0115
TTY: (901) 544-0112

Miami District Office

One Biscayne Tower
2 South Biscayne Boulevard
Suite 2700
Miami, FL 33131
Phone: (305) 536-4491
TTY: (305) 536-5721

Milwaukee District Office

310 West Wisconsin Ave.
Suite 800
Milwaukee, WI 53203-2292
Phone: (414) 297-1111
TTY: (414) 297-1115

Minneapolis Area Office

330 South Second Ave.
Suite 430
Minneapolis, MN 55401-2224
Phone: (612) 335-4040
TTY: (612) 335-4045

Nashville Area Office

50 Vantage Way
Suite 202
Nashville, TN 37228
Phone: (615) 736-5820
TTY: (615) 736-5870

Newark Area Office

1 Newark Center, 21st Floor
Newark, NJ 07102-5233
Phone: (973) 645-6383
TTY: (973) 645-3004

New Orleans District Office

701 Loyola Ave.
Suite 600
New Orleans, LA 70113-9936
Phone: (504) 589-2329
TTY: (504) 589-2958

New York District Office

201 Varick St., Room 1009
New York, NY 10014
Phone: (212) 741-8815,
   (212) 741-2783
TTY: (212) 741-3080

Norfolk Area Office

Federal Bldg., Suite 739
200 Granby St.
Norfolk, VA 23510
Phone: (757) 441-3470
TTY: (757) 441-3578

Oakland Local Office

1301 Clay St.
Suite 1170-N
Oakland, CA 94612-5217
Phone: (510) 637-3230
TTY: (510) 637-3234

Oklahoma Area Office

210 Park Ave.
Oklahoma City, OK 73102
Phone: (405) 231-4911
TTY: (405) 231-5745

Philadelphia District Office

21 South 5th St.
4th Floor
Philadelphia, PA 19106
Phone: (215) 440-2600
TTY: (215) 440-2610

Phoenix District Office

3300 N. Central Ave.
Suite 690
Phoenix, AZ 85012-1848
Phone: (602) 640-5000
TTY: (602) 640-5072

Pittsburgh Area Office

1001 Liberty Ave.
Suite 300
Pittsburgh, PA 15222-4187
Phone: (412) 644-3444
TTY: (412) 644-2720

Raleigh Area Office

1309 Annapolis Drive
Raleigh, NC 27608-2129
Phone: (919) 856-4064
TTY: (919) 856-4296

Richmond Area Office

3600 West Broad St.
Room 229
Richmond, VA 23230
Phone: (804) 278-4651
TTY: (804) 278-4654

San Antonio District Office

5410 Fredericksburg Rd.
Suite 200
San Antonio, TX 78229-3555
Phone: (210) 281-7600
TTY: (210) 281-7610

San Diego Area Office

401 B St.
Suite 1550
San Diego, CA 92101
Phone: (619) 557-7235
TTY: (619) 557-7232

San Francisco District Office

901 Market St., Suite 500
San Francisco, CA 94103
Phone: (415) 356-5100
TTY: (415) 356-5098

San Jose Local Office

96 North 3rd St., Suite 200
San Jose, CA 95112
Phone: (408) 291-7352
TTY: (408) 291-7374

Savannah Local Office

410 Mall Blvd.
Suite G
Savannah, GA 31406-4821
Phone: (912) 652-4234
TTY: (912) 652-4439

Seattle District Office

Federal Office Bldg.
909 First Ave., Suite 400
Seattle, WA 98104-1061
Phone: (206) 220-6883
TTY: (206) 220-6882

St. Louis District Office

Robert A. Young Bldg.
1222 Spruce St., Room 8.100
St. Louis, MO 63103
Phone: (314) 539-7800
TTY: (314) 539-7803

Tampa Area Office

501 East Polk St., 10th Floor
Tampa, FL 33602
Phone: (813) 228-2310
TTY: (813) 228-2003

Washington Field Office

1400 L St. N.W., Suite 200
Washington, D.C. 20005
Phone: (202) 275-7377
TTY: (202) 275-7518

APPENDIX 3
STATE WORKERS' COMPENSATION DIRECTORY

Alabama

Department of Industrial Relations
Workmen's Compensation Division
649 Monroe Street
Montgomery, AL 36131
(334) 242-2868
1-800-528-5166
www.dir.state.al.us//wc.htm

Alaska

Department of Labor
Division of Workers' Compensation
P.O. Box 25512
Juneau, AK 99802-5512
(907) 465-2790
FAX: (907) 465-2797
www.labor.state.ak.us

Arizona

Industrial Commission
800 W. Washington Street
Phoenix, AZ 85007
(602) 542-4411
www.ica.state.az.us

Arkansas

Workers' Compensation Commission
P.O. Box 950
324 Spring Street
Little Rock, AR 72203-0950
(501) 682-3930
Legal Advisor: 1-800-250-2511
www.awcc.state.ar.us/

California

Division of Workers' Compensation
455 Golden Gate Avenue,
2nd Floor
San Francisco, CA 94102
1-800-736-7401
(415) 703-5020
For a list of all California
    WC offices:
www.dir.ca.gov/dwc

Colorado

Department of Labor and
    Employment
Division of Workers'
    Compensation
1515 Arapahoe
Denver, CO 80202-2117
1-888-390-7936
(303) 318-8700
FAX: (303) 318-8710
www.coworkforce.com/DWC/

Connecticut

Workers' Compensation
    Commission
Capitol Place
21 Oak Street
Hartford, CT 06106
(800) 223-9675 (CT only)
(860) 493-1500
FAX: (860) 247-1361
http://wcc.state.ct.us/

Delaware

Department of Labor
Division of Industrial Affairs
P.O. Box 8902
4425 N. Market Street,
3rd Floor
Wilmington, DE 19899-8902
www.delawareworks.com

District of Columbia

Department of Employment
    Services
Office of Workers' Compensation
Labor Standards Bureau
77 P Street NE, 2nd Floor
Washington, DC 20002
(202) 671-1000
*www.does.ci.washington.dc.us/
services/wkr_comp.shtm*

Florida

Department of Labor and
    Employment Security
Division of Workers'
    Compensation
2012 Capital Circle S.E.
211 Hartman Bldg.
Tallahassee, FL 32399-0685
(850) 488-2514
www2.myflorida.com/les/wc/

Georgia

Board of Workers' Compensation
270 Peachtree Street NW
Atlanta, GA 30303-1299
(404) 656-3870
www.state.ga.us/sbwc/

Hawaii

Department of Labor and
    Industrial Relations
830 Punchbowl Street,
Room 209
Honolulu, HI 96813
(808) 586-8865
FAX: (808) 586-9219
www.dlir.state.hi.us

Idaho

Industrial Commission
317 Main Street
Boise, ID 83720
1-800-950-2110
(208) 334-6000
FAX: (208) 334-2321
www2.state.id.us/iic/index.htm

Illinois

Illinois Department of Labor
160 North LaSalle Street, C-1300
Chicago, IL 60601
www.state.il.us/agency/idol/

Indiana

Workers' Compensation of
Indiana
402 West Washington Street
Room W-196
Indianapolis, IN 46204
1-800-824-COMP
www.state.in.us/wkcomp/

Iowa

Division of Workers' Compensation
1000 East Grand
Des Moines, IA 50319
1-800-831-1399
(515) 281-5387
FAX: (515) 281-6501
www.iowaworkforce.org

Kansas

Department of Human Resources
Division of Workers'
Compensation
800 SW Jackson, Suite 600
Topeka, KS 66612-1227
(785) 296-3441
www.hr.state.ks.us/wc/html/wc.htm

Kentucky

Department of Workers' Claims
Perimeter Park West, Building C
1270 Louisville Road
Frankfort, KY 40601
(502) 564-5550
http://dwc.state.ky.us/

Louisiana

Office of Workers' Compensation
Administration
P.O. Box 94090
Baton Rouge, LA 70804-9040
(225) 342-7555
FAX: (225) 342-5665
www.idol.state.la.us/sec2owca.asp

Maine

Workers' Compensation Board
State House Station
Augusta, ME 04333-0027
Toll Free ME Only: 1-888-801-9087
(207) 287-3751
FAX: (207) 287-7198

Maryland

Workers' Compensation
Commission
10 East Baltimore Street
Baltimore, MD 21202-1641
(410) 864-5100
www.charm.net/~ wcc/

Massachusetts

Department of Industrial Accidents
600 Washington Street, 7th Floor
Boston, MA 02111
1-800-323-3249
(617) 727-4900
www.state.ma.us/dia/index.htm

Michigan

Department of Consumer and
Industry Services
Workers' Compensation
P.O. Box 30004
525 W. Ottawa
Lansing, MI 48909
(517) 373-1820
www.cis.state.mi.us/wkrcomp/

Minnesota

Department of Labor and Industry
Workers' Compensation Division
443 Lafayette Road
St. Paul, MN 55155
1-800-342-5354
FAX: (651) 297-4377
www.doli.state.mn.us/

Mississippi

Workers' Compensation Commission
1428 Lakeland Drive
Jackson, MS 39296-5300
(601) 987-4200
www.mwcc.state.ms.us

Missouri

Department of Labor and
Industrial Relations
Division of Workers' Compensation
P.O. Box 58
3315 West Truman Boulevard
Jefferson City, MO 65102-0058
1-800-775-2667
(573) 751-4231
FAX: (573) 751-2012
*www.dolir.state.mo.us/wc/index.
htm*

Montana

Workers' Compensation
Claims Assistance Bureau
P.O. Box 8011
1805 Prospect Ave.
Helena, MT 59604-8011
1-800-332-6102
*http://erd.dli.state.mt.us/Work
CompClaims/WCChome.htm*

Nebraska

Workers' Compensation Court
P.O. Box 98908
Lincoln, NE 68509-8908
(402) 471-6468
www.nol.org/home/WC

Nevada

Division of Industrial Relations
515 East Musser Street
Carson City, NV 89714
(702) 327-2700
http://dirweb.state.nv.us/iirs.htm

New Hampshire

Department of Labor
Division of Workers' Compensation
State Office Park South
95 Pleasant Street
Concord, NH 03301
1-800-272-4353
(603) 271-3176
*www.labor.state.nh.us/workers_
compensation.asp*

New Jersey

Department of Labor Division of
Workers' Compensation
P.O. Box 381
John Fitch Plaza
Trenton, NJ 08625-0381
(609) 292-2525
FAX: (609) 984-2515
*www.state.nj.us/labor/wc/
Default.htm*

New Mexico

Workmen's Compensation
Administration
P.O. Box 27198
2410 Centre Ave. SE
Albuquerque, NM 87125-7198
(505) 841-6000
www.state.nm.us/wca/

New York

Workers' Compensation Board
180 Livingston Street
Brooklyn, NY 11248
(718) 802-6616/6617
FAX: (718) 834-2116
www.wcb.state.ny.us/

North Carolina

Industrial Commission
4319 Mail Service Center
Raleigh, NC 27699-4319
(919) 807-2500
FAX: (919) 715-0282
www.comp.state.nc.us/

North Dakota

Workmen's Compensation
500 E. Front Ave.
State Capitol, 13th Floor
Bismarck, ND 58504-5685
1-800-777-5033
(701) 328-3800
www.ndworkerscomp.com

Ohio

Bureau of Workers' Compensation
30 W. Spring Street
Columbus, OH 43215-2256
1-800-644-6292
FAX: 1-877-520-6446
www.bwc.state.oh.us/

Oklahoma

Department of Labor
Workers' Compensation Division
4001 N. Lincoln Boulevard
Oklahoma City, OK 73105-5212
1-888-269-5353
(405) 528-1500
FAX: (405) 528-5751
www.oklaosf.state.ok.us/

Oregon

Workers' Compensation Division
350 Winter Street NE, Room 27
Salem, OR 97301
1-800-452-0288
(503) 947-7810
www.cbs.state.or.us/external/wcd/

Pennsylvania

Bureau of Workers' Compensation
1171 S. Cameron Street, Room 324
Harrisburg, PA 17104-2501
1-800-482-2383
(717) 772-4447
FAX: (717) 772-0342
www.li.state.pa.us/bwc/index.html

Rhode Island

Department of Labor and Training
Division of Workers' Compensation
P.O. Box 10190
1511 Pontiac Ave., Building 69
2nd Floor
Cranston, RI 02920-0942
(401) 462-8100
*www.dlt.state.ri.us/webdev/wc/
default.htm*

South Carolina

Workers' Compensation
Commission
P.O. Box 1715
1612 Marion Street
Columbia, SC 29202-1715
Claims Dept: (803) 737-5723
FAX: (803) 737-5768
www.state.sc.us/

South Dakota

Division of Labor and Management
Kneip Building
700 Governors Drive
Pierre, SD 57501-2291
(605) 773-3681
FAX: (605) 773-4211
*www.state.sd.us/dol/dlm/
dlm-home.htm*

Tennessee

Department of Labor
Workers' Compensation Division
710 James Robertson Parkway
Nashville, TN 37243
1-800-332-2667
(615) 741-2395
FAX: (615) 532-5929
*www.state.tn.us/labor-wfd/
email.html*

Texas

Workers' Compensation
Commission
4000 South IH-35
Austin, TX 78704-7491
Injured Workers: 1-800-252-7031
(512) 448-7900
www.twcc.state.tx.us/

Utah

Labor Commission
Industrial Accidents
P.O. Box 146610
160 East 300 South,
3rd Floor
Salt Lake City, UT 84114-6610
(801) 530-6800
*www.ind-com.state.ut.us/
indacc/indacc.htm*

Vermont

Department of Labor and
Industry
Workers' Compensation Division
National Life Building,
Drawer 20
Montpelier, VT 05620-3401
(802) 828-2286
FAX: (802) 828-2195
*www.state.vt.us/labind/
wcindex.htm*

Virginia

Workers' Compensation
Commission
1000 DMV Drive
Richmond, VA 23220
(804) 367-8600
FAX: (804) 367-9740
www.vwc.state.va.us/

Washington

Industrial Insurance
P.O. Box 44299
Olympia, WA 98504-4299
1-800-547-8367
(360) 902-5800
www.lni.wa.gov/insurance

West Virginia

Workers' Compensation
4700 McCorkle Avenue
Charleston, WV 25304
(304) 558-3423
Claims Information:
   1-800-628-4265
www.state.wv.us/bep/wc/
   default.htm

Wisconsin

Department of Workforce
   Development
Workers' Compensation
P.O. Box 7901
201 East Washington Avenue
Room C100
Madison, WI 53707-7901
(608) 266-1340
www.dwd.state.wi.us/wc/
   default.htm

Wyoming

Department of Employment
Workers' Safety and
   Compensation Division
122 West 25th Street
Cheyenne, WY 82002
(307) 777-7441
FAX: (307) 777-6552
http://wydoe.state.wy.us/
   doe.asp?1D=9

GLOSSARY

A

Abandonment The suspension of treatment of a patient without justification and proper notification.

Acceptance Agreement to an offer as stated in a contract.

Accessory One who contributes to or aids in the commission of a crime, either by a direct or an indirect act.

Accomplice One who directly participates in the commission of a crime.

Accreditation Official authorization or approval for conforming to a specified standard.

Active Euthanasia A conscious act that results in death.

Administer To instill a drug into the body of a patient.

Administrative Law Enabling statutes enacted to define powers and procedures when an agency is created.

Advance Directive A document that makes one's wishes known concerning medical life-support measures in the event that one is unable to speak for oneself.

Affidavit A sworn, written statement made under oath or an affirmation before an authorized magistrate or officer of the court.

Affirmative Action Programs that use goals and quotas to provide preferential treatment for minority persons determined to have been underutilized in the past.

Affirmative Defenses Defenses used by defendants in medical professional liability suits that allow the accused to present factual evidence that the patient's condition was caused by some factor other than the defendant's negligence.

Age Discrimination in Employment Act A federal act passed in 1967 making it illegal for employers with 20 or more employees working at least 20 weeks a year to discriminate against workers aged 40 years or older.

Age of Majority The age at which full civil rights are accorded.

Agency The relationship between a principal and his or her agent.

Agent One who acts for or represents another, as when an employee acts on behalf of his or her employer.

Alternative Dispute Resolution (ADR) Methods of settling civil disputes between parties using neutral mediators or arbitrators without going to court.

Ambulatory-Care Setting Medical care provided in a facility such as a medical office, clinic, or outpatient surgical center for patients who can walk and are not bedridden.

Amendments to the Older Americans Act A 1987 federal act that defines elder abuse, neglect, and exploitation but does not deal with enforcement.

American Medical Association Principles A code of ethics for members of the American Medical Association, written in 1847.

Americans With Disabilities Act Applying to employers with 15 or more employees who work at least 20 weeks a year, Titles I and III of this act took effect in January 1992 and lessened discrimination toward the disabled in the workplace and mandated full access in all public places.

Amicus Curiae Literally, "friend of the court"; a legal brief in which one that is not a party to a particular litigation is permitted by the court to advise it in some matter of law that directly affects the case in question.

Amniocentesis A test whereby the physician withdraws a sample of amniotic fluid (the fluid surrounding the developing fetus inside the mother's womb) from a woman's pregnant uterus. The fluid is then tested for genetic or other conditions that may lead to abnormal development of the fetus.

Anencephaly A congenital deformity in newborns characterized by absence of the brain and spinal cord.

Anesthesiologist Assistant Assists the anesthesiologist in developing and implementing an anesthesia care plan. Duties can include preoperative and postoperative tasks, as well as operating room assistance.

Appeals Phase The phase of a trial, after the verdict, during which appeals may be submitted.

Arbitration The hearing and determination of a case in controversy by a third party, chosen by the parties concerned or appointed under statutory authority.

Arraigned The process by which a person charged with a crime is allowed to answer the indictment in court by pleading guilty, not guilty, or *nolo contendere*.

Artificial Insemination The mechanical injection of viable semen into the vagina.

Assault The open threat of bodily harm to someone.

Associate Practice A medical management system in which two or more physicians share office space and employees but practice individually.

Assumption of Risk A legal defense that holds the defendant is not guilty of a negligent act, since the plaintiff knew of and accepted beforehand any risks involved.

Athletic Trainer Works with attending and/or consulting physicians as an integral part of the health care team associated with physical training and sports.

Audiologist A health care practitioner who is educated in the science of hearing and is qualified to test patients' hearing and to prescribe some types of therapy for hearing problems.

Autopsy A postmortem examination to determine the cause of death or to obtain physiological

evidence, as in the case of a suspicious death.

B

Battery Any bodily contact without permission.

Bilateral Agreement An agreement between two parties that is mutually acceptable.

Bioethics A discipline dealing with the ethical implications of biological research methods and results, especially in medicine.

Biotechnology Applied biological science.

Bloodborne Pathogen Standard The authority by which OSHA can levy fines, based upon guidelines of the Centers for Disease Control.

Brain Death Final cessation of bodily activity, used to determine when death actually occurs; circulatory and respiratory functions have irreversibly ceased, and the entire brain (including the brain stem) has irreversibly ceased to function.

Breach of Confidentiality Failure to keep private information entrusted to a health care professional by a patient.

Breach of Contract Failure of either party to comply with the terms of a legally valid contract.

Burden of Proof The task of presenting testimony to prove guilt or innocence in a trial.

C

Capital Punishment Government-sanctioned death by execution of those convicted of certain crimes.

Capitation A uniform per capita payment or fee that a managed care plan pays to physicians.

Cardiovascular Technologist Works under the supervision of physicians to perform diagnostic and therapeutic examinations in the cardiology (heart) and vascular (circulation) areas.

Case Law Law established through common law and legal precedent.

Case Manager A health practitioner affiliated with a managed-care health plan who is responsible for coordinating the medical care of individuals enrolled in the plan.

Certification A voluntary credentialing process whereby applicants who meet specific requirements may receive a certificate.

Certiorari A written order issued by a superior court to call up the records of an inferior court or a body acting in a quasi-judicial capacity.

Checks and Balances The system established by the U.S. Constitution that keeps any one branch of government from assuming too much power over the other branches.

Chemical Hygiene Plan The Standard for Occupational Exposures to Hazardous Chemicals in Laboratories, which clarifies the handling of hazardous chemicals in medical laboratories.

Child Abuse Prevention and Treatment Act A federal law passed in 1974 requiring physicians to report cases of child abuse and to try to prevent future cases.

Chiropractor One who is trained to provide a system of manipulative treatments for diseases caused by impingement on spinal nerves.

Chromosome Microscopic structures found within the nucleus of plant and animal cells that carry genes responsible for the organism's characteristics.

Civil Law Law that involves crimes against persons.

Civil Rights Act of 1964 Title VII of the act makes discrimination in the workplace illegal, for reasons of race, color, religion, sex, or national origin; applies to businesses with 15 or more employees who work at least 20 weeks a year.

Claims-Made Insurance A type of liability insurance that covers the insured only for those claims made (not for any injury occurring) while the policy is in force.

Clinical Investigation The process by which research is conducted to produce data that are scientifically valid and significant.

Clinical Laboratory Improvement Amendments (CLIA) Federal statutes passed in 1988 that established minimum quality standards for all laboratory testing.

Cloning The process by which organisms are created asexually, usually from a single cell of the parent organism.

Code of Ethics A system of principles intended to govern the behavior of those entrusted with providing care to the sick.

Commission on Accreditation of Allied Health Education Programs (CAAHEP) Accredits programs in 18 allied health professions and provides information concerning duties, education requirements, and sources for further information about the profession and the location of schools offering the accredited programs.

Common Law The body of unwritten law developed in England, primarily from judicial decisions based on custom and tradition.

Comparative Negligence An affirmative defense claimed by the defendant, alleging that the plaintiff contributed to the injury by only a certain degree.

Compensatory Damages Monetary damages awarded to the plaintiff in a civil suit. May be general—to compensate for injuries or losses due to a violation of the plaintiff's rights—or special—to compensate for losses not directly caused by the wrong.

Competency The state of having requisite or adequate ability, skills, or qualities.

Confidentiality The act of holding information in confidence, not to be released to unauthorized individuals.

Confidentiality of Alcohol and Drug Abuse, Patient Records A federal statute that protects patients with histories of substance abuse regarding the release of information about treatment.

Conflict of Interest A situation in which a person is faced with choosing between financial gain and his or her duty to provide the best possible medical care to patients.

Consent Permission from a patient, either expressed or implied, for something to be done by another. For example, consent is required for a physician to examine a patient, to perform tests that aid in diagnosis, and/or to treat for a medical condition.

Consequential Damages Monetary award to a plaintiff based on losses caused indirectly by a product defect.

Consideration Something of value bargained for as part of a contractual agreement.

Contingent Dependent on or conditioned by something else.

Contract A voluntary agreement between two parties in which specific promises are made for a consideration.

Contributory Negligence An affirmative defense that alleges that the plaintiff, through a lack of care, caused or contributed to his or her own injury.

Controlled Substances Act The federal law giving authority to the Drug Enforcement Agency to regulate the sale and use of drugs.

Coroner A public official who investigates and holds inquests over those who die from unknown or violent causes; he or she may or may not be a physician, depending upon state law.

Corporation A body formed and authorized by law to act as a single person.

Counteroffer An alternative offer made by one who has rejected an earlier, unsatisfactory offer.

Crime An offense against the state or sovereignty, committed or omitted, in violation of a public law forbidding or commanding it.

Criminal Law Law that involves crimes against the state.

Curative Care Treatment directed toward curing a patient's disease.

Cybermedicine A form of telemedicine that involves direct contact between patients and physicians over the Internet, usually for a fee.

Cytology The study of the structure and function of cells.

Cytotechnologist Works with pathologists to microscopically examine body cells, in order to detect changes that may help to diagnose cancer and other diseases.

D

Damages Monetary awards sought by plaintiffs in lawsuits.

Defamation of Character Damaging a person's reputation by making public statements that are both false and malicious.

Defendant The person or party against whom criminal or civil charges are brought in a lawsuit.

Defensive Medicine The practice of ordering and/or performing medical tests and procedures simply to protect against future liability and to construct for patients a medical record that documents the health care provider's judgment.

Denial A defense that claims innocence of the charges or that one or more of the four Ds of negligence are lacking.

Dental Assistant One who serves as a chair-side assistant to a dentist/employer within a dental office.

Dental Hygienist A health care practitioner who performs clinical and educational duties related to hygiene of the mouth and teeth, usually for dentist/employers within a dental office. A dental hygienist may work for one dentist or for several dentists at varying locations.

Deposition Sworn testimony given and recorded outside the courtroom during the pretrial phase of a case.

Diagnostic Medical Sonographer Administers ultrasound examinations under the supervision of a physician responsible for the use and interpretation of ultrasound procedures.

Dietician One who works closely with physicians and other medical practitioners to educate and assist patients with special dietary and nutritional needs.

Discrimination Prejudiced or prejudicial outlook, action, or treatment.

Dispense To deliver controlled substances in some type of bottle, box, or other container to a patient.

DNA Deoxyribonucleic acid; a complex protein that carries genetic information for all organisms except some viruses.

Doctrine of Common Knowledge Literally, "the thing speaks for itself"; also known as the doctrine of *res ipsa loquitur.* Under this principle, an act of negligence was obviously under the control of the defendant, the patient did not contribute to the accident, and it is apparent the patient would not have been injured if reasonable care had been used.

Doctrine of Informed Consent The legal basis for informed consent, usually outlined in a state's medical practice acts.

Doctrine of Mature Minors A principle that allows minors to make their own decisions regarding medical treatment if they are mature enough to comprehend a physician's recommendations and give informed consent.

Doctrine of Professional Discretion A principle under which a physician can exercise judgment as to whether to show patients who are being treated for mental or emotional conditions their records. Disclosure depends on whether, in the physician's judgment, such patients would be harmed by viewing the records.

Do-Not-Resuscitate Orders (DNR) Orders written at the request of patients or their authorized representatives that cardiopulmonary resuscitation not be used to sustain life in a medical crisis.

Drug Enforcement Agency A branch of the U.S. Department of Justice that regulates the sale and use of drugs.

Durable Power of Attorney An advance directive that confers upon a designee the authority to make a variety of legal decisions on behalf of the grantor, usually including health care decisions.

Duty of Care The obligation of health care professionals to patients and, in some cases, nonpatients.

E

E-Health Term used for the use of the Internet as a source of consumer information about health and medicine.

Electrocardiogram (ECG) The recording made by an instrument that measures the electrical activity of the heart.

Electrocardiogram (ECG) Technician A health care practitioner who, under the direct supervision of physicians, operates electrocardiogram equipment to measure and record the electrical activity of the heart.

Electroencephalogram (EEG) The recording made by an instrument that measures the electrical activity of the brain.

Electroencephalogram Technician and Technologist A health care practitioner who works under the supervision of physicians to operate EEG equipment used to perform patient diagnostic tests.

Electroneurodiagnostic Technologist Involves the study and recording of the electrical activity of the brain and nervous system. Electroneurodiagnostic technologists work in collaboration with EEG technicians and technologists.

Emancipated Minor An individual in his or her mid- to late teens who legally lives outside of his or her parents' or guardian's control.

Emergency A type of affirmative defense in which the person who comes to the aid of a victim in an emergency is not held liable under certain circumstances.

Emergency Medical Technician (EMT) A paramedic who most often works from an ambulance or in a hospital emergency room to provide life-support care to critically ill and injured patients.

Employment-at-Will A concept of employment whereby either the employer or the employee can end the employment at any time, for any reason.

Endorsement The process by which a license may be awarded based on individual credentials judged to meet licensing requirements in a new state.

Equal Employment Opportunity Commission (EEOC) A federal agency that enforces provisions of the Civil Rights Act, the Age Discrimination in Employment Act, the Equal Pay Act, and the Rehabilitation Act.

Ethics Standards of behavior, developed as a result of one's concept of right and wrong.

Ethics Committee Made up of individuals involved in a patient's care, including health care practitioners, family members, clergy, and others.

Etiquette Standards of behavior considered good manners among members of a profession as they function as individuals in society.

Eugenic Abortion A medical termination of pregnancy performed because the fetus is severely damaged or deformed.

Euthanasia The practice of willfully ending life in an individual with an incurable disease or condition.

Executive Branch That branch of government responsible for administering the law. The President is the chief executive of the executive branch at the federal level; governors preside at the state level.

Executive Order A rule, or regulation, issued by the President of the United States that becomes law without the prior approval of Congress.

Expert Testimony Trial testimony provided by recognized authorities in a particular field.

Expressed Contract A written or oral agreement in which all terms are explicitly stated.

F

Fair Debt Collection Practices Act A federal statute prohibiting certain unfair and illegal practices by debt collectors and creditors.

False Imprisonment The unlawful violation of the personal liberty of another.

Federal False Claims Act A law that allows for individuals to bring civil actions on behalf of the United States government for false claims made to the federal government, under a provision of the law called *qui tam* (from Latin meaning to bring an action for the king and for one's self).

Federal Register A U.S. government publication that contains all administrative laws.

Federal Trade Commission Act A federal statute that established the Federal Trade Commission (FTC), which prohibits unfair or deceptive acts in advertising and other trade areas.

Federal Unemployment Tax Act (FUTA) The act that requires employers to contribute to a fund that is paid out to eligible unemployed workers.

Fee Splitting Payment by one physician to another solely for the referral of a patient, or payment from a source for using its services or supplies.

Felony An offense punishable by death or by imprisonment in a state or federal prison for more than one year.

Fiduciary Duty A physician's obligation to his or her patient, based upon trust and confidence.

Food and Drug Administration (FDA) A federal agency within the Department of Health and Human Services that oversees drug quality and standardization and must approve drugs before they are released for public use.

Forensics A division of medicine that incorporates law and medicine and involves medical issues or medical proof at trials having to do with malpractice, crimes, and accidents.

Four Ds of Negligence Elements necessary to prove negligence: duty, derelict, direct cause, and damages.

Fraud Dishonest or deceitful practices in depriving, or attempting to deprive, another of his or her rights.

G

Gatekeeper Physician The primary-care physician who directs the medical care of HMO members.

Gene A tiny segment of DNA found on a cell's chromosomes. Each gene holds the formula for making a specific molecule.

Gene Therapy The insertion of a normally functioning gene into cells in which an abnormal or absent element of the gene has caused disease.

General Duty Clause A section of the Hazard Communication Standard which states that any equipment that may pose a health risk must be specified as a hazard.

General Liability The legal responsibility for personal acts borne by all competent adults, both on the job and in their private lives.

Genetic Counseling The process by which prospective parents at risk for passing on genetic disorders to their offspring are screened.

Genetic Discrimination Differential treatment of individuals based on their actual or presumed genetic differences.

Genetic Engineering The synthesis, alteration, or repair of hereditary material.

Genetics The science that accounts for natural differences and resemblances among organisms related by descent.

Genome All the DNA in an organism, including its genes.

Germ Line Therapy A procedure in which a replacement gene is put into human gametes, resulting in expression of the new gene in the patient's offspring.

Good Samaritan Acts State laws protecting physicians and sometimes other health care practitioners and laypersons from charges of negligence or abandonment if they stop to help the victim of an accident or other emergency.

Group Model HMO A type of HMO that contracts with independent groups of physicians to provide coordinated care for large numbers of HMO patients for a fixed, per-member fee.

Group Practice A medical management system in which a group of three or more licensed physicians share their collective income, expenses, facilities, equipment, records, and personnel.

H

Hazard Communication Standard (HCS) An OSHA standard intended to increase health care practitioners' awareness of risks, to improve work practices and appropriate use of personal protective equipment, and to reduce injuries and illnesses in the workplace.

Health Care Integrity and Protection Data Bank (HCIPDB) A national health care fraud and abuse data collection program for the reporting and disclosure of certain adverse actions taken against health care providers, suppliers, or practitioners.

Health Care Practitioners Those who are trained to administer medical or health care to patients.

Health Care Proxy A durable power of attorney issued for purposes of health care decisions only.

Health Care Quality Improvement Act of 1986 A federal statute passed to improve the quality of medical care nationwide. One provision established the National Practitioner Data Bank.

Health Information Technologist or Technician A health care practitioner who may have full responsibility for the records department of a medical office, clinic, hospital, or other health care institution. Duties include organizing, analyzing, and preparing health information about patients, usually for use by patients, patients' physicians, and the health care facility.

Health Insurance Portability and Accountability Act (HIPAA) of 1996 Helps workers keep continuous health insurance coverage for themselves and their dependents when they change jobs, protects confidential medical information from unauthorized disclosure and/or use, and helps curb the rising cost of fraud and abuse.

Health Maintenance Organization (HMO) A health plan that combines coverage of health care costs and delivery of health care for a prepaid premium.

Heredity The process by which organisms pass genetic traits on to their offspring.

Heterologous Artificial Insemination Donor sperm is mechanically injected into a woman's vagina to fertilize her eggs.

Hippocratic Oath A pledge for physicians, developed by the Greek physician Hippocrates circa 400 B.C.

Homologous Artificial Insemination The husband's sperm is mechanically injected into his wife's vagina to fertilize her eggs.

Hospice A facility or program (often carried out in a patient's home) in which teams of health care practitioners and volunteers provide a continuing environment that focuses on the emotional and psychological needs of the dying patient.

Hostile Environment An antagonistic work environment that has been created by, among other things, sexual harassment.

Human Genome Project A scientific project funded by the U.S. government. It was begun in 1990 for the purpose of mapping all of a human's genes, and was successfully completed in 2000.

I

Implied Contract An unwritten and unspoken agreement whose terms result from the actions of the parties involved.

Implied Limited Contract A contract created when a physician or other health care worker treats a patient in an emergency situation. The agreement does not extend to the relationship after the emergency ends.

In Vitro Fertilization (IVF) Fertilization that takes place outside a woman's body, literally, "in glass," as in a test tube.

Incapacity A lack of physical or intellectual power, or of natural or legal qualifications.

Incompetent Lacking the qualities or skills necessary for effective action.

Indemnity A traditional form of health insurance that covers the insured against a potential loss of money from medical expenses for an illness or accident.

Indicted Charged with a crime.

Individual (or independent) Practice Association (IPA) A type of HMO that contracts with groups of physicians who practice in their own offices and receive a per-member payment (capitation) from participating HMOs to provide a full range of health services for HMO members.

Informed Consent The patient's right to receive all information relative to his or her condition and then to make a decision regarding treatment based upon that knowledge.

Intentional Tort *See* "Tort."

Interrogatory A written set of questions requiring written answers from a plaintiff or defendant under oath.

Invasion of Privacy Intrusion into a person's seclusion or into his or her private affairs.

Involuntary Euthanasia The act of ending a terminal patient's life by medical means without his or her permission.

J

Judicial Branch That branch of government responsible for interpreting laws; the court system and judges.

Judicial Council Opinions A publication of the American Medical Association, issued for the purpose of defining ethics for physicians in all situations common to the practice of medicine.

Jurisdiction The power and authority given to a court to hear a case and to make a judgment.

Just Cause An employer's legal reason for firing an employee.

K

Kinesiology The study of muscles and muscle movement.

Kinesiotherapist Work under a physician's supervision, using therapeutic exercise and education to treat the effects of disease, injury, and congenital disorders on body movement.

L

Law Rule of conduct or action prescribed or formally recognized as binding or enforced by a controlling authority.

Law of Agency The law that governs the relationship between a principal and his or her agent.

Legal Precedents Decisions made by judges in the various courts that become rule of law and apply to future cases, even though they were not enacted by legislation.

Legislative Branch The Senate and the House of Representatives, responsible for creating laws.

Liability Insurance Contract coverage for potential damages incurred as a result of a negligent act.

Liable Accountable under the law.

Libel Expressing through publication in print, writing, pictures, or signed statements that injure the reputation of another.

Licensed Practical Nurse (LPN) A health care practitioner who performs many of the same duties as a registered nurse.

Licensure A mandatory credentialing process established by law, usually at the state level, that grants the right to practice certain skills and endeavors.

Lien A charge upon real or personal property for the satisfaction of a debt or duty owed by law.

Limited Practitioner A provider licensed to provide specific treatment or treatments specific to certain body parts.

Litigious Prone to engage in lawsuits.

Living Will An advance directive that specifies an individual's end-of-life wishes.

M

Malfeasance The performance of a totally wrongful and unlawful act.

Managed Care A system in which financing, administration, and delivery of health care are combined to provide medical services to subscribers for a prepaid fee.

Material Safety Data Sheet (MSDS) A sheet that identifies each hazardous chemical used in the workplace and lists safety precautions necessary for its use, storage, and disposal; manufacturers must supply an MSDS upon request for each hazardous chemical used.

Mature Minor An individual in his or her mid- to late teens, who, for health care purposes, is considered mature enough to comprehend a physician's recommendations and give informed consent.

Medical Assistant One who performs administrative and clinical duties for a physician/employer within a medical office.

Medical Boards Bodies established by the authority of each state's medical practice acts for the purpose of protecting the health, safety, and welfare of health care consumers through proper licensing and regulation of physicians and other health care practitioners.

Medical Examiner A physician who investigates suspicious or unexplained deaths.

Medical Illustrator Creates illustrations for science and medical texts and other publications, and may also function in administrative, consultative, and advisory capacities.

Medical Laboratory Technician (MLT) A health care practitioner who performs simple tests in hematology, serology, blood banking, urinalysis, microbiology, and clinical chemistry.

Medical Practice Acts State laws written for the express purpose of governing the practice of medicine.

Medical Record A collection of data recorded when a patient seeks medical treatment.

Medical Technologist (MT) A health care provider who supervises technicians and assistants and performs more complicated, analytical laboratory tests than a medical laboratory technician.

Medical Transcriptionist One who keys material dictated by physicians, to be placed with patients' medical records.

Medical Waste Tracking Act The federal law that authorizes OSHA to inspect hazardous medical wastes and to cite offices for unsafe or unhealthy practices regarding these wastes.

Mentally Incompetent Unable to fully understand all the terms and conditions of a transaction.

Minor Anyone under the age of majority—18 in most states—21 in some jurisdictions.

Misdemeanor A crime punishable by fine or by imprisonment in a facility other than a prison for less than one year.

Misfeasance The performance of a lawful act in an illegal or improper manner.

Moral Values One's personal concept of right and wrong, formed through the influence of the family, culture, and society.

Mutual Assent An understanding and consent to the terms of an agreement by both parties in order for the contract to be legally valid.

N

National Childhood Vaccine Injury Act A federal law passed in 1986 that created a no-fault compensation program for citizens injured or killed by vaccines, as an alternative to suing vaccine manufacturers and providers.

National Organ Transplant Act Passed in 1984, a statute that provides grants to qualified organ procurement organizations and established an Organ Procurement and Transplantation Network.

National Practitioner Data Bank A repository of information about health care practitioners, established by the Health Care Quality Improvement Act of 1986.

Negligence An unintentional tort alleged when one may have performed or failed to perform an act that a reasonable person would or would not have done in similar circumstances.

Nominal Damages A token court-awarded payment, usually one dollar, which recognizes that the legal rights of the plaintiff were violated but that no actual loss was proved.

Nonfeasance The failure to act when one should.

Nurse Practitioner A registered nurse who has completed a graduate degree program and is skilled in physical diagnosis, psychosocial assessment, and primary health care management. He or she may work independently.

Nursing Assistant A health care practitioner who provides routine patient care under the direct supervision of registered nurses.

O

Occupational Safety and Health Act (OSHA) Established by the Occupational Safety and Health Act of 1970, it enforces compulsory standards for health and safety in the workplace.

Occupational Safety and Health Administration Established by the Occupational Safety and Health Act, the organization that is charged with writing and enforcing compulsory standards for health and safety in the workplace.

Occupational Therapist One who works with clients who are mentally, physically, developmentally, and/or emotionally disabled to help these individuals become more independent and productive.

Occurrence Insurance A type of liability insurance that covers the insured for any claims arising from an incident that occurred, or is alleged to have occurred, during the time the policy is in force, regardless of when the claim is made.

Officers of the Court Those individuals charged with specific responsibilities in the conduct of court cases.

Ophthalmic Medical Technician/Technologist Assists ophthalmologists by performing such tasks as collecting data, administering diagnostic tests, and administering some treatments ordered by the supervising ophthalmologist.

Ophthalmologist A physician who specializes in the treatment of disorders and diseases of the eye.

Optician One who is licensed to sell or make optical materials.

Optometrist One who is trained and licensed to examine the eyes in order to determine the presence of vision problems and to prescribe and adapt lenses to preserve or restore maximum efficiency of vision. The optometrist's professional degree is doctor of optometry (O.D.).

Organ Transplantation The process by which a patient (recipient) surgically receives a body organ from a living or dead donor.

Orthotist and Prosthetist Work directly with physicians and others to rehabilitate people with disabilities. The orthotist designs and fits devices (orthoses) for patients with disabling conditions of the limbs and spine. The prosthetist designs and fits devices (prostheses) for patients who have partial or total absence of a limb.

P

Palliative Care Treatment of a terminally ill patient's symptoms in order to make dying more comfortable; also called comfort care.

Parens Patriae A legal doctrine that gives the state the authority to act in a child's best interest.

Partnership A form of medical practice management system whereby two or more parties practice together under a written agreement specifying the rights, obligations, and responsibilities of each partner.

Passive Euthanasia The act of allowing a patient to die naturally, without medical interference.

Patient Self-Determination Act A federal law passed in 1990 that requires hospitals and other health care providers to provide written information to patients regarding their rights under state law to make medical decisions and execute advance directives.

Patient's Bill of Rights A statement approved by the American Hospital Association in 1973, guaranteeing an individual's rights to certain courtesies and considerations while a hospital patient.

Peer Review The process by which professional colleagues may review and judge one another's actions.

Perfusionist Operates transfusion equipment when necessary and consults with physicians in selecting the appropriate equipment, techniques, and transfusion media to be used, depending upon the patient's condition.

Phlebotomist One who draws blood from patients or donors for diagnostic testing or other medical purposes.

Physical Therapist (PT) A health care practitioner who helps patients restore function to muscles, nerves, joints, and bones after impairment due to illness or injury.

Physician-Hospital Organization (PHO) A health care plan in which physicians join with hospitals to provide a medical care delivery system and then contract for insurance with a commercial carrier or an HMO.

Physician's Assistant (PA) One who performs routine diagnostic and treatment procedures for the physician/employer.

Plaintiff The person bringing charges in a lawsuit.

Pleadings Phase That time before a trial when a complaint is filed, a summons is issued, an answer filed, and a counter-complaint made.

Point of Service (POS) Option A type of HMO that allows members to seek care from non-HMO physicians, but at higher premiums, co-payments, and deductibles than for traditional HMOs.

Precedent Decisions made by judges in the various courts that become rule of law and apply to future cases, even though they were not enacted by a legislature; also known as case law.

Preferred Provider Organization (PPO) A network of independent physicians, hospitals, and other health care providers who contract with an insurance carrier to provide medical care at a discount rate to patients who are part of the insurer's plan.

Prepaid Group Practice (PGP) A group model HMO in which physicians are salaried employees, usually practice in facilities provided by the HMO, and share in profits at the end of the year.

Prescribe To issue a medical prescription for a patient.

Pretrial Discovery Phase That period before a trial begins when a trial date is set by the court and pretrial motions are made and decided. Discovery procedures may be used to uncover evidence that will support the charges when the case comes to court, subpoenas are issued, depositions are taken, and pretrial conferences are called by the judge to discuss the issues in the case.

Primary-Care Physician (PCP) The physician responsible for directing all of a patient's medical care and determining whether the patient should be referred for specialty care.

Private Law The range of legal rights defining the relationships between private entities.

Privileged Communication Information held confidential within a protected relationship.

Professional Courtesy The practice of treating other physicians and their families free of charge or at a reduced fee.

Professional Liability One's legal accountability regarding all actions performed as a member of a certain profession.

Proposed Guidelines for Universal Precautions A list of general precautions issued by the Centers for Disease Control to promote safety and prevent contamination in the workplace.

Prosecution The government as plaintiff in a criminal case.

Protocol A code prescribing "correct" behavior in specific situations, such as in a medical office.

Public Law Law that refers to those legal rights defining the relationship between the government (the public sector) and the governed (certain private individuals or institutions, the private sector).

Public Policy The common law concept of wrongful discharge.

Punitive Damages Monetary award to the plaintiff in a lawsuit by the court, intended to serve as punishment for the defendant's act.

Q

Quality Improvement (or Quality Assurance) Measures taken by health care providers and practitioners to uphold the quality of patient care.

Quid Pro Quo Literally, "something for something"; a concept in the commission for sexual harassment in which an employee is expected to exchange sexual favors for workplace advantages.

R

Radiologic, or Medical Imaging, Technologist A health care practitioner who positions patients for X rays, operates the X-ray equipment, develops exposed X-ray film, and maintains records and films.

Reasonable Person Standard That standard of behavior that judges a person's actions in a situation according to what a reasonable person would or would not do under similar circumstances.

Reciprocity The process by which a professional license obtained in one state may be accepted as valid in other states by prior agreement without reexamination.

Referral The act of recommending to a patient the diagnostic or therapeutic services of another physician.

Registered Nurse (RN) A nurse who has completed a university or associate degree program.

Registration A credentialing procedure whereby one's name is listed on a register as having paid a fee and/or met certain criteria within a profession.

Rehabilitation Act of 1973 An act that requires federal contractors to take affirmative action to hire the disabled, requires federal contractors to implement affirmative action plans in hiring and promoting disabled employees, and prohibits discrimination against the disabled in programs that receive federal funds.

Release of Tortfeasor A technical defense to a lawsuit that prohibits a lawsuit against the person who caused an injury (the tortfeasor) if he or she was expressly released from further liability in the settlement of a suit.

Res Ipsa Loquitur "The thing speaks for itself"; also known as the doctrine of common knowledge. Under this doctrine no expert witnesses need to be called.

Res Judicata "The thing has been decided." A claim cannot be retried between the same parties if it has already been legally resolved.

Respiratory Technician or **Therapist** A health care practitioner who works under a physician's supervision to assist patients with breathing disorders.

Respondeat Superior Literally, "Let the master answer," a doctrine under which an employer is legally liable for the acts of his or her employees, if such acts were performed within the scope of the employee's duties.

Revocation The cancellation of a professional license.

Right-to-Know Laws State laws that allow employees access to information about toxic or hazardous substances, employer duties, employee rights, and other workplace health and safety issues.

Risk Contract An arrangement in which a health provider agrees to provide medical services to a set population of patients for a prepaid fee. The physician is responsible for managing the care of these patients and risks losing money if total expenses exceed prepaid fees.

Risk Management Steps taken to minimize danger, hazard, and liability.

S

Sexual Harassment A form of sexual discrimination in the workplace, in which an employee is expected to exchange sexual favors for employment advantages or must work in a hostile environment.

Sexual Misconduct An unethical sexual relationship between medical supervisors and trainees or between health care providers and patients.

Slander The speaking of defamatory words intended to prejudice others against an individual in a manner that jeopardizes his or her reputation or means of livelihood.

Sole Proprietorship A form of medical practice management in which a physician practices alone, assuming all benefits and liabilities for the business.

Somatic Cell Therapy A procedure in which human cells other than germ cells (eggs and sperm) are genetically altered.

Specialist in Blood Bank Technology Performs both routine and specialized tests in blood bank immunohematology and performs transfusion services. Must have a bachelor's degree and certification in medical technology and must have completed the required course of study in blood bank technology.

Staff Model HMO A type of HMO that employs salaried physicians and other health practitioners who provide care solely for members of one HMO.

Staff Privileges The right to practice at a particular hospital.

Standard of Care A level of performance expected of a health care worker in carrying out his or her professional duties.

Statute of Frauds State legislation governing written contracts.

Statute of Limitations That period of time established by state law during which a lawsuit may be filed.

Statutes Laws enacted by state or federal legislatures.

Statutory Law Law passed by the U.S. Congress or state legislatures.

Stem Cells Early embryonic cells that have the potential to become any type of body cell.

Subpoena A legal document requiring the recipient to appear as a witness in court or to give a deposition.

Subpoena Duces Tecum A legal document requiring the recipient to bring certain written records to court to be used as evidence in a lawsuit.

Substantive Law Regulations passed by an agency that pertain specifically to the functions of that agency.

Summary Judgment A decision made by a court in a lawsuit in response to a motion that pleads there is no basis for a trial.

Summons A written notification issued by the clerk of the court and delivered with a copy of the complaint to the defendant in a lawsuit, directing him or her to respond to the charges brought in a court of law.

Surety Bond A type of insurance that allows employers, if covered, to collect up to the specified amount of the bond if an employee embezzles or otherwise absconds with business funds.

Surgical Technologist Works closely with surgeons, anesthesiologists, nurses, and other surgical personnel before, during, and after surgery.

Surrogate Mother A woman who becomes pregnant, usually by artificial insemination or surgical implantation of a fertilized egg, and bears a child for another woman.

Suspension The temporary withdrawal of a professional license.

T

Technical Defenses Defenses used in a lawsuit that are based upon legal technicalities.

Telemedicine Remote consultation by patients with physicians or other health professionals via telephone, closed-circuit television, or the Internet.

Terminally Ill Referring to patients who are expected to die within six months.

Termination The ending of a contract between a physician and a patient, usually because all treatment has been completed and the bill has been paid.

Testimony Statements sworn to under oath by witnesses testifying in court and giving depositions.

Thanatology The study of death and of the psychological methods of coping with it.

Therapeutic Abortion A medical termination of pregnancy performed to save the life of the mother.

Third Party Payor Contracts A written agreement signed by a party other than the patient who promises to pay the patient's bill.

Title VII of the Civil Rights Act of 1964 A law that makes discrimination in the workplace illegal.

Tort A civil wrong committed against a person or property, excluding breach of contract.

Tortfeasor The person guilty of committing a tort.

Trial Phase That point in a lawsuit when the actual court trial begins, wherein evidence is heard and a verdict reached.

Truth-in-Lending Act A law that specifies those collection agreements that must be in writing and lists items that must be included in such contracts; also known as Regulation Z of the Consumer Protection Act of 1968.

U

Unemployment (or Reemployment) Insurance Under the Federal Unemployment Tax Act (FUTA), employers contribute to a fund that is paid out to eligible unemployed workers. Each state also provides for unemployment insurance.

Uniform Anatomical Gift Act A national statute allowing individuals to donate their bodies or body parts, after death, for use in transplant surgery, tissue banks, or medical research or education.

Uniform Determination of Death Act A proposal that established uniform guidelines for determining when death has occurred.

Uniform Rights of the Terminally Ill Act A federal statute passed in 1989 to guide state legislatures in constructing laws to address advance directives.

Unintentional Tort *See* "Tort."

Universal Precautions Guidelines of the Centers for Disease Control and Prevention (CDC) that deal with handling body fluids.

V

Vital Statistics Numbers collected for the population of live births, deaths, fetal deaths, marriages, divorces, induced terminations of pregnancy, and any change in civil status that occurs during an individual's lifetime.

Void Without legal force or effect.

Voidable Able to be set aside or to be revalidated at a later date.

Voluntary Euthanasia The act of ending a patient's life by medical means with his or her permission.

W

Waiver The act of intentionally relinquishing a known right, claim, or privilege.

Withholding Deductions made from an employee's paycheck.

Workers' Compensation A form of insurance established by federal and state statutes that provides reimbursement for workers who are injured on the job.

Wrongful Death Statutes State statutes that allow a person's beneficiaries to collect for loss to the estate of the deceased for future earnings when a death is judged to have been due to negligence.

Wrongful Discharge A concept established by precedent that says an employer risks litigation if he or she does not have just cause for firing an employee.

X

Xenotransplantation Transplanting animal tissues and organs into humans.

INDEX

research and, 228–233
   unethical experimentation and,
      246
Ethics committees, 12–13
Etiquette, 12–13
Euthanasia, 242–243, 291
Executive branch of government, 53
Experimental treatment, 229
Expert testimony, 105, 108
Expressed contracts, 65–67

F

Fact testimony, 105
Fair Debt Collection Practices Act, 66
Fair Labor Standards Act of 1938, 183
False imprisonment (false arrest),
   58–59
Family Leave Act of 1991, 183
Fax machines, as threats to confiden-
   tiality, 136
Federal courts, 61
Federal False Claims Act, 41
Federal Trade Commission Act, 257
Fees, of physicians, 264–265
Fee splitting, 265
Felonies, 55–56
Fetal research, 230
Fetal tissue transplantation, 239
Fetal umbilical cord blood, 240
Fiduciary duty, 136
Firing
   laws affecting, 179
   wrongful discharge and, 179, 229
Food and Drug Administration
   (FDA), 169
Foreign language speakers, lack of
   ability to give informed consent,
   140
Forensic medicine, 157
Formularies, 37
Fraud, 4, 58–59, 74
   controlling, 41–42
Frozen preembryos, ethics and, 236
Funeral customs and rites, 282–283
Futile care, 226–227

G

Gatekeeper physicians, 38
Gatekeeper plans, 38
General compensatory damages, 100
General Duty Clause, 186
Genes, 201
Gene therapy, 207
   ethics and, 230–231
Genetic counseling, 202

ethics and, 231
   nurses' roles in, 231
Genetic discrimination, 204–205
Genetic engineering, 205–206
   ethics and, 233
Genetics, 201–207
   gene therapy and, 207
   genetic engineering and, 205–207
   genetic testing and, 202–205
   research in, 203, 206–207
Genetic testing, 202–205
   of children, 232–233
   discrimination based on, 204–205
   by employers, 232
Genome, 201–202
   patenting of, 230
Germ line therapy, 231
Good Samaritan Acts, 143–144
Government, branches of, 53
Grief, 292–295
   definition of, 292
   stages of, 293–294
   support and, 294–295
Grounds, liability for, 85
Group practices, 35

H

Hazard Communication Standard
   (HCS), 186
Health care abuse, controlling, 41–42
Healthcare Integrity and Protection
   Data Bank (HIPDB), 41
Health care plans. *See also* Managed
   care
   legislation affecting, 40–43
Health care practitioners, 26–30. *See
   also specific practitioners*
   definition of, 3
   dilemmas of, 271
   interprofessional relationships of,
      253–257
   successful, qualities of, 13
Health care proxy, 289
Health Care Quality Improvement
   Act of 1986 (HCQIA), 40
Health information administrators, 28
Health information technicians/tech-
   nologists, 28
Health insurance
   coinsurance and, 37
   experimental treatment and, 229
   genetic information and, 232
   portability of, 40–41, 204
   release of information for, 137
   third-party indemnity, 36

Health Insurance Portability and
   Accountability Act of 1996
   (HIPAA), 40–41, 204
Health maintenance organizations
   (HMOs), 37–38
   coverage for high-dose
      chemotherapy, 39
   liability for physician malpractice,
      70
Heart valve defect, 6
Heredity, 201
Heterologous artificial insemination,
   209
Hippocratic oath, 9
Hiring, 192–193
   laws affecting, 179
HIV status, notification to sexual
   partners, 163
HIV testing, 246
   ethics and, 246
Homologous artificial insemination,
   209
Hospice care, 285–286
Hospital(s)
   negligence by, 94
   physicians' contracts with,
      256–257
Hospital relations, 256–257
Housestaff services, billing for, 256
Human genome, 201–202
   patenting of, 230
Human Genome Project, 202
Human stem cell research, 206–207

I

Images, in medical records, 132–133
Implied contracts, 65, 68–69
Imprisonment, false, 58, 59
Indemnity, 36
Indian Child Welfare Act, 211
Individual (independent) practice
   associations (IPAs), 37–38
Infants. *See* Minors; Newborns
Infertility, 209
Informed consent, 140–143
   doctrine of, 140
Injuries
   to hospital patient, 5
   lack of, court case on, 60
   of patient in parking lot, 85
   reportable, 166–169
   workers' compensation for,
      188–191
Instructions, failure to follow, termi-
   nation of contract for, 75

National Organ Transplant Act of 1984, 147
National Practitioner Data Bank (NPDB), 40
Negligence, 60, 94-102
   comparative, 119
   contributory, 119-120
   court cases on, 60-61, 94-99, 101-102, 190
   damage awards and, 100-102
   research ipsa loquitur doctrine and, 97-99
Newborns
   anencephalic, as organ donors, 240
   rights of, 212-213
   seriously ill, treatment decisions for, 243-244
Nominal damages, 100
Nonfeasance, 95
Nonscientific practitioners, relationships with, 253
Notifiable diseases, 160-164
Nuisance, 59
Nurse(s)
   interprofessional relationships of, 253
   license revocation and, 32
   role in genetic counseling, 231
Nurse practitioners, 29
Nursing assistants, 29
Nutritionists, 27

O

Occupational Exposure to Blood-borne Pathogen Standard, 186-187
Occupational Safety and Health Act of 1970, 183
Occupational Safety and Health Administration (OSHA), 184-188
   health standards of, 186-188
Occupational therapists (OTs), 29
Occurrence insurance, 125
Open access plans, 38
Ophthalmic medical technicians/technologists, 29
Opticians, 29
Optometrists, 29
Organ donation, 145-147
   from anencephalic neonates, 240
   directives for, 289
   ethics and, 237-241
   financial incentives for, 238
   hospital conditions of participation in programs for, 240-241

Organ Procurement and Transplantation Network (OPTN), 147, 241
Organ procurement organizations (OPOs), 147, 240-241
Organ transplantation, ethical guidelines for, 239
Orthotists, 29
Ownership, of medical records, 134

P

Palliative care, 284
Paramedics, 28
Parens patriae doctrine, 212
Parents, consent to abortion and, 223
Partnerships, 35
Passive euthanasia, 291
Patient(s)
   award to, court increase of, 96
   communication with, preventing liability suits and, 116-117
   with mental or emotional disorders, showing medical records to, 134
   referral of. *See* Referrals
   rights and responsibilities of, 71-72
   unhappy, dealing with, 126
Patient contacts, documentation of, 118
Patient-physician arbitration agreement, 106, 107
Patients' Bill of Rights Act of 1999, 42-43
Patient Self-Determination Act of 1990, 286
Payment, lack of, termination of contract for, 75
Payment agreements, written, 66, 67
Percival, Thomas, 9
Percival's Medical Ethics (Percival), 9
Perfusionists, 29
Phlebotomists, 29-30
Photographs, in medical records, 132-133
Physical therapists (PTs), 30
Physical therapists, advertising by, 260
Physician(s)
   advertising by, 257-258
   advisory services provided by, 258-259
   antitrust case, 36
   contracts with managed care, 69
   discipline by medical board, 25-26
   disclosure of medical mistakes by, 93

   duty to protect others from contaminated tissue samples, 163
   education of, 31-32
   fees of, 264-265
   with foreign medical education, 32
   gatekeeper, 38
   hospital relations and, 256-257
   interprofessional relationships of, 253-257
   licensure of, 31-34
   as medical examiners, 157
   medical practice types of, 34-35
   primary care, 38
   rights and responsibilities of, 69-71, 270-271
   specialization by, 32
   standard of care for, 86-88
   switching of, by patient, termination of contract for, 75
   transfer between, release of information for, 137
Physician-assisted suicide, 243, 291-292
Physician's assistants, 30
Plaintiffs, 56
Pleading phase of lawsuit, 102-103
Point-of-service (POS) plans, 38
Practice
   ethical guidelines for, 267-270
   types of, 34-35
Preembryos
   frozen, 236
   splitting of, 236-237
Preferred provider associations (PPAs), 38
Preferred provider organizations (PPOs), 38
Pregnancy Discrimination Act of 1976, 183
Prescribing, 169
   unlawful, of controlled substances, 172
Prescription drugs. *See* Drug(s)
Pretrial discovery phase of lawsuit, 103
Primary care physicians (PCPs), 38
Printers, as threats to confidentiality, 136
Prisoner treatment, ethics and, 227
Privacy, invasion of, 59
   imaging and, 132
Privileged communication, 89
Profession(s), 26-30
Professional corporations, 35